# CLINICAL INTERVIEWING

# *Preface*

> *I advise teachers to cherish mother-wit. I assume that you will keep the grammar, writing, reading, and arithmetic in order, 'tis easy, and of course you will. But smuggle in a little contraband wit, fancy, imagination, thought.*
> —Ralph Waldo Emerson, *Selected Prose and Poetry*

In the following pages, we aim to take Emerson's advice. This text is a serious examination of clinical interviewing as a professional activity; it includes the "grammar, writing, reading, and arithmetic" of professional interviewing. But in the spirit of Emerson, we have also smuggled in some contraband, and we encourage you to do the same. For our part, we include occasional humor, the practical application of fantasy through skill-building activities, and stories of our own and our colleagues' pitfalls and successes. For your part, we hope you learn clinical interviewing with all the seriousness that an enterprise dedicated to evaluating and helping people who come to you in emotional pain and distress deserves. We also hope you will smuggle a little contraband into the learning process. In particular, we hope the contraband you smuggle in is yourself.

Clinical interviewing is a practical, hands-on activity. It's hard to imagine learning to sit with, listen to, evaluate, and provide professional help to another human being simply by reading a book. Nevertheless, that's exactly the purpose of this book. We hope that by reading it—in combination with classroom activities, practicum or prepracticum experiences, and feedback from peers and supervisors—budding mental health professionals will learn the art and science, the intimacy and objectivity of clinical interviewing.

This, the third edition of *Clinical Interviewing,* marks the 10th anniversary of its original publication. This fact not only makes us 10 years older, but also, we hope, 10 years wiser. If nothing else, it means we've had a decade to reflect on what we originally wrote. We've made numerous positive changes and updates, which include:

- A stronger multicultural emphasis, with 13 new "Individual and Cultural Highlights" sprinkled throughout the text.
- A continued emphasis on contemporary literature in psychiatry, psychology, counseling, and social work as reflected by over 100 new citations.
- New sections in Chapters 6 and 10 on the science of clinical interviewing.
- A new section in Chapter 7—Intake Interviewing and Report Writing—that includes information on writing intake reports—complete with an intake outline and sample report.
- New sections in Chapter 7 on interviewing clients with chemical dependency problems and trauma victims (with a special emphasis on using motivational interviewing principles and strategies).

- A new section on individual and cultural considerations when conducting mental status examinations in Chapter 8.
- A completely revised section on interviewing for depression in Chapter 9.
- Inclusion of new risk factors for suicide and new suicide intervention approaches in Chapter 9.
- One fewer chapter—we have shortened and integrated Chapters 2 and 3 from the second edition so readers get to the meat and potatoes of clinical interviewing more quickly.
- New case examples throughout the book, with five new case examples in Chapter 13, the multicultural interviewing chapter.
- A revised and expanded instructor's manual and test bank available online at www.wiley.com.
- A method for contacting the authors with questions, comments, or suggestions at sommersflanagan@hotmail.com.

Despite the changes, we hope this edition continues to be as learner-friendly as earlier versions. Throughout the text, we've tried to maintain an accessible voice; we want students to not only learn about clinical interviewing (and about themselves), but also to enjoy reading this text, and we want them to treasure the learning process. Above all, we hope this edition lives up to the comments made by Hood (2000) in his review of the second edition published in *Contemporary Psychology:*

> Its use will depend on the instructor's teaching philosophy, but when it is used, I expect graduate students will consider it [*Clinical Interviewing*] one of their favorite texts. (p. 457)

## HOW THIS BOOK IS ORGANIZED

This text is divided into four parts. Part One, "Becoming a Mental Health Professional," includes two chapters. Chapter 1, "Introduction: Philosophy and Organization," begins by orienting readers to our general philosophy toward clinical interviewing. In this chapter, we cover basic, state-of-the-art practices in clinical interviewing and encourage readers to begin their own theoretical and philosophical development. In Chapter 2, "Foundations and Preparations," we outline the definition of *clinical interviewing,* discuss physical setting variables common to clinical interviewing, and review crucial professional and ethical issues.

Part Two, "Listening and Relationship Development," includes three chapters covering a wide range of listening, directive, and relationship-enhancing responses that can occur in a clinical setting. For many people—including mental health professionals—listening is neither easy nor natural; therefore, we review key listening components in Chapter 3, "Basic Attending, Listening, and Action Skills." Chapter 4, "Directives: Questions and Action Skills," includes a description of numerous directive statements and techniques—including questioning—available to clinical interviewers. In Chapter 5, "Relationship Variables and Clinical Interviewing," the nature and purpose of the interview is explored from a variety of different theoretical perspectives.

Part Three, "Structuring and Assessment," includes five chapters designed to guide interviewers in more directive interviewing procedures; these procedures are specifically designed to gather assessment information via the clinical interview. Chapter 6,

"An Overview of the Interview Process," provides a guide for understanding and managing the generic stages of all clinical interviews, followed by a brief section on the science of clinical interviewing. Chapter 7, "Intake Interviewing and Report Writing," specifically addresses intake interviewing, report writing, and other demands inherent in that first therapist-client encounter. Chapter 8, "The Mental Status Examination," provides a succinct overview of the mental status examination (MSE). Knowledge and skills for conducting an MSE are necessary for any mental health professional working in hospital, medical, or chemical dependency treatment settings. Chapter 9, "Suicide Assessment," gives readers a detailed look at suicide assessment interviewing strategies, including a review of risk factors, technical procedures, and potential personal reactions interviewers may have to suicidal clients. The final chapter in this section, Chapter 10, "Diagnosis and Treatment Planning," offers interviewing trainees an informative overview of psychiatric diagnosis and treatment planning. With the prevalence of managed care and time-limited therapies, diagnosis and treatment planning have become activities essential to competent clinical interviewing.

Part Four, "Interviewing Special Populations," consists of three chapters. Chapter 11, "Interviewing Young Clients," includes a description of basic procedures for interviewing child and adolescent clients. In Chapter 12, "Interviewing Couples and Families," issues facing interviewers who work with couples and families are reviewed. And finally, in Chapter 13, "Multicultural and Diversity Issues" (coauthored by Dr. Darrell Stolle), we focus on issues and strategies for interviewing clients from diverse cultural backgrounds. Each of the populations covered in this section represents specialty areas in mental health work. The chapters are intended to provide a foundation for dealing with these special populations; additional study, supervised experience, and training are necessary to become competent in working with these populations.

Throughout the book, we share examples from our clinical work and personal experiences. Please note that, when necessary, we have changed information to protect the identities and privacy of people with whom we've worked. In addition, we intermittently use both masculine and feminine pronouns to maintain gender balance when describing individual clients and interviewers.

Not surprisingly, we have had significant help and encouragement from many important people. First and foremost, our editor, Tracey Belmont, has been an absolute pleasure to work with. She is a person who can provide writers with that unusual, but ideal, blend of enthusiastic support and attention to detail. We look forward to working with her on additional Wiley projects and to conducting essential restaurant research with her at professional conferences. Thanks also to Kerstin Nasdeo of Wiley whose organizational skills helped us to enjoy online copyediting as much as humanly possible.

A number of our professional colleagues provided support and inspiration for our lives and for our professional writing aspirations. In particular, Christine Fiore (a Montana professor who teaches Clinical Interviewing, who provides us with great support and insight), Jan Wollersheim (our initial guiding influence in the field of suicide assessment interviewing), Phil Bornstein (the guy who taught us not to "fly by the seat of our pants"), Scott Meier and Susan Davis (coauthors of *The Elements of Counseling,* who coined the oft-cited phrase "only confront as much as you've supported"), Paul Silverman (a developmental and clinical psychologist who reviewed an initial draft of the chapter on interviewing young clients), Sherry Cormier (lead author of the nearly classic *Interviewing Strategies for Helpers*), Jack Watkins (the famous hypnotherapist who provided us with an excellent education about psychoanalytic constructs), and

Darrell Stolle (a professional colleague who enthusiastically threw himself into revising and updating the multicultural interviewing chapter) all deserve a generous thank-you.

There are, of course, many supportive friends, family members, and colleagues not mentioned here. We hope you know how crucial you are to making it all worthwhile.

# Contents

# PART ONE

# BECOMING A MENTAL HEALTH PROFESSIONAL

# Chapter 1

# *INTRODUCTION*
## *Philosophy and Organization*

> *You cannot hope to build a better world without improving the individuals. To that end each of us must work for his (sic) own improvement, and at the same time share a general responsibility for all humanity, our particular duty being to aid those to whom we think we can be most useful.*
>
> —Marie Curie

---

**CHAPTER OBJECTIVES**

This chapter welcomes you to the professional field of clinical interviewing and orients you to the philosophy and organization of this book. In addition, you will learn:

- How clinicians from different theoretical orientations approach the interviewing task.
- Basic requirements for clinical interviewers.
- Advantages and disadvantages of being a non-directive interviewer.
- The goals and objectives of this book.

---

Imagine you are sitting face-to-face with your first client. You have carefully chosen your wardrobe and seating arrangements, set up the video camera, and completed the introductory paperwork. You are doing your best to communicate warmth and helpfulness through your body posture and facial expressions. Now, imagine your client refuses to talk, or she talks too much, or he asks if he can smoke, or she starts crying. How will you respond to these situations? What will you say? What will you do?

From the first client forward, every client you meet will be different. Your challenge or mission (if you choose to accept it) is to make human contact with each of these different clients, to build a working alliance, gather information, instill hope, and, if appropriate, provide clear and helpful recommendations. To top it off, you must gracefully end the interview on time. These are no small tasks.

If you are interested in clinical interviewing, you probably want to learn how to—in Marie Curie's words—build a better world by helping improve individuals. So when you imagine yourself sitting with your first client, we believe you would like to know how to respond if he or she doesn't talk, talks too much, asks to smoke, or starts crying.

As a prospective psychologist, counselor, social worker, or psychiatrist, you face a challenging future. Becoming a mental health professional requires intellect, interpersonal maturity, a balanced emotional life, ongoing skill attainment, compassion, authenticity, and courage. Many classes, supervision, workshops, and other training experiences will pepper your life in the coming years. In fact, you need to be a lifelong learner to stay current and skilled in mental health work.

The clinical interview is the most fundamental area of mental health training. The interview constitutes first contact with clients. It is the basic unit of connection between helper and the person seeking help. It is the beginning of a counseling or psychotherapy relationship. It is the cornerstone of psychological assessment. And it is the focus of this book.

## WELCOME TO THE JOURNEY

This book is designed to teach you basic and advanced clinical interviewing skills. The chapters guide you through elementary listening skills onward to more advanced, complex enterprises such as intake interviewing, mental status examinations, and suicide assessment. We enthusiastically welcome you as new colleagues and fellow lifelong learners. Although becoming a mental health professional is a challenging career choice, it is a fulfilling one. As Norcross (2000) states:

> . . . the vast majority of mental health professionals are satisfied with their career choices and would select their vocations again if they knew what they know now. Most of our colleagues feel enriched, nourished, and privileged. . . (p. 712)

For many of you, this text will accompany your first taste of practical, hands-on, mental health training experience. For those with substantial clinical experience, this book will help you better understand your previous experiences by placing them into a more systematic learning context. Whichever the case, we hope this text challenges you and helps you develop skills needed for conducting competent and professional clinical interviews.

In the 1939 book *The Wisdom of the Body,* Walter Cannon wrote:

> When we consider the extreme instability of our bodily structure, its readiness for disturbance by the slightest application of external forces . . . its persistence through so many decades seems almost miraculous. The wonder increases when we realize that the system is open, engaging in free exchange with the outer world, and that the structure itself is not permanent, but is being continuously broken down by the wear and tear of action, and as continuously built up again by processes of repair. (p. 20)

This observation seems equally applicable to the psyche. The structure itself is impermanent, and, as most of us would readily agree, life brings many experiences—some that psychologically break us down and some that build us up. The clinical interview is the entry point for most people who have experienced psychological or emotional difficulties and who are looking for a therapeutic experience to build themselves up again.

## TEACHING PHILOSOPHY

Like all authors, we have underlying philosophies and beliefs that shape what we say and how we say it. Throughout the text, we try to identify our biases and stances, explain them, and allow you to weigh them for yourself.

We have important central beliefs about the activity of clinical interviewing. First, we consider clinical interviewing to be both art and science. This means you need to exercise your brain through study and critical thinking. Further, you need to develop and expand personal attributes required for effective clinical interviewing. We encourage academic challenges for your intellect and fine-tuning of the most important instrument you have to exercise this art: yourself. Second, with reference to the Cannon quote, we believe, from the client's perspective, the clinical interview should *always* be on the building-up or reparative side in the ledger of life's experiences. Reasons for interviews vary. Experience levels vary. But as Hippocrates implied to healers many centuries ago: As far as it is in your power, never allow the clinical interview experience to harm your client.

We also have strong beliefs and feelings about *how* clinical interviewing skills are best learned and developed. These beliefs are based on our experiences as students and instructors and on the state of scientific knowledge pertaining to clinical interviewing (Hill, 2001).

The remainder of this chapter outlines our teaching approach, philosophical orientation, and the book's goals and objectives.

## Learning Sequence

We believe many, but not all, students can learn to conduct competent clinical interviews. Further, we believe interviewing skills are acquired most efficiently when students learn, in sequence, the following skills and procedures:

1. How to quiet yourself and focus on what your clients are communicating (instead of focusing on what *you* are thinking or feeling).
2. How to develop rapport and positive working relationships with a wide range of clients—including clients of different ages, cultural backgrounds, sexual orientation, social class, and intellectual functioning.
3. How to efficiently obtain diagnostic or assessment information about clients and their problems.
4. How to identify and appropriately apply individualized counseling or psychotherapy methods and techniques.
5. How to evaluate client responses to your counseling or psychotherapeutic methods and techniques.

This text is limited in focus to the first three skills listed. Extensive information on implementing and evaluating counseling or psychotherapeutic methods and techniques is not in the scope of this text, but we do touch on them as we cover situations that beginning clinical interviewers may face.

## Quieting Yourself and Listening to Clients

Professional interviewers need to quiet themselves; they need to rein in their natural urges to help, their egos, and their anxieties. Listening nondirectively is the first order of the day. This is especially true during beginning stages of an interview. For example, as Shea (1998) notes, ". . . in the opening phase, the clinician speaks very little . . . . there exists a strong emphasis on open-ended questions or open-ended statements in an effort to get the patient talking" (p. 66).

The purpose of quieting yourself and listening nondirectively is to help your client find his or her voice and tell his or her story. Unfortunately, staying quiet and listening well is difficult because, when cast in a professional role, you will find it hard to turn off or turn down your mental activity. It is common to feel pressured and hyper, because you want to help clients resolve problems immediately. However, this can cause you to unintentionally become too authoritative or even bossy with new clients.

When students (and experienced practitioners) become prematurely active and directive, they run the risk of being insensitive and nontherapeutic. This viewpoint echoes the advice that Strupp and Binder (1984) give to mental health professionals: ". . . the therapist should resist the compulsion to do something, especially at those times when he or she feels under pressure from the patient (and himself or herself) to intervene, perform, reassure, and so on" (p. 41).

In a majority of professional interview situations, managed mental health care notwithstanding, the best start allows clients to explore their own thoughts, feelings, and behaviors (Daniels, 2001). When possible, interviewers should help clients follow their own leads and make their own discoveries (Meier & Davis, 2001; Strupp & Binder, 1984). We consider it the clinical interviewer's professional task to *encourage* client self-expression. On the other hand, given time constraints commonly imposed on therapeutic activities, it is also the interviewer's task to *limit* client self-expression. Whether you are encouraging or limiting client self-expression, the big challenge is to do so skillfully and professionally.

### Developing Rapport and Positive Therapeutic Relationships

Before developing assessment and intervention skills, interviewers must learn rapport and therapeutic relationship development skills. This involves learning active listening, empathic responding, and other behavioral skills leading to the development and maintenance of positive rapport (Othmer & Othmer, 1994). Counselors and psychotherapists from virtually every theoretical perspective agree on the importance of developing a positive relationship with clients before implementing treatment procedures (Goldfried & Davison, 1976; Luborsky, 1984; C. H. Patterson & Watkins, 1996). Some theorists refer to this as *rapport*—others discuss the importance of establishing strong therapeutic relationships (J. Sommers-Flanagan & Sommers-Flanagan, 1997). It can be challenging to develop skills for establishing rapport with clients from divergent cultural backgrounds and situations (A. Ivey, D'Andrea, Ivey, & Simek-Morgan, 2002; Vontress, Johnson, & Epp, 1999).

Most interviewers want to help their clients. They also feel a natural desire to know exactly what to do to be maximally beneficial. These desires sometimes cause interviewers to be impatient and to focus on what to *do* with clients rather than how to *be* with clients. Focusing first on how to be with clients facilitates the development of good working relationships between interviewers and clients (Dickson & Bamford, 1995). In Part Two of this text (Chapters 3 and 4), we focus squarely on the skills needed to develop positive psychotherapy or counseling relationships.

### Learning Diagnostic and Assessment Skills

After learning to listen well and develop positive relationships with clients, professional interviewers should learn diagnostic and assessment skills and procedures. Although the need for assessment and the validity of diagnosis is controversial along many lines (J. Sommers-Flanagan & Sommers-Flanagan, 1998; Szasz, 1961, 1970; Wakefield,

1997), initiating counseling or psychotherapy without adequate assessment is ill-advised, unprofessional, and potentially dangerous (Corey, 2001; Hadley & Strupp, 1976). Think about how you would feel if, after taking your automobile to the local repair shop, the mechanic simply began fixing various engine components without first asking you questions designed to understand the problem. Of course, clinical interviewing is much different from auto mechanics, but the analogy speaks to the importance of completing assessment and diagnostic procedures before initiating clinical interventions. Over a decade ago, Phares (1988) concluded that the need for diagnosis before intervention is no longer a controversial issue in psychology:

> Intuitively, we all understand the purpose of diagnosis or assessment. Before physicians can prescribe, they must first understand the nature of the illness. Before plumbers begin banging on pipes, they must first determine the character and location of the difficulty. What is true in medicine and plumbing is equally true in clinical psychology. Aside from a few cases involving blind luck, our capacity to solve clinical problems is directly related to our skill in defining them. (p. 142)

Interviewers should begin using specific counseling or psychotherapy methods and techniques only after three conditions have been fulfilled:

1. They have quieted themselves and listened to their clients' communications.
2. They have developed positive relationships with their clients.
3. They have identified their clients' individual needs and therapy goals through diagnostic and assessment procedures.

Additionally, beginning interviewers should obtain professional supervision when using therapeutic methods (C. Watkins, 1995).

## THEORETICAL ORIENTATIONS

Professional interviewers should obtain a broad range of training experiences, both in a variety of settings and from a variety of theoretical orientations. In our own training, we learned important lessons from different theoretical perspectives, even those with which we tended to disagree. As Freud, a person not often remembered for his openness and flexibility, once said: "There are many ways and means of conducting psychotherapy. All that lead to recovery are good" (in Trilling & Marcus, 1961).

In some ways, at the treatment level, we are staunchly eclectic. We believe therapists need to be flexible, changing therapeutic approaches depending on the client, the problem, and the setting. However, as noted previously, when it comes to *learning* clinical skills, we advocate an approach that focuses first on less directive interviewing approaches and later on more directive approaches. Therefore, in early chapters of this text, we emphasize person-centered and psychodynamic approaches. By beginning nondirectively, we hope to emphasize the depth and richness of human interaction. Later, as we focus on interview assessment procedures, more directive behavioral, cognitive-behavioral, and solution-oriented approaches to interviewing receive greater emphasis.

Although person-centered and psychodynamic approaches are usually considered philosophically dissimilar, both teach that interviewers should initially allow clients to freely talk about their concerns with minimal external structure and direction

(S. Freud, 1940/1949; Luborsky, 1984; Rogers, 1951, 1961). In other words, person-centered and psychodynamically oriented interviewers are alike in that they allow clients freedom to discuss whatever personal issues or concerns they want to discuss. Consequently, these interviewing approaches have been labeled *nondirective* and heavily emphasize listening techniques. (It would be more appropriate to label person-centered and psychodynamic approaches *less directive,* because all interviewers, intentionally or unintentionally, influence and therefore direct their clients some of the time.)

Person-centered and psychodynamic interviewers are nondirective for very different reasons. Briefly, person-centered interviewers believe that by allowing clients to talk freely and openly in an atmosphere characterized by acceptance and empathy, personal growth and change occur. Carl Rogers (1961), the originator of person-centered therapy, stated this directly: "If I can provide a certain type of relationship, the other person will discover within himself the capacity to use that relationship for growth, and change and personal development will occur" (p. 33).

For Rogers, an interviewer's expression of unconditional positive regard, congruence, and accurate empathy constitutes the necessary and sufficient ingredients for positive personal growth and healing. We look more closely at how Rogers defines these three ingredients and other theoretical orientations in Chapter 5.

Psychoanalytically oriented interviewers advocate nondirective approaches because they believe that letting clients talk freely—through free association—allows unconscious conflicts to emerge during the therapeutic hour (S. Freud, 1940/1949). Eventually, through interpretation, psychoanalytic interviewers bring underlying conflicts into awareness so they can be dealt with directly and consciously.

Similar to person-centered therapists, psychoanalytic therapists acknowledge that empathic listening may be a powerful source of healing in its own right: "Frequently underestimated is the degree to which the therapist's presence and empathic listening constitute the most powerful source of help and support one human being can provide another" (Strupp & Binder, 1984, p. 41). However, for psychoanalytically oriented clinicians, empathic listening is usually viewed as a necessary, but not sufficient, ingredient for client personal growth and development (Brenneis, 1994; Meissner, 1991).

In contrast to person-centered and psychodynamic interviewers, behavioral, cognitive, or solution-oriented interviewers are more inclined to take an expert role from the beginning of the first clinical interview. They believe that specific thoughts, personal frameworks, and maladaptive behaviors cause mental and emotional distress (Beck, 1976; Hoyt, 1996; Kazdin, 1979). Therefore, their main therapeutic work involves identifying and modifying or eliminating maladaptive thinking and behavioral patterns, replacing them with more adaptive patterns as quickly and efficiently as possible, thereby alleviating the client's social and emotional problems. Kendall and Bemis (1983) describe the cognitive-behavioral therapist's directive orientation:

> The task of the cognitive-behavioral therapist is to act as a diagnostician, educator, and technical consultant who assesses maladaptive cognitive processes and works with the client to design learning experiences that may remediate these dysfunctional cognitions and the behavioral and affective patterns with which they correlate. (p. 566)

Despite this description, most cognitive-behavioral clinicians also recognize the importance of empathic listening as a necessary, although not sufficient, factor in adaptive behavior change (Meichenbaum, 1997; Wright & Davis, 1994). Michael Mahoney (1991), a renowned cognitive-behavioral therapist, has stated that "a secure and caring relationship" constitutes one of the most basic "general principles of human helping" (p. 270). Other cognitive-behavioral practitioners have made similar statements. Notably, Wright and Davis, in the inaugural issue of the journal *Cognitive and Behavioral Practice,* state: "We find strong consensus in the conclusion that the relationship is central to therapeutic change" and "Even in specific behavioral therapies, patients who view their therapist as warm and empathetic will be more involved in their treatment and, ultimately, have a better outcome" (1994, p. 26).

We are not suggesting that person-centered and psychodynamic approaches are more effective than cognitive, behavioral, or other clinical approaches. In fact, controlled studies indicate that cognitive and behavioral therapies are at least as effective, and perhaps more so, than psychodynamic and person-centered approaches (Luborsky, Singer, & Luborsky, 1975; M. Seligman, 1995; Smith, Glass, & Miller, 1980; Stiles, Shapiro, & Elliott, 1986). Instead, our intent is to assert, as Corsini and others (1989; Hubble, Duncan, & Miller, 1999) have suggested, that developing nondirective interviewing skills provides an excellent foundation for building positive therapy relationships and learning more advanced and more active/directive psychotherapy strategies and techniques. A number of important facts support this assertion (see Putting It in Practice 1.1).

## BASIC REQUIREMENTS FOR CLINICAL INTERVIEWERS

You must meet four basic requirements to become an effective interviewer:

1. You must master the technical knowledge associated with clinical interviewing. This means you must know the range of interviewing responses available to you and their likely influence on clients. For example, you must know different types of questions interviewers can ask and how clients typically respond or react to them. You must know when the interview situation dictates structured information gathering and when less directive approaches are warranted. You must know ethical guidelines associated with professional clinical interviewing. In other words, you must have an intellectual grasp of the basic tools of the trade.

2. You must be self-aware. You need to know how you affect other people and how others affect you, both those in your own cultural and socioeconomic class and those outside your familiar surroundings. You need to be aware of the sound and range of your own voice, your body or physical presence, perceived level of interpersonal attractiveness, and usual patterns of eye contact and interpersonal distance, because all of these variables influence your clients. Further, you must constantly be willing to learn and grow, addressing blind spots and shortcomings you may have because of your personal and social background.

    It is also important that you be aware of how your own culture and social class have shaped your personal values and ways of behaving. You need to become aware that others, both in and outside your culture, may have been taught values and behaviors very different from yours. It is incumbent on you as interviewer to realize when cultural, class, and gender differences may be influencing or hampering effective communication between you and your client. To be a culturally insensitive clinical interviewer is unprofessional and unethical (Essandoh, 1996; Vontress et al., 1999).

## Putting It in Practice 1.1

# Why Be Nondirective?

Many famous psychotherapists began with a psychoanalytic orientation—Karen Horney, Aaron Beck, Albert Ellis, Fritz Perls, Carl Rogers, and Nancy Chodorow. These respected theorists and therapists developed their unique approaches after years of listening nondirectively to distressed individuals. An underlying philosophy of this book is that beginning interviewers should begin by listening nondirectively to distressed individuals. Although it is natural for beginning interviewers to feel impatient and eager to help their clients, their safest and probably most helpful behavior is effective listening. As Strupp and Binder (1984) note, "Recall an old Maine proverb: 'One can seldom listen his way into trouble'" (p. 44). Some advantages of nondirective interviewing follow:

1. It's much easier to begin interviewing someone in a nondirective mode and later shift to a more directive mode than to begin interviewing in an active or directive mode and then change to a less directive approach (Luborsky, 1984; Wolberg, 1995).
2. Strategies designed to deliberately influence clients in a particular manner require that interviewers have knowledge of the psychopathology involved to make sound judgments regarding how a given strategy can help clients change. Most beginning interviewers don't have the foundational training in psychopathology and the supervised psychotherapy experiences needed to implement more directive therapeutic strategies.
3. Nondirective interviewing is an effective means for helping beginning interviewers enhance their self-awareness and learn about themselves (J. Sommers-Flanagan & Means, 1987). Through self-awareness, beginning interviewers become capable of choosing a particular theoretical orientation and effective clinical interventions.
4. A nondirective listening approach, properly implemented, helps reduce the tension that beginning interviewers feel to perform, to help, and to prove something to their initial clients. In short, nondirective approaches help beginning interviewers effectively cope with that urge to "do something and do it right."
5. Nondirective approaches have less chance of offending or missing the mark with early clients (Meier & Davis, 2001). Although clinical interviewers often start out working with volunteers, even analogue or role-play clients are real people, with either real or role-played reasons for being interviewed. Nondirective interviewers, who are there only to listen, place more responsibility on clients' shoulders and can therefore lessen their own fears (as well as the real possibility) of asking the wrong questions or suggesting an unhelpful course of action. In addition, beginning interviewers tend to feel too responsible for their clients; a nondirective approach can help prevent interviewers from feeling too much responsibility.
6. A nondirective listening stance helps clients establish feelings and beliefs of independence and self-direction. This stance also communicates respect for the client's personal attitudes, behaviors, and choices. Such respect is rare, gratifying, and possibly healing (W. Miller, 2000; Strupp & Binder, 1984).

========================= **Putting It in Practice 1.1 (continued)** =========================

Specific helping strategies developed from all major theoretical orientations can be important tools for professional interviewers. Evidence indicating that some forms of psychotherapy may be better than others for particular clients and particular problems is beginning to accumulate (Beck, Rush, Shaw, & Emery, 1979; Hubble et al., 1999; Lazarus, Beutler, & Norcross, 1992; Nathan, 1998). The day when every therapist rigidly adheres to a single theoretical orientation may be drawing to an end (Goldfried, 1990; C. Watkins & Watts, 1995). Although we welcome psychotherapy integration, theoretical rapprochement, and the identification of specific treatment strategies for specific clinical problems, too often, therapists are tempted to employ powerful therapeutic interventions before they have received basic clinical training and supervision.

Our belief that interviewers should begin from a foundation of nondirective listening is articulated by the following excerpt from C. H. Patterson and Watkins (1996, p. 509; quoting Lao Tzu): "Lao Tzu, a Chinese philosopher of the fifth century B.C., wrote a poem titled *Leader*, which applies when *therapist* is substituted for *leader* and *clients* is substituted for *people.*"

### A Leader (Therapist)

A leader is best when people hardly know he [sic] exists;
Not so good when people obey and acclaim him;
Worst when they despise him.
But of a good leader who talks little,
When his work is done, his aim fulfilled,
They will say, "We did it ourselves."

The less a leader does and says,
The happier his people;
The more he struts and brags,
The sorrier his people.

[Therefore,] a sensible man says:
If I keep from meddling with people, they take care of themselves.
If I keep from preaching at people, they improve themselves.
If I keep from imposing on people, they become themselves.

3. Clinical interviewing requires observational and assessment skills (to acquire "other-awareness"). Having these skills means that you know of and are sensitive to various individual and cultural values, behaviors, and norms. You also must be able to recognize and appreciate the perspectives of others (this skill is also known as an "empathic way of being," Rogers, 1961).

    Awareness of others is a basic principle underlying interviewing assessment and evaluation. Clinical interviewers must objectively observe client behavior and evaluate for psychopathology. Assessment and evaluation can involve highly structured procedures such as mental status examinations, suicide assessments, and diagnostic interviewing. Clinical interviewers must be aware not only of client cultural issues, but also of psychological, behavioral, historical, and diagnostic status (Matthews & Walker, 1997; Mezzich & Shea, 1990).

4. To be an effective clinical interviewer, you need practice and experience. As you begin to learn about interviewing and how you affect others, you must also begin practice interviews. This usually involves extensive role-playing with fellow students or actors or arranged interview experiences with people you do not know (Balleweg, 1990; J. Sommers-Flanagan & Means, 1987; Weiss, 1986). Practice interviewing is designed to prepare you for the real thing—the actual clinical interview. To reduce your anxiety and increase your competence, you should have extensive supervised practice before beginning actual interviewing or counseling sessions. As you expand your basic skills, begin reading about and working on understanding people who are culturally, sexually, physically, and socioeconomically different from you (S. Sue, 1998; see Individual and Cultural Highlight 1.1).

The more diverse interviewing and supervision experiences you obtain, the more likely you are to develop the broad, empathic perspective you need to understand clients (Speight & Vera, 1997; Vacc, Wittmer, & DeVaney, 1988). In some ways, this process is similar to becoming acculturated (Heinrich, Corbine, & Thomas, 1990).

## The Perfect Interviewer

What if you could be a perfect clinical interviewer? Of course, this is impossible. But if you could be a perfect interviewer, you would be able to stop at any point in a given interview and outline: (a) what you are doing (based on technical expertise); (b) why you are doing it (based on technical knowledge and assessment or evaluation information); (c) whether any of your personal issues or biases are interfering with the interview (based on self-awareness); and, perhaps most importantly, (d) how your client, regardless of his or her age, sex, or culture, is reacting to the interview (based on other awareness).

Put another way, if you were a perfect interviewer, you could "tune in" to each client's personal world so completely that you would resonate with the client, as a sensitive violin string begins to move when a matching tone is played in the room (J. Watkins & Watkins, 1997). You would be able to use this resonance to determine where every interview needed to go.

You would also assess each client's needs and situation and carry out appropriate therapeutic actions to address the client's needs and personal situation, from initiating a suicide assessment to beginning a behavioral analysis of a troublesome habit—all during the clinical interview. One can only imagine the vast array of skills and the depth of wisdom necessary for a clinical interviewer to approach perfection.

We readily acknowledge that perfection is unattainable. However, clinical interviewing is a professional endeavor based on scientific research and supported by a long history of supervised training (Hill, 2001). As a consequence, it is inappropriate and unprofessional to, as an old supervisor of ours used to say, "fly by the seat of your pants" in an interview session (P. H. Bornstein, personal communication, January 1982).

In the end, as a human and imperfect interviewer, you may not be able to explain every clinical nuance or every action and reaction. You may not feel as aware and tuned in as you could be, but your interviewing behavior will be guided by sound theoretical principles, humane professional ethics, and basic scientific data pertaining to therapeutic efficacy. Additionally, once you have become grounded in psychological theory,

====  INDIVIDUAL AND CULTURAL HIGHLIGHT 1.1  ====

## Pitfalls of Nondirectiveness

Most swords are double-edged. And nondirective listening is no exception. To be blunt (no pun intended), some people simply detest nondirective listening. For example, if you practice too many nondirective listening techniques on them, your friends and family will quickly become annoyed. They will be annoyed partly because you may be unskilled, but also because, in most social and cultural settings, nondirective listening is inappropriate.

As we discuss in Chapter 13, some cultural groups, for the most part, prefer directiveness from health and mental health professionals. This does not mean that you must never listen nondirectively to people of these cultural groups. Instead, it speaks to the importance of recognizing that different techniques help or hinder relationship building in different individuals who come to you seeking assistance.

Additional pitfalls of nondirectiveness include:

1. Clients can perceive nondirective interviewers as manipulative or evasive.
2. Too many nondirective responses can leave clients feeling lost and adrift, without any guidance.
3. If clients come to therapy expecting expert advice, they may be deeply disappointed when you steadfastly refuse to do anything but listen nondirectively.
4. If you never offer a professional opinion, you may be viewed as unprofessional, ignorant, or weak.

When it comes to interviewing clients, often, too much of any response or technique is ill advised. We say this despite the fact that we are beginning by emphasizing nondirective listening skills. Don't worry. We recognize that too much nondirectiveness can be just as troublesome as too much directiveness— especially when it comes to interviewing clients outside mainstream American culture.

professional ethics, and empirical research, you will be able to add clinical intuition and spontaneity to your clinical repertoire.

## GOALS AND OBJECTIVES OF THIS BOOK

The basic objectives of this book are to:

1. Guide you through an educational and training experience based on the previously described teaching approach.
2. Provide technical information about clinical interviewing.
3. Introduce methods for interviewer self-awareness, cultural awareness, and personal growth.
4. Introduce client assessment and evaluation methods (i.e., facilitate acquisition of diagnostic skills).

5. Describe procedures for interviewing culturally diverse clients and special client populations.
6. Provide suggestions for experiential interviewer development activities.

## SUMMARY

This book's underlying philosophy emphasizes a particular approach to learning how to become a competent clinical interviewer. Specifically, students should begin learning interviewing skills from a nondirective perspective, gradually adding more directive skills as they master the basics of listening. Beginning interviewers should focus on learning to: (a) quiet themselves and listen to clients, (b) develop a positive therapeutic relationship with clients, and (c) obtain diagnostic and assessment information.

Interviewers can benefit from obtaining a broad range of training experiences. It is especially important to learn and practice interviewing from different theoretical perspectives, including person-centered, psychoanalytic, behavioral, cognitive, feminist, and solution-oriented viewpoints. Diverse experiences help interviewers learn about how technical interviewer responses, self-presentational styles, cultural background, and gender affect each client, taking into account the client's own particular set of problems, biases, cultural background, and gender. Although perfection is impossible, if interviewers base their behavior on sound theoretical principles, professional ethics, and scientific research, they will become competent and responsible mental health professionals.

This book is organized into four parts, moving the beginning clinical interviewer through stages designed for optimal skill development. Because actual practice is necessary for interviewer skill development, each chapter offers suggested experiential activities to help interviewers become more self-aware, more culturally sensitive, and to develop greater technical expertise.

## SUGGESTED READINGS AND RESOURCES

It helps if you have some knowledge of personality theory and psychopathology before studying the interviewing process. We recognize, however, that not all interviewing and counseling courses have personality theory and psychopathology prerequisites. For those lacking such background, the following textbooks, articles, and recreational readings on theories of personality, theories and approaches to counseling and psychotherapy, and psychopathology provide a worthwhile foundation for professional skill development.

Corey, G. (2001). *Theory and practice of counseling and psychotherapy* (6th ed.). Monterey, CA: Brooks/Cole. Corey's text is clear and excellent for beginners who have not read about various theoretical approaches to counseling and psychotherapy.

Corsini, R., & Wedding, D. (2000). *Current psychotherapies* (6th ed.). Itasca, IL: E. E. Peacock. This latest edition of an edited volume contains specific chapters on many different approaches to psychotherapy. Corsini and Wedding's textbook is a classic and is often adopted for graduate-level theories courses. We especially like Corsini's efforts to define the differences between counseling and psychotherapy in the introductory chapter.

Giordano, P. J. (1997). Establishing rapport and developing interviewing skills. In J. R. Matthews & C. E. Walker (Eds.), *Basic skills and professional issues in clinical psychology* (pp. 59–82).

Needham Heights, MA: Allyn & Bacon. This chapter offers readers an alternative review of essential components for developing clinical interviewing skills. The author describes a wide range of "pitfalls" common to beginning interviewers.

Goldfried, M. (Ed.). (2001). *How therapists change: Personal and professional recollections.* Washington, DC: American Psychological Association. This book gives you an insider's look into how professionals have undergone personal change. It gives you a feel for how the profession of counseling and psychotherapy might affect you personally.

Hubble, M. A., Duncan, B. L., & Miller, S. D. (1999). *The heart and soul of change: What works in therapy.* Washington, DC: American Psychological Association. This book, recipient of a Menninger Writing Award, focuses squarely on the common factors associated with positive change in counseling and psychotherapy. It provides practical suggestions for integrating these common factors into your interviewing practice.

Ivey, A. E., D'Andrea, M., Ivey, M. B., & Simek-Morgan, L. (2002). *Theories of counseling and psychotherapy: A multicultural perspective* (5th ed.). Boston: Allyn & Bacon. Ivey and his colleagues provide a multicultural slant to the traditional theories of counseling and psychotherapy.

Miller, P. H. (2001). *Theories of developmental psychology* (4th ed.). San Francisco: W. H. Freeman. Miller provides excellent descriptions of the various theories of psychological development. Her chapters on Piaget and Freud are especially clear and easy to read.

Roukema, R. (1998). *What every patient, family, friend, and caregiver needs to know about psychiatry.* Washington, DC: American Psychiatric Press. This book is written for laypersons but makes a nice introduction to psychiatry for budding mental health professionals. Be forewarned that it has a clear medical model, as illustrated by its discussions of emotional versus mental illness.

Sommers-Flanagan, J., & Sommers-Flanagan, R. (1989). A categorization of pitfalls common to beginning interviewers. *The Journal of Training and Practice in Professional Psychology, 3,* 58–71. We describe common beginning interviewer pitfalls, including adequacy, activity, atmosphere, and attentiveness. The article is designed to help beginning interviewers see potential problems and thereby control them more effectively.

# Chapter 2

# *FOUNDATIONS AND PREPARATIONS*

*What infants yearn for is the reassurance that they will never lose their caretaker's love, that no matter what, she (or he) will keep them safe from any lurking hazard. Although female caretakers are more fluent in high-pitched babyese . . . fathers should not sell short their own ability to reassure—or harm.*

From *Mother Nature* by Sarah Blaffer Hrdy, p. 540

---

### CHAPTER OBJECTIVES

When building a house, you must first define what you mean by *house*. In addition, you must prepare by gathering together your design plan, your tools, and your resources. This chapter focuses on what we mean by *clinical interviewing* and how to prepare yourself for meeting with clients. After reading this chapter, you will know:

- A comprehensive definition of clinical interviewing.
- The nature of a professional relationship between interviewer and client.
- Common client motivations for seeking professional assistance.
- How you can both improve your effectiveness and make yourself uncomfortable by becoming more self-aware.
- Expectations and misconceptions common to beginning interviewers.
- How clinical interviewing can be compared to seven different vocational activities.
- How to handle essential physical dimensions of the interview, such as seating arrangements, note taking, and videotape and audiotape recording.
- Practical approaches for managing professional and ethical issues, including how to present yourself to clients, time management, discussing confidentiality and informed consent, documentation procedures, and personal stress management.

---

To compare the framework of a clinical interview with parenting an infant is an exaggeration. Nevertheless, as you read this chapter, consider the following concept. As a professional interviewer, your first task is to build a secure base for clients—and this secure base serves as a foundation from which therapeutic work can grow.

When questioned about early graduate school memories, a former student shared the following:

Probably because of too little practice and too few role plays, what I remember most about my first clinical interview is my own terror. I don't remember the client. I don't remember the problem areas, the ending, or the subsequent treatment plan. I just remember breathing deeply and engaging in some very serious self-talk designed to calm myself. All my salient memories have to do with me, not the person who was coming for help. Ironic, isn't it?

It is understandable and even likely that in your first therapy interviews, you will sweat more than a few proverbial bullets. But our hope is that by reading this book, thinking (and breathing) deeply, and practicing faithfully with anyone who will let you, you will quickly advance past the self-conscious stage articulated by our student and be able to focus on your client and your interviewing tasks.

Discerning the difference between what happens in a formal interview and what happens in normal social relationships can be hard. Nonetheless, clinical interviews are much different from ordinary conversation. This chapter delineates these differences and describes the physical surroundings and professional and ethical considerations essential to preparing for your first interview.

## TOWARD A DEFINITION OF CLINICAL INTERVIEWING

Clinical interviewing has been defined in many different ways. Some prefer a narrow, straightforward definition:

> An interview is a controlled situation in which one person, the interviewer, asks a series of questions of another person, the respondent. (Keats, 2000, p. 1)

Others are more ambiguous:

> An interview is an interaction between at least two persons. Each participant contributes to the process, and each influences the responses of the other. However, this characterization falls short of defining the process. Ordinary conversation is interactional, but surely interviewing goes beyond that. (Trull & Phares, 2001)

Still others combine specificity with ambiguity:

> An interview represents a verbal and nonverbal dialogue between two participants, whose behaviors affect each other's style of communication, resulting in specific patterns of interaction. In the interview one participant who labels himself or herself as the "interviewer" attempts to achieve specific goals, while the other participant generally assumes the role of "answering the questions." (Shea, 1998, pp. 6–7)

From our perspective, an adequate definition of clinical interviewing should include the following factors:

1. A professional relationship between interviewer and client is established.
2. The client is motivated, at least to some degree, to accomplish something by meeting with the interviewer.
3. The interviewer and client work together, to some extent, to establish and achieve mutually agreeable goals for the client.

4. In the context of the professional relationship, interviewer and client interact, both verbally and nonverbally, as the interviewer applies a variety of active listening skills and psychological techniques to evaluate, understand, and help the client achieve his or her goals.

5. The quality and quantity of interactions between interviewer and client are influenced by many factors, including interviewer and client personality style, attitudes, and mutually agreed on goals.

## The Nature of a Professional Relationship

A professional relationship involves an explicit agreement for one party to provide services to another party or entity. This may sound awkward, but it is important to emphasize that a professional relationship includes an agreement for service provision. In counseling or psychotherapy, this agreement is usually referred to as *informed consent* (Beahrs & Gutheil, 2001). Essentially, informed consent means the client has been given all the important information about services to be provided to him or her during the interview. Further, informed consent indicates the client has freely consented to treatment (Welfel, 2002). Informed consent is discussed in detail later in this chapter.

---

**Putting It in Practice 2.1**

### Just How Much Is Your Professional Help Worth?: The Value of Therapy

Many counselors, social workers, psychologists, and psychiatrists who are in training react strongly to charging a fee for their services. Take a moment to think about this issue. Then discuss the following questions with your classmates:

1. How much do counselors, social workers, psychologists, and psychiatrists who are in private practice charge for providing mental health services in your town or city? What is the top fee? What are your reactions to the top fee charged by mental health providers?
2. Are there any places in your town or city where clients can obtain free or low-cost mental health services? If so, how long is the wait for such services? What do people think of the relative quality of services at the low-cost clinic versus the high-cost private practitioner?
3. How much do you imagine being paid for providing mental health services?
4. Imagine for a moment how you will feel charging someone who receives your professional services. How much will you feel comfortable charging? How much or how little payment would make you uncomfortable?
5. If the training clinic where you are employed requires at least $25 from each client, how might receiving such a fee influence how you handle yourself during the session? What if your client asks for a discount? How will you feel if he or she consistently "forgets" to pay you?

If the idea of receiving payment for your services as a counselor or therapist is uncomfortable, don't worry because you're not alone. One of our colleagues back in graduate school once commented: "I should be paying my clients to see me because I'm totally inexperienced and they're letting me practice on them!"

Professional relationships are also characterized by payment or compensation for services. This is true whether the therapist receives payment directly (as in private practice) or indirectly (as when payment is provided by a mental health center, Medicaid, or other institution). Professional interviewers provide a service to someone in need—a service that should be worth its cost (see Putting It in Practice 2.1).

Some writers have cynically labeled psychotherapy *the purchase of friendship* (Korchin, 1976, p. 285), but there are many differences between a therapy relationship and friendship. Your friends do not schedule appointments to meet with you in an office setting; they do not regard their own self-expression, personal growth, and the resolution of their problems as the sole objective of your time together (or if they do, you may begin considering alternative friendships). Friends usually don't carry liability insurance to be friends; and although there are many benefits of friendship, such benefits are not subjected to outcome and efficacy research, discussed in scholarly journals, or taught in graduate training programs.

Although there are social and friendly aspects to a professional relationship, professional interviewers control their friendliness. Part of becoming a mature professional is learning to be warm, interactive, and open with clients, while at the same time staying within professional relationship boundaries (see Putting it in Practice 2.2).

---

**Putting It in Practice 2.2**

## Defining Appropriate Relationship Boundaries

Although we don't often stop to think about it, boundaries define most relationships. Most boundary breaks have ethical implications. Being familiar with role-related expectations, responsibilities, and limits is an important part of being a good interviewer. Consider the following professional relationship boundary "breaks." Rate, evaluate, and discuss the seriousness of each one. Is it a minor, somewhat serious, or a very serious boundary violation?

- Having a cup of coffee with the client at a coffee shop after the interview.
- Asking your client for a ride to pick up your car.
- Offering to take your client out to dinner sometime.
- Accepting an offer to go to a concert with a client.
- Asking your client (a math teacher) to help your children with their homework.
- Borrowing money from a client.
- Sharing a bit of gossip with a client about someone you both know.
- Talking with one client about another client.
- Fantasizing having sex with your client.
- Giving your client a little spending money because you know your client faces a long weekend with no food.
- Inviting your client to your church, synagogue, or mosque.
- Acting on a financial tip your client gave you by buying stock from your client's stockbroker.
- Dating your client.
- Giving your client's name to a volunteer agency.
- Writing a letter of recommendation for your client's job application.
- Having your client write you a letter of recommendation for a job application.

## Client Motivations

Most clients come to a mental health professional for one of the following reasons:

- They are experiencing subjective distress, discontent, or personal-social impairment.
- Someone, perhaps a spouse or probation officer, has insisted they obtain treatment. Usually this means the client has been misbehaving, breaking the law, or irritating others.
- They are seeking personal growth and development.

When clients come to therapy because of personal distress or impairment, they often feel defeated because they have been unable to independently cope with their problems. At the same time, these clients, feeling the pain or cost of their problems, unless profoundly depressed, also may be highly motivated. Their strong motivation can translate into considerable cooperation, general hopefulness, and receptivity to what the therapist has to say (Frank & Frank, 1991; Glasser, 1998).

In contrast, sometimes clients show up in the therapist's office with little motivation. They may have been cajoled or coerced into attending therapy sessions by someone else. In such cases, the client's primary motivation may be to terminate therapy or to be pronounced "well" (J. Sommers-Flanagan & Sommers-Flanagan, 1997). Obviously, if clients are poorly motivated for therapy, it is challenging for interviewers to establish and maintain a professional therapist-client relationship.

Clients who come to therapy for personal growth and development are often highly motivated to engage in a therapeutic process. Because they come by choice and for positive reasons, these clients can be particularly eager for therapy and easy to work with.

## Establishing Common Goals

To establish common therapy goals with clients, therapists must use evaluation and assessment procedures. This means getting clients to participate in or articulate a personal self-assessment. Early in the counseling hour, the therapist needs to interact with the client to help identify what the client thinks is wrong and what the client thinks might help. When the client and therapist agree on the client's problem(s), establishing therapy goals is relatively easy and painless.

On the other hand, sometimes clients and therapists disagree about what should be accomplished in therapy. These disagreements may stem from a variety of sources including, but not limited to: (a) poor client motivation or insight and (b) questionable therapist motives or insight. Historically, more directive approaches to psychotherapy (e.g., psychoanalytic, behavioral) usually considered client motivation and insight as limited or suspect, while therapist motivation and insight was considered relatively infallible. More recently, perhaps because of an emphasis on ethical issues such as informed consent and therapist accountability, most therapy approaches place greater value on the client's perspective than in years past.

Inconsistency between a client's and the therapist's therapy goals is illustrated in the movie (and book) *Ordinary People* (Guest, 1982). In this case, during the initial session, the teenage client tells his psychologist that his goal is to "have more control." In contrast, the psychologist views the client as overcontrolled, needing to loosen up, let go, and relax more. Popular books and movies, perhaps for purposes of mounting conflict and excitement, frequently portray therapists and clients as having different (and sometimes incompatible) therapy goals (see *Girl, Interrupted,* Kaysen, 1993; *Lying on the Couch,* Yalom, 1997).

As an interviewer, it is important for you to value the client's perspective, while at the same time providing a professional opinion regarding appropriate goals and strategies. Striking this balance requires sensitivity, tact, and excellent communication skills.

Clinical interviewers are designated experts in the area of mental health and, therefore, have the responsibility to professionally evaluate or assess client problems before proceeding with treatment. The purpose of evaluating clients is to facilitate the intervention or helping process. A minimal first-session evaluation includes a thorough assessment of your client's presenting problem, an analysis of his or her expectations or goals for therapy, and a review of previous efforts at solving the problem or problems that bring him or her to seek therapy. In most cases, if an initial assessment reveals that client and therapist goals are incompatible, it is incumbent on the therapist to offer the client an opportunity to work with a different therapist.

Premature interventions based on inadequate assessment have been linked to negative therapy outcomes (Hadley & Strupp, 1976; Lynn, Martin, & Frauman, 1996). If a premature intervention is offered before adequate assessment is conducted and mutual goals are formulated, a number of negative outcomes might occur. These include, but are not limited to, the following:

- The interviewer may choose an inappropriate therapeutic approach or technique that is potentially damaging to the client's condition (e.g., one that increases rather than decreases anxiety).
- The client may feel misunderstood and rushed, concluding either that the problem is too bad for even a professional to understand, or that the interviewer is not very bright or competent.
- The client may follow the therapist's incorrect or inappropriate guidance and become frustrated with therapy. As a result, the client's openness to subsequent therapy interventions, and possibly subsequent therapists, is significantly diminished.
- The therapist may not have taken time to listen to strategies the client has already employed to solve the problem. Consequently, he or she may suggest a remedy that the client has already tried without success. The therapist's credibility is thereby diminished.

A clinical interview may produce less-than-positive effects. Negative effects often result from misguided, inappropriate, or premature efforts to help clients. This is why interviewers carefully listen to and evaluate clients, establishing reasonable and mutual treatment goals, before implementing specific change strategies.

## Applying Listening Skills and Psychological Techniques

The common element underlying both evaluation/assessment and intervention/helping is sensitive and effective listening. Whether your primary role is evaluator or interventionist, you must demonstrate to your client that you are a good listener.

It is commonly assumed that one of the best ways to listen to clients is to ask carefully crafted questions; however, this assumption is incorrect. Asking good questions is very important to interviewing, but it is also a directive activity that does *not* always allow clients to freely express themselves. Questions guide and restrict client verbalizations so that the material produced is what the interviewer thinks the client should produce. It may or may not actually represent what clients really want to tell you. Although asking questions is an integral part of interviewing, establishing listening as a priority will assist you in evaluating and helping your clients more effectively (advantages and disadvantages of questions are discussed in Chapter 3).

Skillful interviewers listen, evaluate, and apply psychological interventions in a manner that makes these three activities seem simultaneous. Students, on the other hand, usually should restrain themselves from applying specific psychological techniques until they've adequately listened (nonjudgmentally) and evaluated (clinically). Therefore, the following guideline may be useful for you: No matter how backward it seems, begin by resisting the urge to help your client. Instead, listen more deeply, fully, and attentively than you have ever listened in your life. Doing so will probably help the client more than if you actually try to help (Rogers, 1961; Strupp & Binder, 1984).

## CASE EXAMPLE

*Jerry Fest, a therapist who works with street youth in Portland, Oregon, wrote of the following encounter in a manual for persons working with street youth (Boyer, 1988). One night, he was working in a drop-in counseling center. A young woman came in obviously agitated and in distress. Jerry knew her from other visits, so he greeted her by name. She said, "Hey, man, do I ever need someone to listen to me." He showed her to an office and listened to her incredibly compelling tale of difficulties for several minutes. He then made what he thought was an understanding, supportive statement. The young woman immediately stopped talking. When she began again a few moments later, she stated again that she needed someone to listen to her. The same sequence of events played out again. After her second stop and start, however, Jerry decided to take her literally, and he sat silently for the next 90 minutes. The woman poured out her heart, finally winding down and regaining control. As she prepared to leave, she looked at Jerry and said, "That's what I like about you, Jer. Even when you don't get it right the first time, you eventually catch on."*

Jerry learned an important lesson from this experience. The young woman's need *to be listened to, without interruption,* was clearly articulated. The moral of the story is obvious: Sometimes, active listening *is* the intervention (see Putting It in Practice 2.3).

### Unique Interactions between Interviewer and Client

One reason for the complexities of clinical interviewing is that it involves two (or more) humans interacting, which, by definition, includes a certain amount of unpredictability. Every client and every interviewer brings into the room a new mix of DNA, personality traits, attitudes, and expectations. This makes coming up with a perfect definition of clinical interviewing an improbable task.

Every interview involves at least three distinct variables: the client, the interviewer, and their interactions. Although most of this book focuses on the client and client-interviewer interactions, the following section focuses on you—the interviewer—and your unique contribution to the interviewing process.

╔══════════════════════════════════════════════════════════════╗

═══════════════  **Putting It in Practice 2.3**  ═══════════════

## Self-Statement for Beginning Clinical Interviewers

Listening should be your primary function as a clinical interviewer. If you do not listen adequately, you have no right to suggest helping strategies to a client. If you do listen adequately, you may not need to offer advice because your clients may tell you themselves which strategies would be most helpful. In fact, avoid giving advice or asking too many questions until you've developed your listening skills. Questions tend to reduce the client's freedom of expression. Try reciting the following self-statement to keep this learning goal firmly in mind before and during your initial interviews: "The goal of my interview is to listen well. If I do this, I will be providing an essential service to the client and learning what I need to learn."

She who speaks sows, and she who listens harvests.
—Guy A. Zona,
*Eyes That See Do Not Grow Old*

╚══════════════════════════════════════════════════════════════╝

## SELF-AWARENESS

*Our own image looking back at us in a mirror carries a very different attraction and energy than the image of someone else. We are drawn to it in a half-embarrassed way, excited and intensely involved. Do you remember the last time someone showed you a picture of yourself, or you watched yourself on video? Wasn't there a surge of feeling and a deep curiosity about how you appear to others?*
—Seymour Fisher, *Body Consciousness: You Are What You Feel*

We fondly recall an old college baseball coach who, with great enthusiasm, discussed the difficulty of hitting a baseball. He claimed that using a round bat to make solid contact with a round ball leaves virtually no room for miscalculation; it requires the player's body to be an instrument that can constantly respond and adjust to a small, round, spinning object traveling at varying high speeds.

The process of becoming a good hitter in baseball requires knowledge, practice, excellent body awareness, and good hand-eye coordination. Clinical interviewing also requires knowledge, practice, and self-awareness. (The eye-hand coordination is optional.)

To stretch the analogy a bit further, as a professional interviewer, you must consistently make solid psychological, social, and emotional contact with individuals you have never met. Ordinarily, you are required to accomplish this task in the short span of 50 minutes. To make contact, you must be sensitive to and tolerant of the limitless number of ways people can present themselves and be just as sensitive to and aware of your own physical, psychological, social, cultural, and emotional presence. (Which of these processes seems more difficult—hitting a baseball or conducting clinical interviews? One ray of hope: After a certain age, efficiency at hitting a baseball rapidly deteriorates, whereas effective interviewing enjoys a much longer efficiency curve.)

Self-awareness (not to be confused with self-absorption) is a positive trait and can be especially important for clinical interviewers. Self-awareness helps interviewers know how their personal biases and emotional states influence and potentially distort their understanding of clients. In addition, working with clients can produce emotional reactions in you (e.g., anxiety, depression, or euphoria). An ability to quickly recognize your own emotional reactions toward clients is an advantage. Good interviewers work to understand themselves and their own relationships before entering into interviewer-client relationships (R. Greenberg & Staller, 1981; Macaskill & Macaskill, 1992; Norcross, 2000; Strupp, 1955). Just as accomplished athletes possess a high level of body awareness to perform effectively, interviewers must possess superior psychological, emotional, and social self-awareness to perform optimally.

## Objective Self-Awareness

Listening to your voice and speech patterns and watching your facial expressions and physical manner through audio- and videotaping helps you see yourself from a new perspective. This increased awareness can be personally and professionally valuable.

Unfortunately, self-awareness can be uncomfortable and paralyzing. The problem is how to increase self-awareness without producing too much discomfort and self-consciousness. One potential solution to this dilemma is to embrace self-consciousness and view it as a positive step toward enhancing your clinical skills (Fenigstein, Scheier, & Buss, 1975; see Putting It in Practice 2.4).

## Forms of Self-Awareness

Forms of self-awareness include physical self-awareness, psychosocial self-awareness, developmental self-awareness, cultural self-awareness, and awareness of interviewing expectations and misconceptions.

### Physical Self-Awareness

Physical self-awareness involves becoming conscious of your voice quality, body language, body size, and other physical aspects of self. It is particularly important to be aware of how you affect others—on the physical dimension. Some people have especially soft, warm, and comforting voices; others come across more authoritatively. Try listening to yourself on audiotape or ask others to listen and give you feedback (see Individual and Cultural Highlight 2.1).

Clients' perceptions of their interviewers are sometimes influenced by the interviewer's gender. For example, male interviewers are commonly described as more rational and authoritarian and females as more warm and compassionate (Basow, 1980). Although this stereotyping may be accurate, it may also have more to do with a client's history of male-female relationships than with the interviewer's actual style (Witt, 1997). Similarly, interviewers may also stereotype their male and female clients (Morshead, 1990).

### Psychosocial Self-Awareness

Psychosocial self-awareness refers to how you view yourself as relating to others. As suggested by C. Bennett (1984), it is a slippery concept: "The social self is . . . elusive. There is no mirror in which we may actually examine interpersonal relations. Most of the feedback, most of the self-percepts come from others" (p. 276).

Not only does psychosocial self-awareness involve perceptions of and feedback about how others view us, but also our psychological, social, and emotional needs and how they influence our lives. In his oft-cited hierarchy of needs, Maslow (1970) contends that all humans have basic physiological needs; safety needs; self-esteem needs;

## Desensitization and Objective Self-Awareness

*Objective self-awareness* is the term coined by researchers to describe feelings of discomfort associated with listening to or viewing yourself on audio- or video-tapes (Fenigstein, 1979). Discomfort comes from viewing physical aspects of yourself (e.g., voice quality, physical appearance, idiosyncratic mannerisms). To watch or listen to yourself produces increased self-awareness, which also increases self-consciousness and inhibition. Expect to experience moderate discomfort as you play back and review recordings of your interviews. Put bluntly, most of us hate watching ourselves on video—especially at first.

Take advantage of every opportunity to observe yourself on tape. Repeatedly viewing yourself will help you get over your discomfort at watching yourself. You may even eventually be able to identify attractive aspects of yourself on tape. The following advice can help you work through objective self-awareness:

1. Videotape or audiotape your interviewing sessions as often as possible.
2. Watch or listen to the tapes by yourself first, if you prefer. This can help you feel more comfortable (or unfortunately, less comfortable) when you present your work to your class.
3. Admit to someone, perhaps to the whole class that will view your recorded session, that you feel uncomfortable. Many in the group will likely acknowledge their own discomfort and support you for the brave act of presenting your tape to the class. In addition, talking about your feelings to people you trust is a good coping strategy.
4. Be open to positive and negative feedback from others, but if you don't want feedback, feel free to request there be none.
5. If someone gives you feedback you don't completely understand, ask for clarification.
6. Be sure to thank people who have given you feedback, even if you did not like or agree with some of the feedback. It is rare in our culture to receive direct feedback about how we come across to others. Take advantage of the opportunity and use it for personal growth.
7. As C. Rogers (1961) and Maslow (1970) suggested, the self-actualized or fully functioning person is "open to experience" (Rogers, 1961, p. 173). We believe good interviewers possess similar qualities. There is nothing to be gained by defensiveness. Adopt an open attitude toward feedback. If this is too difficult, look for support from people you trust.
8. If you cannot identify anyone in your class whom you trust, you have several choices. First, keep trying. Sometimes, persistence pays off and you'll begin trusting some classmates. Second, find someone outside the group (friend, colleague, or therapist) in whom you can confide, with the eventual goal of also identifying someone in your class. Third, find a new group or individual you trust. Sometimes, pathological groups or classes form that do not provide empathy or support for their members. If you are sure this is the case, move on to more healthy surroundings. On the other hand, always scrutinize yourself before leaving a class or group. You may be able to modify your own attitudes and successfully stay.
9. Learn a relaxation technique. Many methods of physical and mental relaxation can help you manage the stress and anxiety that accompany self-awareness (see Davis, McKay, & Eshelman, 2000; Kabat-Zinn, 1995).

---

INDIVIDUAL AND CULTURAL HIGHLIGHT 2.1

## Discovering Your Accent

We once had an African student in an interviewing class who indicated privately that he believed others were uncomfortable with his accent. After securing his permission to do so and after he presented an audiotaped interview, we asked the class to give him feedback about his voice. Much to his surprise, his classmates were uniformly positive about the pleasant aspects of his voice. This supportive feedback helped Amhad relax a little more about his accent and voice.

Recently, while on a teaching exchange in Great Britain, we came to understand Amhad's perspective more deeply. During our Britain experience, nearly everyone we met commented on our accents. The usual comments were: "Oh, it's obvious you're American" or our more sarcastic British friends might say, when introducing us, "As you can tell by their accents, John and Rita were born and raised here in England." This experience of being pigeonholed based on an accent even affected our 12-year-old daughter, who, throughout her stay at a local British middle school, was approached by other children who would ask, "Would you say something so we can hear your accent?"

The point is that we all have accents, and others can often quickly detect these accents. Furthermore, people will judge you based on your accent.

From time to time, while taking your interviewing course, remember to ask others about your voice. In particular, be sure to ask individuals who are culturally or regionally different from you. Do your best to discover your accent and to understand its potential effect on others.

---

self-actualization needs; and needs for love, acceptance, and interpersonal belongingness. Good clinical interviewers are aware of their own particular psychological and interpersonal needs and how such needs can affect their interviewing and counseling behavior. One way of enhancing your psychosocial self-awareness is to intentionally reflect on your life and career goals. Ask yourself:

- What are my most important personal values?
- What are my life goals? What do I really want out of life, and why? Does my everyday behavior move me toward my life goals?
- What are my career goals? If I want to be a counselor or psychotherapist, how will I achieve this goal? Why do I want to be a counselor or psychotherapist?
- How would I describe myself in only a few words? How would I describe myself to a stranger? What do I particularly like and what do I especially dislike about myself?

It is also important to regularly get feedback from trusted friends and colleagues regarding how you come across to others. Having a clear sense of how others perceive you can help you avoid taking a client's inaccurate evaluation of you at face value.

## CASE EXAMPLE

*A client periodically accused her therapist of being too unemotional. She would say, "You never seem to have any feelings. I'm pouring my heart out to you in here and you're just stiff as a board. Don't you care about me at all?" To stay secure about his social-emotional identity, the therapist asked his colleagues for feedback, and they assured him that he was a kind and caring person. Additionally, at the same time, he was seeing another female client who consistently accused him of "being too emotional," complaining that he was overreacting to what she told him. Both of these clients were extremely disturbed (i.e., inpatients on a psychiatric unit), and their perceptions were distorted by their own problems. However, even less disturbed clients can have distorted perceptions of your physical, social, and emotional presentation; this can be disconcerting if you have not received other feedback from peers and supervisors about your interpersonal style. We discuss this process, also known as transference or parataxic distortion, in Chapter 5.*

Another way to evaluate your psychosocial self involves traditional psychological testing. Many tests are available that can provide you with insight regarding your psychosocial needs and tendencies. Some tests commonly used by therapists to become more familiar with their psychosocial selves include the Minnesota Multiphasic Personality Inventory, 2nd edition (MMPI-2; Butcher, Dahlstrom, Graham, Tellegen, & Kaemmer, 1989) and the Myers Briggs Type Indicator (MBTI; Myers, 1962).

## Developmental Self-Awareness

Although developmental self-awareness is closely linked to psychosocial self-awareness, it merits separate discussion. Developmental self-awareness refers to a consciousness of one's personal history, of specific events that significantly influenced personal development. Everyone has at least a few vivid memories that characterize and capture very personal aspects of self. These memories usually mark personal struggles, victories, or traumas that occurred during particular developmental transitions (e.g., adolescence).

In the tradition of both psychoanalysis and most Adlerians (Adler, 1937), we suggest that you explore your own history of interpersonal relationships, beginning with childhood. Reviewing and perhaps uncovering consistencies in your patterns of relating to others can provide you with insight regarding how you will react to clients. You can begin this exploration by sitting quietly and recalling all the people (and events) in your life who made a pivotal difference in where you are today. Go back as far as you can, picturing each person or scenario in as much detail as possible. You may even want to list them chronologically and fashion a psychosocial developmental map of your history. Another way of exploring your developmental history is through personal psychotherapy (R. Greenberg & Staller, 1981; Norcross, 2000).

## Cultural Self-Awareness

The belief in the innate superiority of one's own tribe to neighboring tribes, or one's own nation or race to other nations or races, is probably as old as our species (Zuckerman, 1990, p. 1297). Geographical isolation and consequent inbreeding resulted in similarities among the members of human groups that laypeople refer to as *characteristics of race*. Zuckerman points out that these characteristics lie along a continuum and constitute only surface differences with regard to species distinction. Commonality among the races overrides the distinctions, just as commonalities among cultures are more numerous than are differences among them.

So why do we advocate caution when you work with clients whose background is different from yours? Why the admonitions to know yourself culturally? Why the belief that to be effective interviewers, therapists must pursue knowledge of other cultures and backgrounds to the extent that they strive to be multicultural? Slowly, we are beginning to awaken to the truth that our ideas about what is proper and improper, right and wrong, appropriate and inappropriate—even normal and abnormal—are highly influenced by our particular cultural, religious, political, and gender-typed upbringing. Whether two people can understand each other depends not so much on racial or cultural backgrounds, but on how strongly each of them believes in the correctness or even the superiority of what is personally familiar. Truly understanding someone from another culture begins with acceptance of differences as normal, interesting aspects of being human.

Social scientists have explored the phenomenon we refer to as *stereotyping* from numerous perspectives. One important finding is that, in general, stereotyping others varies inversely with the person's experience with individual members of other groups. Although simple exposure to different cultures is not sufficient to end stereotyping, it can improve attitudes and decrease anxiety between individuals from different racial backgrounds (Stephan, Diaz-Loving, & Duran, 2000; see Individual and Cultural Highlight 2.2).

Multiculturalism remains a hot issue in psychology and counseling. Not infrequently, discussion of multicultural theory and practice results in heated argument. One example is an article published in the *American Psychologist* titled "Why Is Multiculturalism Good?" (Fowers & Richardson, 1996). The article emphasized a European American tradition and was subsequently attacked by numerous authors on a variety of grounds, including claims that Fowers and Richardson minimized the extent of contemporary discrimination and racism, portrayed multiculturalism as inherently adversarial, and were insufficiently realistic (Hall et al., 1997; Teo & Febbraro, 1997). What this series of articles demonstrates, aside from intellectual controversy surrounding multicultural issues, is that cultural and ethnic issues are inherently emotional. The implication for clinical interviewers is that individual clients' cultural roots need to be explored and understood on an emotional level. More specific guidelines for multicultural interviewing are provided in Chapter 13.

---

**INDIVIDUAL AND CULTURAL HIGHLIGHT 2.2**

### Discovering Your Personal Biases

We suggest that you and your classmates take time to consider your own cultural, religious, and political biases. It is helpful to explore these, even among yourselves. How many in your class were raised to believe in a God referred to as masculine? How many were raised to believe that to care for the poor is a high and honorable calling in life? How many were raised to believe that being on time and standing in line are signs of weakness? The list of varying beliefs and values is endless. To further complicate matters, it is not only how we were raised or even what we believe now that we need to explore, but also the interaction of our cultural beliefs with another person's beliefs. How have we matured? How do we now respond to those who believe as we once did? There is no easy way to become culturally self-aware, but exposure, introspection, discussion, reading, and even personal therapy to uncover your biases and blind spots will help you work more effectively and sensitively with people of different cultures (Paniagua, 1998; D. W. Sue, Ivey, & Pedersen, 1996; D. Sue & Sue, 1987).

*Awareness of Interviewing Expectations and Misconceptions*

Before you begin conducting interviews, explore your expectations in some depth. Specifically, think about the expectations you hold for yourself as a clinical interviewer. Do you expect you will easily be effective and successful or that you will struggle and even potentially fail miserably? What thoughts or images come to mind when you think of interviewing someone for the first time? What preconceived ideas do you have about how to act in an interview? Do you believe a good clinician must be a certain type of person? Write down your thoughts, feelings, and expectations about entering this profession.

## EFFECTIVE INTERVIEWING: SEVEN VOCATIONAL PERSPECTIVES

Many factors make becoming a competent clinical interviewer a challenging process. Nonetheless, learning effective interviewing is not only possible, but also fun and entertaining. For a lighter look at the demands of interviewing, consider the following similarities between clinical interviewing and other human activities.

1. You must know what famous philosophers know: the importance of knowing thyself (C. Bennett, 1984). Because you are the instrument through which you hear and respond to clients, you must be keenly aware of your physical presence, personality style, and individual biases. In other scientific enterprises, scientists calibrate their instruments before using them for research or practice. Checking in with your most central instrument, your self, is one of your essential duties.

2. You must know what good landscapers know: the terrain. You must learn how to set up an environment that is maximally conducive to your objective. A number of situational factors can make clients more—or less—willing to discuss their personal concerns. It is your job to establish an environment that allows clients to be comfortable and open.

3. You must have what successful music teachers have: a good ear. You must know how to listen to your client with all your senses. You must have knowledge of which behaviors effective listeners use and which they avoid. Good interviewers listen so well that their clients have no doubts that they have been heard.

4. You must do what successful athletes do: practice. Dedicated practice moves skills from brain to body and from theory to practice. Without accumulating many interviewing experiences, the knowledge you obtain about clinical interviewing and a dollar will buy you a cup of coffee. Only through direct experience will you become more self-aware and learn how to apply the principles discussed in this text.

5. You must know what good office managers know: how to prioritize information. As an interviewer, you must quickly sort through many verbal and nonverbal messages given to you by clients so you can focus on important clinical material. Some client information may require immediate attention and action. For example, if your client reports suicidal thoughts, you need to act quickly. On the other hand, some client information requires a much different kind of attention. As a novice interviewer, you should develop evaluation and prioritization skills as soon as possible because you can't predict when you will face your first major clinical decision.

6. You must know what efficient wardrobe managers know: how to mix and match. Good interviewers apply evaluation and listening skills to a variety of situations.

Conducting intake interviews, suicide assessments, and mental status exams in preparation for choosing clinical techniques and assisting clients with referrals are all applications of the interviewer's evaluation and listening skills.

7. You must know what good car mechanics know: how to troubleshoot. Just as car mechanics recognize sounds indicative of bad wheel bearings or troubled fuel injectors, you need to know the signs and symptoms of depression, anxiety, paranoia, and more. Even beginners need a rudimentary knowledge of psychopathology to judge whether clients require a regular tune-up or a major overhaul.

## THE PHYSICAL SETTING

*The environment not only prods or lashes, it selects. Its role is similar to that in natural selection, though on a very different time scale, and was overlooked for the same reason. It is now clear that we must take into account what the environment does to an organism not only before but after it responds. Behavior is shaped and maintained by its consequences. Once this fact is recognized, we can formulate the interaction between organism and environment in a much more comprehensive way.*
—B. F. Skinner, *Walden Two*

When interviewer and client sit down to talk, many environmental factors influence their behavior. Although the interviewer is the most important stimulus affecting client behavior, other physical or external variables influence clinical interviewing process and outcome. Interviewers should be conscious of these variables and carefully consider them before conducting clinical interviews.

### The Room

What kind of room is most appropriate for clinical interviewing?

Of course, circumstances beyond your control can determine what kind of room you use for your interviews. Many undergraduate programs and some graduate programs do not have a therapy clinic complete with private offices. In fact, some interviewers do not have a room at all; Alfred Benjamin (1981), a renowned client-centered therapist, reported conducting interviews in a tent on the desert. We hope most readers of this book will have better facilities, but no matter what the circumstances, certain features require your close attention.

Usually, counseling and psychotherapy interviews take place in a room, but there are some exceptions. Behavioral therapists sometimes take clients to a scene that produces anxiety to implement anxiety-reduction or response-prevention techniques (Fones, Manfro, & Pollack, 1998; Wells, 1997). Other counseling and psychotherapy activities have been reported as taking place while interviewer and client were outside jogging, walking, dancing, or sitting in a comfortable setting, such as under a tree on a pleasant day (Abt & Stuart, 1982; Hayes, 1999; O'Kelly, Piper, Kerber, & Fowler, 1998). We take a fairly traditional and conservative approach for students in clinical training. We require a room, especially for the beginning interviewer.

The minimum requirement for the room is privacy. Some practitioners are very particular about room specifications, believing that for optimal communication to occur, a soundproof room with covered windows and a private exit is *required* (Langs, 1973,

1986). We do not go quite that far, partly because there are real-world limits to what's possible in many settings. However, as suggested in the preceding quote from Skinner (1972), do not underestimate the importance of physical surroundings.

Ordinarily, people are not inclined to reveal their deepest fears or secrets at the student union building over coffee—at least not to someone they have just met. Privacy and comfort are central to a good interview. On the other hand, when attempting to present yourself professionally, it is not necessary to hide behind a massive oak desk with a backdrop of velvet curtains and 27 framed professional degrees. As is true regarding many variables associated with interviewing, when choosing a room, it is useful to strike a balance between professional formality and casual comfort. Consider the room an extension of your professional self. In an initial interview, your major purpose is to foster *trust* and *hope* in your client, build rapport, and help the client talk openly. Your room choice should reflect that purpose.

Control is a central issue in setting up and planning the atmosphere in which the interview takes place (see Putting It in Practice 2.5). The client may be given small choices such as chair selection, but overall, the interviewer should be in control of the surroundings.

Numerous elements distinguish the clinical interview from other social encounters. One such distinction is that time devoted to the interview is set aside and its exclusive purpose respected. Although interruptions during a business or social encounter may be permissible or even welcome, this is not true in counseling or psychotherapy. In our view, interruptions are nearly intolerable. At our training clinic, everyone from the janitor to the supervisors realize that while interviewers are in session, they are not to be disturbed. The secretary would never dream of interrupting and, in fact, guards the students' client hours with a fierce loyalty to both student and client. After moving out of his tent, Benjamin (1981) commented on interruptions:

> Outside interruptions can only hinder. Phone calls, knocks on the door, people who want "just a word" with you, secretaries who must have you sign this document "at once," may well destroy in seconds what you and the interviewee have tried hard to build over a considerable time span. (p. 4)

This statement would hold true even if Dr. Benjamin were speaking about interviews held in his tent. A place and time set aside for clinical interviews should be just that: set aside. If you do not have access to rooms in which privacy is assured, you should place a *Do Not Disturb* or *Session in Progress* sign on the door to reduce the probability of interruptions. Additionally, phone ringers and answering machines should be turned down so that a voice stating "Hello, you've reached . . ." doesn't blare out just as your client begins sharing something deeply personal.

One word of caution is in order. Although interviewers should take every reasonable measure available to assure they are not interrupted, we *do not* recommend locking the door to the room. There are many reasons to avoid locking the room. For example, if you are interviewing someone with poor impulse control and he or she gets angry, it is best to have a fairly direct exit available. We hope that you will never need to use such an exit, but you will feel better knowing it exists. Also, a locked door conveys a sort of intimacy that could lead some people to impute a message you did not intend. To summarize: Quiet, comfortable, protected—yes. Locked—no.

Sometimes, despite our best efforts, an interruption occurs. Essentially, there are three types of interruptions. First, there are inadvertent and brief interruptions. For

---

**Putting It in Practice 2.5**

## Staying in Control of the Interview Setting

Imagine yourself confronted with the following scenario: An interviewing student calls a volunteer interviewee:

"Hello, is Sally Sampson there?"

*"Yes, this is she."*

"Sally, my name is Beth McNettle and I'm taking Interviewing 443. I believe you signed up to be interviewed for extra credit in your Psychology 101 class. I got your name, so I'm calling to set up a time."

*"Oh sure. No problem . . . but it's almost finals week. I'm pretty busy."*

"Uh, yeah. I wanted to do this sooner in the semester, but uh, well, let's see if we can find a time."

After much searching, they find a mutually agreeable time. Unfortunately, Beth forgot to check the room schedule and finds no rooms are available at the time chosen. She calls Sally back:

"Sally, this is Beth McNettle again. I'm sorry, but there are no rooms available at the time we decided."

Sally is a bit irritated, and it shows in her voice. Beth is feeling apologetic, indebted, and a little desperate. There is only one week left in the semester. They discuss their limited options. Beth suggests, "Maybe I should call someone else."

Sally counters with:

*"Hey, look, I really want to do this. I need the extra credit. Why don't you just come to my room? I live in University Hall, right here on campus."*

Knowing she is violating the rules, Beth reluctantly agrees to do the interview in Sally's dorm room. After all, it's just a class assignment, right? What's wrong with a nice, quiet dorm room? Who will ever know where the interview was conducted? Besides, it's better than inviting Sally to *her* house, isn't it? Beth asks Sally to make sure they will have the room to themselves. "No problem," says Sally, sounding distracted.

The next day, Beth arrives. It is late afternoon. It just happens to be the one hour designated as the time when residents can make as much noise as they please to compensate for quiet hours and finals stress. The Grateful Dead, Madonna, and Pearl Jam compete for air space. Sally's friend from across the hall is getting her hair permed, which, except for the odor, should not be all that relevant, but somehow, Sally's digital clock is being used to time the perm. No one besides Beth and Sally are actually in the room, but there are numerous interruptions and the phone rings six times, twice with calls for Sally.

Unfortunately, this is a true story. Beth had the courage to report her rule violation and "horrible" experience. She shared with us her dismal failure in establishing any kind of meaningful communication with Sally and admitted feeling out of control. Although this example is extreme, it illustrates the importance of controlling the interview setting. Loss of control can happen easily.

example, a new office manager or untrained staff member may knock on the door or enter without understanding the importance of privacy. In such cases, the interviewer should gently inform the intruder that the meeting is private.

Second, there are legitimate interruptions that take a few minutes to manage. For example, the secretary at your seven-year-old daughter's school telephones your office, indicating your child is ill and needs to be picked up from school. This interruption may require five minutes for the interviewer to contact a friend or family member who is free to pick up the child. In this situation, the interviewer should inform the client that a short break from their session is necessary, apologize, and then make the telephone calls. On returning to the session, the interviewer should apologize again, offer restitution for the time missed from the session (e.g., ask the client "Can you stay an extra five minutes today?" or "Is it okay to make up the five minutes we lost at our next session?"), and then try, as smoothly as possible, to begin where the interview had been interrupted.

Third, an interruption may bring information of some kind of personal or professional emergency that requires your immediate presence somewhere else. If so, the interviewer should apologize for having to end the session, reschedule, and provide the rescheduled appointment at no charge (or refund the client's payment for the interrupted session). Depending on one's theoretical orientation, it may or may not be necessary or appropriate to disclose the nature of the emergency to your client. Usually, a calm, explanatory statement should suffice:

> "I'm sorry, but I need to leave because of an urgent situation that can't wait. I hope you understand, but we'll need to reschedule. This is very unusual, and I'm terribly sorry for inconveniencing you."

Often, giving clients general information about your leaving allays both their concern and their curiosity.

Overall, key issues for handling interruptions are (a) modeling calmness and problem-solving ability, (b) apologizing for the interruption, and (c) compensating the client for any interview time lost because of the interruption. In addition, if the interviewer is taking notes when an interruption occurs, he or she should make certain the notes are placed in a secure file or given to the office manager before leaving the counseling office.

## Seating Arrangements

When teaching interviewing, we routinely ask students how two people should sit during an interview. The variety of student responses to this question is surprising. Some students suggest a face-to-face seating arrangement, others like having a desk between themselves and clients, and still others prefer sitting at a 90- to 120-degree angle so that client and interviewer can look away from each other without discomfort. A few students usually point out that some psychoanalytically oriented psychotherapists still place clients on a couch, with the therapist seated behind the client and out of view.

Some training clinics have predetermined seating arrangements. For example, our old clinic had a single, soft reclining chair along with two or three more austere wooden chairs available. Theoretically, the soft recliner provides clients with a comfortable and relaxing place from which they can freely express themselves. The recliner is also an excellent seat to use for hypnotic induction, for teaching progressive relaxation, and for free association. Unfortunately, having a designated seat for clients can produce dis-

comfort, especially during early sessions. In training facilities using such an arrangement, clients notoriously avoid the selected seat or complain of feeling they are on the
throne or hot seat.

Several factors dictate seating arrangement choices. Interviewer theoretical orientation is one factor. Psychoanalysts often choose couches, behaviorists often choose recliners, and person-centered therapists usually emphasize the importance of having
chairs of equal status and comfort. In classes, we consistently notice a connection between students' suggestions for seating arrangements and their personality styles.
More assertive students tend to prefer the face-to-face arrangement, and students with
needs for control more frequently like their clients on couches or recliners. You might
try out a number of different seating arrangements to get a sense for what feels best.
This does not necessarily mean you always *choose* whatever arrangement feels best to
you, but discovering your preference may be enlightening. You should also remain sensitive to your clients' preferences, as there are certain arrangements that feel better and
worse to each of them.

Generally, interviewer and client should be seated at somewhere between a 90- and
150-degree angle to each other during initial interviews. Benjamin (1981) states the rationale for such a seating arrangement quite nicely:

> [I] prefer two equally comfortable chairs placed close to each other at a 90-degree angle
> with a small table nearby. This arrangement works best for me. The interviewee can face
> me when he wishes to do so, and at other times he can look straight ahead without my get-
> ting in his way. I am equally unhampered. The table close by fulfills its normal functions
> and, if not needed, disturbs no one. (p. 3)

The 90-degree-angle seating arrangement is safe and conservative. It usually does
not offend anyone. Nonetheless, many interviewers (and clients) prefer a less extreme
angle so they can look at the client more directly but not quite face-to-face (perhaps at
a 120-degree angle).

In some cases, clients disrupt your prearranged seating by moving the chair to a different position. Generally, we recommend that interviewers *not* insist on any given seating arrangement. If a client appears comfortable with an unplanned or unusual seating
arrangement, simply allow the client to choose, make a mental note of this behavior,
and proceed with the interview. An exception to this general rule can occur when a
client (usually a child or adolescent) blatantly refuses to sit in an appropriate or re-
sponsive position in the interviewer's office.

## Note Taking

Many therapists and writers have discussed note taking (Benjamin, 1987; Pipes & Davenport, 1999; Shea, 1998). Although some experts recommend that interviewers take
notes only after a session has ended, others point out that interviewers do not have
perfect memories and thus some ongoing record of the session is desirable (Benjamin, 1987; Shea, 1998). The bottom line is that, in some cases, note taking may offend clients, whereas in other cases, it may enhance rapport and interviewer credibility
(Hickling, Hickling, Sison, & Radetsky, 1984). Clients' reactions to note taking are usually a function of their intrapsychic issues, interpersonal dynamics, previous experiences with note-taking behavior, and the tact of the interviewer while taking notes. Because you cannot predict a client's reaction to note taking in advance, you should offer
an explanation when you begin taking notes during a session. Shea (1998) recommends
the following approach:

I frequently do not even pick up a clipboard until well into the interview. When I do begin to write, as a sign of respect, I often say to the patient, "I'm going to jot down a few notes to make sure I'm remembering everything correctly. Is that alright with you?" Patients seem to respond very nicely to this simple sign of courtesy. This statement of purpose also tends to decrease the paranoia that patients sometimes project onto note-taking, as they wonder if the clinician is madly analyzing their every thought and action. (p. 180)

We agree that whenever interviewers take notes, they should introduce note taking in a courteous manner and proceed tactfully (i.e., the interviewer should always pay more attention to the client than to the notes). However, we recommend practicing your interviews both with and without taking notes. It is important to explore how it feels to take notes and how it feels not to take notes during a session.

### Rules for Note Taking

The following list summarizes general rules for note taking.

- Never allow note taking to interfere with interview flow or with rapport; always pay more attention to your client than to your notes.
- Explain the purpose of note taking to clients. Usually, a comment about not having a perfect memory suffices. Alternatively, some clients are disappointed if you do not take notes; explain to them why you are choosing not to take notes.
- Never hide or cover your notes or act in any manner that might suggest to clients that they do not or should not have access to your notes.
- Never write anything on your notepad that you do not want your client to read. This means you should stick to the facts. If you write down personal observations you intended to keep to yourself, rest assured that your client will want to read what you have written. Clients with paranoid qualities will be suspicious about what you've written and may ask to read your notes or, in extreme cases, simply stand up and grab your notes (or read the notepad over your shoulder).
- If clients ask to see what you've written, explore their concerns and offer to let them read your notes. Only occasionally do clients accept such an offer. However, when a client does, you'll be glad you followed the previous rule.

### Videotape and Audiotape Recording

If you record a session with video or audio equipment, you should do so as unobtrusively as possible. In general, the more comfortable and matter-of-fact you are in discussing the recording equipment, the more quickly clients become comfortable being recorded. This is easier said than done because as the interviewer, you will be more closely observed on the subsequent review of the tape; therefore, you may be even more nervous than your client about being tape-recorded. To reassure the client (but not yourself), you might say:

"The main reason I have to record our session is so that my supervisor can watch me working. It's to help make sure you get the best service possible and to make sure I'm using my counseling skills effectively."

When planning to audiotape or videotape a session, you must obtain the client's permission before turning on the recorder. Usually, permission is obtained on a written consent form. This is important for a number of reasons. Recording clients without their knowledge is an invasion of privacy and violates their trust. It is also important for ethical and legal reasons to explain possible future uses of the recording and how it will be stored, handled, and eventually destroyed.

## CASE EXAMPLE

*In an effort to obtain a fresh recording of interactions he was about to have with a new client, a student decided to start his audiotape recorder before the client entered the interviewing room. He assumed that, after preserving the important initial material on tape, he could then discuss the issue of tape recording with the client. Not surprisingly, when the client discovered she was being recorded, she was angry about her privacy being violated and refused to continue the interview. Furthermore, she delivered to the young man a punishing tirade against which he had no defense (and, of course, he conveniently recorded this tirade for himself). The student had unwittingly pinpointed one of the best ways of destroying trust and rapport early in an interview: He failed to ask permission to record the interview on tape.*

We have one final observation about taping. When you have conducted your best interview ever, you will inevitably discover there was a minor problem with the equipment and, consequently, your session either did not record properly or did not record at all. On the other hand, when you've conducted a session you'd rather forget, the equipment always seems to work perfectly and the session turns out to be the one your supervisor wants to examine closely. Because of this particular variation of Murphy's Law, we recommend that you carefully test the recording equipment before all your sessions.

## PROFESSIONAL AND ETHICAL ISSUES

Before conducting real or practice interviews, interviewers should consider numerous professional and ethical issues. Beginning interviewers often struggle with dressing professionally, presenting themselves and their credentials (or lack thereof) comfortably, handling time boundaries, and discussing confidentiality. The remainder of this chapter focuses on how to deal with professional and ethical issues comfortably and effectively.

### Self-Presentation

*You* are your own primary instrument for a successful interview. Your appearance and the manner in which you present yourself to clients are important components of professional clinical interviewing.

#### Grooming and Attire

Deciding how to dress for your first clinical interviews can be difficult. Some students ignore the issue; others obsess about wearing just the right outfit. The question of how to dress may reflect a larger developmental issue: How seriously do you take yourself as a professional? Is it time to take off the Salvation Army sweats, or stop trying to capture the title of Most Likely to Be on the Cover of *Seventeen*? Is it time to don the dreaded three-piece suit and come out to do battle with mature reality, as your parents or friends may have suggested? Don't worry. We are not interested in telling you how you should dress. Our point again involves self-awareness. Be aware of how your clothes may affect others. Even if you ignore this issue, your clients—and your supervisor—will not. Your choice of clothing and grooming communicates a great deal to clients and can be a source of conflict between you and your supervisor.

We knew a student whose distinctive style included closely cropped, multicolored hair; large earrings likely to elongate his earlobes over time; and an odd assortment of scarves, vests, sweaters, runner's tights, and sandals. He easily stood out in most crowds. Imagine his effect on, say, a middle-aged dairy farmer referred to the clinic for depression, or a mother-son dyad having trouble with discipline, or the local mayor's son or daughter. No matter what effect you imagined, the point is that there is likely to be an effect. Clothing is not neutral; it nearly always provokes a reaction. An unusual fashion statement by an interviewer can be overcome, but it may use up time and energy better devoted to other issues (see Putting It in Practice 2.6).

Although it is unfortunate that people quickly form first impressions and that these impressions may be inaccurate, your clients will judge you by the way you look and dress (Lennon & Davis, 1990). The first impression often takes the form of a vague positive or negative emotional reaction:

> Typically, a first impression of a stranger . . . is poorly differentiated and hard to put into words; yet it often yields a distinct emotional flavor of liking or dislike. This affective reaction may be a source of both useful information and error. (Holt, 1969, p. 20)

Your goal as a clinical interviewer is to present yourself in a way that takes advantage of first impressions. Dress and grooming that fosters rapport, trust, and credibility should be a useful source of information for the client (Strong, 1968). Err on the conservative side, at least until you have a firm understanding of the effects of your presentation.

---

**Putting It in Practice 2.6**

## Dressing for Success

When it comes to fashion, everyone has an opinion and everyone (almost) has his or her particular taste. Unfortunately, the clinical interview may not be the best place for you to really let loose by expressing your own unique fashion statement.

Just for fun, if your professor or supervisor doesn't bring up the topic of what's appropriate and what's not appropriate to wear for a professional interview, be sure to do it yourself. Here are a few questions that might stimulate a discussion with your professor/supervisor or with your classmates.

- Is it acceptable for male interviewers to wear earrings or ponytails?
- When should males wear neckties?
- Are shorts ever appropriate therapeutic attire?
- Is it a problem for female interviewers to wear pants?
- When it comes to skirt length and women interviewers, how short is too short?
- How about women's blouses and tops—how low of a neckline is appropriate, and is Erin Brockovich a reasonable standard?

*Presenting Your Credentials*

Students notoriously have difficulty introducing themselves to clients. Referring to yourself as a student may bring forth spoken or imagined derogatory comments such as, "So, I'm your guinea pig?" Our advice to student interviewers is to state clearly and firmly your full name and an accurate description of your training status to your clients. For example: "My name is Holly Johnson and I'm in the graduate training program in clinical psychology," or "I'm working on my master's degree," or "I'm enrolled in an advanced interviewing course." You should pause after this description to provide the client a chance to ask questions about your credentials. If the client asks questions, answer them directly and nondefensively. Always represent your status clearly and honestly with clients, whether they are role-play volunteers or actual clients referred for counseling. It is an ethical violation to misrepresent yourself by overstating your credentials. No matter how inexperienced or inadequate you feel inside, do not try to compensate by fraudulent misrepresentation.

Practicing simple introductory portions of the clinical interview is important. Before reading further, formulate exactly how you want to introduce yourself in the clinical setting. You may want to write out your introduction or say it into a tape recorder. We also recommend practicing introductions while role-playing with fellow students. Practicing your introduction helps you to avoid making statements like: "Well, I'm just a student and um, I'm taking this interviewing course, and I have to um, practice, so . . . uh, here we are."

There is nothing wrong with being a student and no need to behave apologetically for being inexperienced. An apologetic action or attitude can quickly erode your credibility and rapport. If you have a tendency to feel guilt over "practicing" your interviewing skills, try a small dose of cognitive therapy: Remind yourself that people usually enjoy a chance to talk about themselves. It is rare in our culture for people to receive 100% of someone's undivided attention. By listening well, you provide a positive experience for clients and, at the same time, learn more about interviewing.

Student interviewers are usually supervised. This fact should be included when you present your credentials. Say something like:

> "As I mentioned, I haven't completed my degree, so my work here at the clinic is being supervised by Dr. Walters. This means I will be reviewing what we talk about with Dr. Walters to ensure you are receiving high-quality professional services. Dr. Walters is a licensed clinical psychologist and will keep what you say confidential in the same way I will."

## Time

As is often said, time is of the essence. This is certainly true with clinical interviewing. Most likely, if the client is paying a fee, the fee is based on your time. Although clinical interviewing is a rich, involved, and complicated process, time is one measure of the commodity you are selling. Therefore, you should always attend to and be respectful of time boundaries.

Clinical interviews typically last 50 minutes. This time period, though somewhat arbitrary, is convenient; it allows the interviewer to meet with clients on an hourly basis, with a few minutes at the end and beginning of each session to write notes and read files. Despite this usual and customary time period, some situations warrant briefer contacts and other situations require longer sessions. For example, initial (intake) or assessment interviews are sometimes longer than the traditional psychotherapy hour because it's difficult to obtain all the information needed to conceptualize a case and establish treatment goals. Depending on the setting, up to 90 minutes or even two hours may be provided for an initial interview. On the other hand, crisis situations can require more flexibility. For example, Wollersheim (1974) recommends shorter but more frequent sessions for suicidal clients.

*Start the Session on Time*

The guiding principle for starting sessions is punctuality. If you are late, apologize to the client and offer to extend the session or somehow compensate for the lost time. You may want to say something like: "I apologize for being late; I had another appointment that lasted longer than expected. Because I missed 10 minutes of our session, perhaps we can extend this session or our next session an additional 10 minutes."

Although many students aren't required to collect fees, another option professionals use for repaying clients for lost time is to offer to prorate the fee for whatever portion of the usual interview hour remains.

You should also avoid beginning sessions early, as in cases in which the client arrives before the scheduled time and you are not committed to meeting with someone else. Pipes and Davenport (1999) state this position succinctly: "Clients will show up early and may ask if you are free. The answer is no, unless there is a crisis" (p. 18).

Punctuality communicates respect to clients. Clients appreciate professionals who begin sessions at the scheduled time. Many times, our classes have discussed the contrast between the attitudes of psychotherapists and physicians (excluding psychiatrists) when it comes to punctuality. Physicians are notoriously late for patient appointments, and such lateness provides a clear message about the nature of typical physician-patient relationships (Siegel, 1986). One student of ours commented in class, "It doesn't matter if physicians offend you by being late because they would never take the time to talk about it with you afterward anyway" (V. Hayes, personal communication, April 1990). This comment captures an important value that good therapists uphold: respect for the client's time and feelings.

When clients are late for a session, an interviewer may have an impulse to extend the session's length or to punish the client by canceling the session entirely. Neither of these options is desirable. Clients should be held responsible for their lateness and experience the natural consequences of their behavior, which is an abbreviated session. This is true regardless of the reason the client was tardy. The client may sincerely regret his or her lateness and ask you for additional time. Be empathic but firm. Say something like:

> "I'm also sorry this session has to be brief, but it really is important for us to stick with our scheduled appointment time. I hope we can have a full session next week."

Unless your client is in crisis, whether or not you have an appointment scheduled for the next hour is irrelevant; stick with your time boundaries. The key point is that clients should be held responsible for their lateness (and similarly, interviewers should be held responsible for *their* lateness).

One option professional interviewers use in cases of client lateness is to offer to schedule an additional appointment at another time during the week so clients don't feel they are falling behind, or being cheated, in terms of therapy or assessment progress. For example, you might suggest: "If you want to make up the time we've lost today, we can try to schedule another appointment for later this week." But keep in mind that, not surprisingly, when clients schedule an additional session (to make up for missed time), they sometimes complicate the problem by "no-showing" for their make-up appointment as well.

It is not unusual for interviewers to feel angry or irritated at clients who are late for a session or who miss a session. As with many emotional reactions toward clients, you should notice and reflect on them, but refrain from acting on them. For example, even though you desperately want to leave the office after waiting only 10 minutes for your chronically late client, do not give in to that desire. Instead, clarify your policy on lateness (e.g., "If you're late, I'll wait around for 20 minutes and then I may leave the office."). If your client completely misses an appointment, you must decide whether to call to reschedule, whether to send a letter asking if he or she wants to continue therapy, or whether to wait for the client to call for a new appointment. Be sure to discuss how to handle this situation with your supervisor.

In some cases, your agency may have a policy of charging clients for a full hour if they do not cancel appointments 24 hours in advance. If so, you must inform your clients—in advance—of this policy. Similarly, inform volunteer clients of consequences associated with missing their scheduled appointments (e.g., loss of extra credit).

## End the Session on Time

Clinical interviews should end on time. Clinicians have many excellent excuses for consciously letting sessions run over, but rarely do these excuses adequately justify breaking prearranged time agreements. Some reasons we have heard from our students (and ourselves) follow:

- We were on the verge of a breakthrough.
- She brought up a clinically important issue with only five minutes to go.
- He just kept talking at the end of the hour, and I felt uncomfortable cutting in (i.e., he seemed to need to talk some more).
- I thought I hadn't been very effective during the hour and felt the client deserved more time.
- I forgot my watch and couldn't see the clock from my chair.

In most of the preceding situations, the interviewer should calmly and tactfully point out that time is up for the day, but that if the client wishes, the session can continue along similar lines next time. Additionally, you should sit in a position that affords you direct visual contact with a clock. It is rude and distracting to glance repeatedly at your watch or to look over your shoulder at the clock during an interview.

There are very few situations in which it is acceptable to extend the clinical hour. These situations are usually emergencies. For example, when the client is suicidal, homicidal, or psychotic, time boundaries may be modified. A colleague of ours was once held overtime—at gunpoint—by one of his clients for about 40 minutes. This is certainly a situation when time boundaries become irrelevant (although we know our friend wished he could have simply said, "Well, it looks like our time is up for today" and had the client put away his gun and leave the office).

Sometimes we fail to uphold time boundaries, despite our best intentions. We recall with affection a session when a colleague of ours, seated in a position where he could clearly view the clock on the wall, started thinking that time on that particular day was passing exceptionally slowly. It turned out that the clock on which our friend was depending had really begun slowing down. Eventually, time actually stood still when the clock stopped because of dead batteries. Our friend ended up having, despite his best intentions, a "73-minute hour."

## Confidentiality

A big part of clinical interviewing involves helping clients talk about very personal information. This is not only a difficult task (people are often uncomfortable disclosing personal information to someone they hardly know) but also a heavy burden. Clients are entrusting interviewers with private information, some of which they may never have told anyone before. Of course, the assumption in counseling and psychotherapy is that whatever is shared is kept confidential.

There are legal and ethical limits of confidentiality. Some information must not be kept secret. For example, a client could say:

> "I'm very depressed and am sick and tired of life. I've decided to quit dragging my family through this miserable time with me . . . so I'm going to kill myself. I have a gun and ammunition at home and I plan to blow myself away this weekend."

In this case, you are legally and ethically obligated to break confidentiality and report your client's suicidal plans to the proper authorities (e.g., police, county mental health professional, or psychiatric hospital admission personnel) and possibly family members.

The central statements regarding confidentiality from the American Psychological Association's (APA; 1992) Ethical Principles are included in Table 2.1. For a contrasting perspective, key statements from the Codes of Ethics for the American Counseling Association (ACA; 1995) are provided in Table 2.2. We should note that the National Association of Social Workers (NASW; 1996) and the American Association for Marriage and Family Therapy (AAMFT; 1991) also have ethical guidelines pertaining to confidentiality. Welfel (2002) summarizes the concept of confidentiality by stating:

> The term *confidentiality* refers to the ethical duty to keep client identity and disclosures secret. It is a moral obligation rooted in the ethics code, the ethical principles, and the virtues that the profession attempts to foster. (p. 74)

Unfortunately, all statements in the various professional codes pertaining to confidentiality are open to interpretation. To better clarify the standards, Putting It in Practice 2.7 provides you with examples of situations in which professional therapists are obligated to break confidentiality.

Confidentiality constitutes an ethical, legal, and clinical issue in professional interviewing. Additional discussion of this crucial issue is provided intermittently throughout this book.

One final point should be made regarding the APA and ACA ethical standards of confidentiality. The APA specifically states: "Unless it is not feasible or is contraindicated, the discussion of confidentiality occurs at the outset of the relationship and thereafter as new circumstances may warrant" (APA, 1995). Concerning this standard, Pipes and Davenport (1999) wrote:

> Although it has been argued that clients deserve information about the legal limits of confidentiality and privileged communication, in actual practice the majority of psychotherapists probably give limited information until specifically asked by the client. (p. 14)

**Table 2.1.    Ethical Statements Regarding Confidentiality of the American Psychological Association**

5.       Privacy and Confidentiality
         These standards are potentially applicable to the professional and scientific activities of all psychologists.

5.01    Discussing the Limits of Confidentiality
         a. Psychologists discuss with persons and organizations with whom they establish a scientific or professional relationship (including, to the extent feasible, minors and their legal representatives) (1) the relevant limitations on confidentiality, including limitations where applicable in group, marital, and family therapy or in organizational consulting, and (2) the foreseeable uses of the information generated through their services.
         b. Unless it is not feasible or is contraindicated, the discussion of confidentiality occurs at the outset of the relationship and thereafter as new circumstances may warrant.
         c. Permission for electronic recording of interviews is secured from clients and patients.

5.05    Disclosures
         a. Psychologists disclose confidential information without the consent of the individual only as mandated by law, or where permitted by law for a valid purpose, such as (1) to provide needed professional services to the patient or the individual or organizational client, (2) to obtain appropriate professional consultations, (3) to protect the patient or client or others from harm, or (4) to obtain payment for services, in which instance disclosure is limited to the minimum that is necessary to achieve the purpose.
         b. Psychologists also may disclose confidential information with the appropriate consent of the patient or the individual or organizational client (or of another legally authorized person on behalf of the patient or client), unless prohibited by law.

The APA also has confidentiality statements pertaining to maintaining confidentiality, minimizing intrusions on privacy, maintenance of records, consultations, confidential information in databases, and other issues.

This table is reprinted from the APA, Ethical Principles of Psychologists and Code of Conduct, with permission from the American Psychological Association. No further reproduction is authorized without permission from the American Psychological Association.

Inform clients, at the outset of the interview, of the legal limits of confidentiality. This should be done both orally and in writing. It is important for clients to clearly understand this most basic ground rule in the professional helping relationship.

Imagine a scenario where a client who was not initially informed of the legal limits of confidentiality begins talking about suicide. At that point, the interviewer needs to consider whether the client's suicidal thoughts are serious enough to warrant breaking confidentiality. As a result, the interviewer may suddenly feel compelled (and rightly so) to inform the client that he or she must break confidentiality. However, to inform a client *after* he or she begins talking about suicide that this information will not be held in confidence is like changing the rules of a game after it has begun. Clients deserve to know in advance the rules and ethics that guide your interactions. Informing clients of confidentiality limits may result in their choosing to be more selective in what they disclose. This is a natural side effect of the legal and ethical limits of confidentiality.

Undoubtedly, situations arise in which your ethical and/or legal responsibilities with respect to confidentiality are unclear. In such cases, you should seek professional or collegial consultation. For example, if the situation involves whether to report child abuse and you are unclear regarding your legal-ethical responsibilities, ask your supervisor for guidance (Corey, Corey, & Callanan, 2003). If you find your supervisor is

**Table 2.2.    Ethical Statements Regarding Confidentiality of the American Counseling Association**

B.1.    Right to Privacy

    a. Respect for Privacy.

    Counselors respect their clients' right to privacy and avoid illegal and unwarranted disclosures of confidential information

    b. Client Waiver.

    The right to privacy may be waived by the client or their legally recognized representative.

    c. Exceptions.

    The general requirement that counselors keep information confidential does not apply when disclosure is required to prevent clear and imminent danger to the client or others when legal requirements demand that confidential information be revealed. Counselors consult with other professionals when in doubt as to the validity of an exception.

    d. Contagious, Fatal Diseases.

    A counselor who receives information confirming that a client has a disease commonly known to be both communicable and fatal is justified in disclosing information to an identifiable third party, who by his or her relationship with the client is at a high risk of contracting the disease. Prior to making a disclosure the counselor should ascertain that the client has not already informed the third party about his or her disease and that the client is not intending to inform the third party in the immediate future.

    e. Court Ordered Disclosure.

    When court ordered to release confidential information without a client's permission, counselors request to the court that the disclosure not be required due to potential harm to the client or counseling relationship.

    f. Minimal Disclosure.

    When circumstances require the disclosure of confidential information, only essential information is revealed. To the extent possible, clients are informed before confidential information is disclosed.

    g. Explanation of Limitations.

    When counseling is initiated and throughout the counseling process as necessary, counselors inform clients of the limitations of confidentiality and identify foreseeable situations in which confidentiality must be breached.

    h. Subordinates.

    Counselors make every effort to ensure that privacy and confidentiality of clients are maintained by subordinates including employees, supervisees, clerical assistants, and volunteers.

    i. Treatment Teams.

    If client treatment will involve a continued review by a treatment team, the client will be informed of the team's existence and composition.

The ACA also has additional confidentiality guidelines associated with group and family work, counseling with minor or incompetent clients, record keeping, research and training, and consultation.

---

This table is reprinted from the ACA Code of Ethics and Standards of Practice, pp. 1–19, with permission from the American Counseling Association. No further reproduction is authorized without permission from the American Counseling Association.

unclear regarding the best course of action, contact your local department of family services or child protection services and inquire, without providing specific identifying information, about your legal and ethical responsibilities. In especially tricky cases, you may want to consult an attorney for legal advice. In addition, most professional organizations (e.g., AAMFT, ACA, APA, NASW) have ethics committees or legal experts with whom you can consult (see Putting It in Practice 2.7).

## Informed Consent

On the surface, informed consent is a simple, self-evident concept. It involves the ethical and sometimes legal mandate to inform clients about the nature of their treatment. Further, once clients understand the treatment they will receive, they can agree to or refuse treatment.

Considered more fully, it is apparent that authentic informed consent is challenging to offer and obtain. First, for many human service, medical, and mental health providers, it can be difficult to describe client problems and available treatments in a clear and straightforward manner. Often, we speak in professional jargon (e.g., "It looks like you need some systematic desensitization for your phobia"). Additionally, clients are usually in physical or psychological pain. They may consent to anything the professional says will help, even though they do not fully understand the procedure.

As a mental health professional, you have a responsibility to explain your theoretical orientation, training, techniques, and likely treatment outcomes to your clients. You must do so in plain language and must welcome interactions and questions from clients who need more time or explanation. Even if you anticipate seeing the client for only one or two interviews, the interview should be explained in a way that allows the client the right to consent to or decline participation. In longer term therapy, informed consent needs revisiting as counseling continues.

At the very least, you should have two or three written paragraphs explaining your background, theoretical orientation, training, and the rationale for your usual choice of techniques. Use of diagnosis, potential inclusion of family members (especially in the case of marital work or work with minors), consultation or supervision practices, policies regarding missed appointments, and the manner in which you can be contacted in an emergency should be included. Many professionals include a statement or two about the counseling process and emotional experiences that might accompany this process.

A single written document cannot fully satisfy the spirit of informed consent, but it does start things off on the right foot. Written informed consent gives clients the message that they have important rights in the therapy relationship. It also helps educate clients about the therapy process—which has a positive effect on overall counseling efficacy (Luborsky, 1984). Finally, research suggests that well-written, readable, and personable consent forms increase the client's impression of therapist expertise and attractiveness (Wagner, Davis, & Handelsman, 1998).

## Documentation Procedures

Most of us have heard the saying, "If it isn't written down, it didn't happen" (to really get the point, try imagining a roomful of grim-faced attorneys, all chanting this slogan in unison).

Note taking and responsible documentation are not usually the highlight of anyone's day. On the other hand, failure to do the requisite documentation can certainly

======= **Putting It in Practice 2.7** =======

## Confidentiality and Its Limits

It is very important for clinical interviewers to understand the practical implications of ethics and laws pertaining to confidentiality. The following guidelines should be followed:

1. You must respect the private, personal, and confidential nature of communications from your client. This means that you do not share personal information about the client unless you have his or her permission. For example, if someone telephones your office and asks if you are working with John Smith, you should simply state something like: "I'm sorry, our policy restricts me from saying whether someone by that name receives services here." If the person persists, you may politely add: "If you want to know if a particular person is being seen here, then you have to get a signed release of information form so that we can legally and ethically provide you with information. Without a signed release of information form, I cannot even tell you if I have ever heard of anyone named John Smith." Additionally, upholding your client's right to confidentiality requires keeping your client records in a secure place.
2. You may disclose information (or break confidentiality) in the following situations:
   a. You have the client's (or his or her legal representative's) permission.
   b. The client is suicidal and you determine there is a clear danger of suicide.
   c. The client is homicidal or is threatening to engage in behaviors where significant danger to others is likely. For example, your client tells you of detailed plans to sabotage a local nuclear plant and you determine there is significant danger to others' lives if he or she carries out such an activity.
   d. The client is a child, and you have evidence to suggest he or she is being sexually or physically abused or neglected.
   e. You have evidence to suggest the client is sexually or physically abusing a minor.
   f. You have evidence to suggest that elder abuse is occurring (either from working with an elderly client or because your client discloses information indicating he or she is abusing an elderly person).
   g. You have been ordered by the court to provide client information.
3. Be sure to tell your client about the legal limits of confidentiality at the beginning of your initial session.

After reviewing confidentiality standards associated with your prospective profession as well as the preceding information, take time to brainstorm with your class potential difficult situations where your need to break confidentiality might be unclear. Discuss what you should do in situations where your ethical and legal responsibilities are unclear. Consider contacting the American Psychological Association at (202) 955-7600 or the American Counseling Association at (703) 823-9800 if you need consultation on specific ethical dilemmas.

ruin your day. People who make a profession of talking with and offering help to emotionally distressed clients need to clearly and carefully record what happens. There are many positive aspects of taking good notes. Obviously, you are more likely to remember the details of what was said and planned. Reviewing your progress notes facilitates the counseling process. In addition, when asked to send your notes to another professional or if your client wishes to review the notes, you are expected to have legible and coherent notes available. If your interactions with the client take unexpected turns, you can go back through your notes and perhaps see patterns you missed before. Finally, on a less positive note, if things do not go well with a client and you are accused of malpractice, your notes become an essential part of your defense.

Most experienced interviewers have a favorite note-taking format. Many use some rendition of the S-O-A-P acronym, which stands for subjective, objective, assessment, and plan. S-O-A-P guides the note taker to document the following:

**S:** The clients' subjective descriptions of their distress.

**O:** The interviewer's objective observations of the client's dress, presentation, and so on.

**A:** The interviewer's assessment of progress.

**P:** The plan for next time, or comments regarding progress on the overall treatment plan.

The form of note taking used by clinicians is less important than regularity, inclusion of the right materials, and neutrality (see Table 2.3). Obviously, everything discussed during a session cannot be documented in the client's file. Interviewers must discern the important or pivotal information of each session and record it in succinct, professional ways that are neither insulting nor overly vague. A colleague of ours recommends following the ABCs of documentation—Accurate, Brief, Clear (D. G. Scherer, personal communication, October, 1998).

Documentation, once it exists, must be stored responsibly. At the least, it should be

**Table 2.3.   Example of SOAP Note**

**S:** Joyce indicated her head hurt; her nose was stuffy, and she felt this was the cause of her extreme irritation. She said, "I wouldn't be so worn out and crabby except for those Russian teachers dancing so late. I just can't say no. I wanted to go home, but it was fun, and they were so cute. It's my same old pattern."

**O:** Joyce arrived on time but appeared tired and distracted. She was dressed in her usual jeans and sweater but kept a scarf wrapped around her neck the entire session. She sneezed and rubbed her nose. She spoke of her ongoing wish to have more peace and quiet in her life, but her inability to set any kind of limits without feeling guilty. She appeared to be sincerely distressed, both by her tiredness and her inability to set any kind of limits.

**A:** During the session, Joyce achieved further insight into the reasons she gives in so easily to the demands of others. She was able to begin making a schedule that gave her some free time every other day. Joyce's continued struggle with her need to please others and other dependent tendencies were evident, but also, she seemed determined to gain insight and make changes.

**P:** Joyce will monitor her use of time in her notebook. We will analyze time use and further clarify goals for balance. She made a goal of saying no to at least one social request and will report back on this next week. We noted that we have two sessions left before her insurance will no longer cover therapy.

filed in a locking file cabinet or locked office, safe from curious perusal by those coming and going in the setting. The length of time such records should be kept depends on your setting and purpose. For instance, in professional practice settings, guidelines suggest that complete materials be saved from between 7 and 12 years. The file may then be reduced to a summary sheet (ACA, 1995; APA, 1995). In public schools, materials generated in interviews with counselors and students are often thought to be the property of the counselor rather than the school. Make sure you understand the documentation, storage, and access policies and procedures of your agency.

### Stress Management for Clinical Interviewers

All mental health workers are exposed to high stress, and stress levels are particularly high for student interviewers (Norcross, 2000; Pearlman & Mac-Ian, 1995; Rodolfa, Kraft, & Reilley, 1988). It is especially common for students to have fears about making mistakes and damaging their clients. Unfortunately, these fears have a basis in reality. You will make mistakes—everyone does—and your mistakes may cause or increase client distress (Lambert & Bergin, 1994). The challenge is to recover from your mistakes and perhaps even use them for learning and growth. Sometimes, an interviewer's mistakes can even humanize the process for the client, because the client sees that even the interviewer is not perfect.

Shea (1998), a nationally renowned psychiatrist and workshop leader, comments on mistakes he makes while conducting interviews:

> Mistakes were made, but I make mistakes every time I interview. Interviews and humans are far too complicated not to make mistakes . . . . With every mistake, I try to learn. (p. 694)

We knew one student interviewer who reported high levels of anxiety accompanied by a tendency to pick at the skin around the edges of his fingers. During his first session, he picked at his fingers until he began feeling some moisture, which prompted him to think that he was so nervous his fingers were sweating. Eventually, he peeked down at his hands and discovered that, much to his horror, one of his fingers had begun to bleed. He spent the rest of the session trying to cover up the blood and worrying that the client had seen his bleeding finger. Though this example is unusual, it illustrates how nervousness and anxiety can interfere with interviewing. Managing stress effectively so that it does not interfere with your interviews is an important professional issue.

Interviewers may be affected by stress before, during, or after the interview. Stress reactions can result in physical, mental, emotional, social, or spiritual symptoms. Consequently, if you are feeling overstressed, it makes sense to seek stress management resources. Relevant stress management readings are included in the Suggested Readings and Resources at the end of this chapter.

## SUMMARY

Clinical interviewing involves a systematic modification of normal social interactions. Although the relationship established between interviewer and client is a friendly one, it is much different from friendship. Clinical interviews serve a dual function: to evaluate and to help clients.

Clinical interviewing is defined in different ways by different writers. Our definition includes the following components: (a) A professional relationship between interviewer and client is established; (b) a client is motivated, at least to some extent, to accomplish something by meeting with the interviewer; (c) the interviewer and client work to establish and achieve mutually agreed on goals; (d) in the context of a professional relationship, interviewer and client interact, both verbally and nonverbally, as the interviewer applies a variety of active listening skills and psychological techniques to evaluate, understand, and help the client achieve his or her goals; and (e) the quality and quantity of interactions between interviewer and client are influenced by a wide variety of factors, including personality traits and mutually agreed on interview goals.

It is important for clinical interviewers to have a high level of self-awareness and insight. There are many forms of self-awareness, including physical, psychosocial, developmental, and cultural. Interviewers should be aware of their preconceived biases and beliefs about themselves and others during the interviewing process.

A number of practical, professional, and ethical factors need to be considered by clinical interviewers. The more practical factors include the room, seating arrangements, note taking, and video- and audiotaping. Professional and ethical issues include interviewer self-presentation, time boundary maintenance, confidentiality, informed consent, documentation, and interviewer stress management. These issues are basic and foundational—they support the interviewing activity and without them, the entire interviewing structure may suffer or collapse.

Clinical interviewing is a very stressful activity, both for beginners and experienced clinicians. Consequently, stress management is a professional issue for most interviewers. Interviewers who are having adverse reactions to stress should seek methods for coping with stress more effectively. Suggested readings at the end of this chapter provide useful information regarding stress management for clinical interviewers.

## SUGGESTED READINGS AND RESOURCES

Benjamin, A. (1987). *The helping interview* (3rd ed.). Boston: Houghton Mifflin Co. This classic text includes information in Chapter 1 on physical conditions such as the room, and in Chapter 4 on recording interviews.

Davis, M., McKay, M., & Eshelman, E. R. (2000). *The relaxation and stress reduction workbook.* Oakland, CA: New Harbinger. This practical and clearly written workbook is primarily for use with clients. However, because providing therapy is stressful, it makes sense for clinicians to apply the strategies outlined in this book to themselves.

Diller, J. V., Murphy, E., & Martinez, J. (1998). *Cultural diversity: A primer for the human services.* London: International Thomson Publishing. This book offers both clinical and theoretical material designed to help professionals provide cross-cultural human services effectively. It includes interviews with professionals from four ethnic backgrounds: Latino/Latina, Native American, African American, and Asian American.

Kabat-Zinn, J. (1995). *Wherever you go there you are: Mindfulness meditation in everyday life.* New York: Hyperion. Mindfulness meditation is an excellent stress management technique for clients and counselors. Kabat-Zinn writes in an easy-to-digest style that makes for relaxing reading.

Paniagua, F. (1998). *Assessing and treating culturally diverse clients: A practical guide.* This book provides general guidelines for assessing and treating multicultural clients. It also includes specific information for working effectively with African American, Hispanic, Asian, and American Indian clients.

Pipes, R. B., & Davenport, D. S. (1999). *Introduction to psychotherapy: Common clinical wisdom* (2nd ed.). Englewood Cliffs, NJ: Prentice Hall. Chapter 2 of this text consists of "questions beginning therapists ask." Many of the questions address the physical interview setting, as well as professional and ethical interviewing issues.

Wolberg, B. (1995). *The technique of psychotherapy* (5th ed.). New York: Grune & Stratton. Chapter 62 of this 1568-page tome provides extended answers to common questions asked by beginning counselors and therapists.

Zeer, D. (2000). *Office yoga: Simple stretches for busy people.* San Francisco: Chronicle Books. This short book provides basic yoga stretching postures for busy professionals. It includes illustrations and easy to implement stress-reducing stretching exercises.

Zuckerman, M. (1990). Some dubious premises in research and theory on racial differences: Scientific, social, and ethical issues. *American Psychologist, 45,* 1297–1303. This article provides a good analysis of theory and research on racial differences.

# PART TWO

# LISTENING AND RELATIONSHIP DEVELOPMENT

# Chapter 3

## *BASIC ATTENDING, LISTENING, AND ACTION SKILLS*

> *Meryt listened in stillness, watching my face as I recounted my mother's history, and the story. . . . My friend did not move or utter a sound, but her face revealed the workings of her heart, showing me horror, rage, sympathy, compassion.*
>
> —Anita Diament, *The Red Tent*

---

**CHAPTER OBJECTIVES**

For the most part, we all know a good listener when we meet one. However, it's not quite so easy to figure out exactly what good listeners do to make it so comfortable for other people to talk openly and freely. This chapter analyzes the mechanics of effective attending and listening skills. After reading this chapter, you will know:

- The difference between positive and negative attending behavior.
- How ethnocultural background and diversity can affect client comfort with specific interviewer attending and listening behaviors.
- How and why interviewers use a range of nondirective listening responses, including silence, paraphrase, clarification, nondirective reflection of feeling, and summarization.
- About the natural inclination many interviewers feel to reassure clients.
- How and why interviewers use a range of directive listening responses, including interpretive reflection of feeling, interpretation, feeling validation, and confrontation.

---

When it comes to human communication, we generally think of two possible roles: the sender of the message or the receiver of the message. When someone is speaking to you, your mission is to be a good listener. It sounds simple enough. The truth is, very little about human communication is simple. Even if your job is to be the listener, you are also simultaneously in the role of sender. This is part of what makes human communication so complex. Communication professors like to express this complexity by citing the old adage: *You cannot not communicate.*

Think about it. No matter what you say (even if you say nothing), you are communicating something. Recall a time when you were talking with a friend on the telephone. Perhaps you said something and then there was a brief silence—a pause. Is it not true that your friend's pause, when he or she said nothing at all, was noticed and interpreted by you as communicating something?

The opening quote to this chapter is another illustration. The listener doesn't move or utter a sound, but she still manages to communicate understanding and empathy (or at least the speaker interprets the listener's facial expressions as empathic).

Much of your client's first impression of you is based on what he or she observes *as he or she speaks.* Your attending behavior is a message to your client—a message that, ideally, is interpreted as an invitation to speak openly and freely. This chapter focuses primarily on how you can learn to look, sound, and act like a good listener.

It may seem ingenuous or phony to suggest that you practice *looking like* a good listener. Nevertheless, good interviewers consciously and deliberately engage in specific behaviors that clients interpret as signs of interest and concern. These behaviors are referred to in the interviewing and counseling literature as *attending behaviors* (A. Ivey & Ivey, 1999, p. 27).

Ideally, interviewers are always *genuinely* interested in their clients' problems and welfare. In reality, there are times, at least moments, when even the best interviewers become bored or distracted and are temporarily uninterested in their clients. Exploring why interviewers become uninterested in their clients and how they should handle such feelings is important, but we review that later (see sections on congruence and countertransference in Chapter 5). For now, we focus our discussion on attending behavior.

## ATTENDING BEHAVIOR

A. Ivey and Ivey (1999) consider *attending behavior* the foundation of interviewing. They define attending behavior as "culturally and individually appropriate . . . eye contact, body language, vocal qualities, and verbal tracking" (p. 15). To succeed, interviewers must pay attention to their clients in culturally and individually appropriate ways. If interviewers fail to look, sound, and act attentive, they will not have many clients. Most clients quit going to counseling if they think their interviewer is not listening to them.

It is refreshing to find a concrete principle in psychology and counseling on which virtually everyone agrees. Attending behavior, and the importance of listening well, is spectacularly uncontroversial (Cormier & Nurius, 2003; Goldfried & Davison, 1994; Wright & Davis, 1994). Perhaps the only helping professionals who minimize the importance of body language are staunch psychoanalysts who continue to use the couch in psychotherapy. Yet, even psychoanalysts pay very close attention to their own vocal qualities, to tracking client verbal behavior, and to the general principle of listening well (Chessick, 1990; Geller & Gould, 1996).

Attending behavior is primarily nonverbal. Edward T. Hall claimed that communication is 10% verbal and 90% a "hidden cultural grammar" (1966, p. 12). Others suggest that 65% or more of a message's meaning is conveyed nonverbally (Birdwhistell, 1970). With respect to interviewing and counseling, Gazda, Asbury, Balzer, Childers, and Walters (1977) claim, "When verbal and nonverbal messages are in contradiction, the helpee will usually believe the nonverbal message" (p. 93). As an interviewer, you must use these powerful nonverbal channels when communicating with clients.

### Positive Attending Behavior NON-VERBAL

Many authors have described different positive and negative attending behaviors (A. Ivey & Ivey, 1999; Pipes & Davenport, 1999; Shea, 1998). Positive attending behaviors open up communication and encourage free expression. In contrast, negative attending behaviors inhibit expression. When it comes to identifying positive and negative attending behaviors, there are few universals because cultural background and previous experiences affect whether clients view a particular attending behavior as positive or negative. Although there are some fundamentals, what works with one client may not work with the next. Therefore, the way you pay attention to clients must vary to some degree depending on each client's individual needs, personality style, and family and cultural background. In some cases, you must be overtly quite attentive, and in others, you need to be less directly attentive—to "turn down the heat."

Ivey and Ivey (1999) identify four dimensions of attending behavior, which are simple and have been studied, to some extent, cross-culturally. They include:

- Eye contact
- Body language
- Vocal qualities
- Verbal tracking

### Eye Contact

The eyes have been called the windows of the soul. Cultures vary greatly in what they regard as appropriate eye contact. There is also much individual variation in eye contact patterns. For some interviewers, sustaining eye contact during an interview is natural. For others, it can be difficult; there may be a tendency to look down or away from the client's eyes because of shyness. The same is true for clients; some prefer more intense and direct eye contact; others prefer looking at the floor, the wall, or anywhere but into your eyes.

Generally, for Caucasian clients, interviewers should maintain eye contact most of the time. In contrast, Native American, African American, and Asian clients generally prefer less eye contact. In addition, some interviewers naturally look at the client's mouth or face rather than into the eyes; you may want to observe yourself to determine your own natural visual style with clients (for more information, see Individual and Cultural Highlight 3.1).

For most clients, it is appropriate to maintain more constant eye contact when they are speaking and less constant eye contact when you are speaking. Some research suggests that clients' pupils tend to dilate when they are emotionally aroused or interested and constrict when they are bored or uncomfortable (Hess, 1975; A. Ivey & Ivey, 1999). However, for most people, eye contact is just a method of making personal contact with someone else. It usually does not involve intense scrutiny of the other person's physical characteristics.

### Body Language

Aspects of communication that involve what most people, refer to as body language are known technically as *kinesics* and *proxemics* (Birdwhistell, 1952; E. Hall, 1966; Knapp, 1972). *Kinesics* denotes variables associated with physical features and physical movement of any body part, such as eyes, face, head, hands, legs, and shoulders. *Proxemics* refers to personal space and environmental variables such as the distance between two people and whether any objects are between them. As most people know from personal experience, a great deal is communicated through simple, and sometimes subtle, movements. When we discussed client-interviewer seating arrangements in Chapter 2, we were analyzing proxemic variables and their potential effect on the interview.

Positive interviewer body language includes the following (derived from Walters, 1980). These positive body language examples are based on mainstream cultural norms. In practice, you will find both individual and cultural variations on these behaviors:

- Leaning slightly toward the client.
- Maintaining a relaxed but attentive posture.

---

**INDIVIDUAL AND CULTURAL HIGHLIGHT 3.1**

## Cultural Background and Personal Space

You should be sensitive to cultural differences in eye contact, body language, vocal qualities, and verbal tracking. Although most Whites in North America interpret eye contact as a positive sign of interest, people from other cultures (e.g., Asian and Native American) tend to prefer less direct eye contact and may view excessive eye contact as disrespectful or invasive.

During a visit to Europe and North Africa, we became acutely aware of cultural differences in body language. We had a limited ability to speak other languages, and therefore our multicultural experiences were based largely on nonverbal perception. Our trip began in central Germany and northern Switzerland, where we hardly noticed any body language differences among the German, Swiss, and our own dominant North American culture. However, as we proceeded south to southern Switzerland and Italy, the average personal space and distance between people shrank. We found ourselves observing much more nose-to-nose communication. In addition, hand gestures were more vigorous and emphatic.

Perhaps our greatest discovery occurred while lining up for tickets at railway stations. In Germany and Switzerland, the lines were organized and polite, with little cutting or verbal exchanges between those waiting to be served. In contrast, lines in southern Italy and Tunisia were characterized by intense masses of bodies near the entrance or destination. Eventually, we discovered that waiting patiently in line was viewed as passive and low class in Southern European and Northern African cultures. People were respected for being what we, in mainstream North American culture, might describe as pushy and aggressive in obtaining services.

It's usually accurate to assume clients from other cultures will have different social habits from your own, but that doesn't mean different interviewing methods or attending behaviors are required (e.g., C. H. Patterson, 1996; Pedersen, 1996). It's acceptable to discuss what's comfortable and uncomfortable—in terms of attending behaviors—directly with clients. You're more likely to offend clients by assuming they've adopted your values and norms than by discussing these issues with them. When possible, read about and experience other cultures to increase your multicultural sensitivity.

---

- Placing your feet and legs in an unobtrusive position.
- Keeping your hand gestures unobtrusive and smooth.
- Minimizing the number of other movements.
- Making your facial expressions match your feelings or the client's feelings.
- Seating yourself at approximately one arm's length from the client.
- Arranging the furniture to draw you and the client together, not to erect a barrier.

*Mirroring,* as an aspect of body language, involves synchrony or consistency between interviewer and client. When mirroring occurs, the interviewer's physical movements and verbal activity is "in sync with" the client. Mirroring is a relatively advanced nonverbal technique that potentially enhances rapport and empathy, but when done poorly, can be disastrous (Banaka, 1971; Maurer & Tindall, 1983). Specifically, if mirroring is obvious, clients may think the therapist is mimicking or mocking them. Therefore, intentional mirroring is best used in moderation. Its benefits are small, but the costs can be great. Generally, mirroring is more of a product of rapport and effective communication than a causal factor in establishing positive communication.

## Vocal Qualities

In Chapter 2, we recommended having your friends or classmates listen to and describe your voice. If you followed this advice, your friends were giving feedback on your vocal quality or paralinguistics (as it is referred to in the communication field). *Paralinguistics* consists of voice loudness, pitch, rate, and fluency. Think about how these vocal variables might affect clients. Interpersonal influence is often determined not so much by *what* you say, but by *how* you say it.

Effective interviewers use vocal qualities to enhance rapport, communicate interest and empathy, and emphasize specific issues or conflicts. In general, interviewers' voices should be soft yet firm, indicating both sensitivity and strength. As with body language, it is often useful to follow the client's lead, speaking in a volume and tone similar to the client. Meier and Davis (2001) refer to this practice as "pacing the client" (p. 9).

On the other hand, interviewers can use voice tone, as with all interviewer responses and directives, to lead clients toward particular content or feelings. For example, speaking in a soft and gentle tone encourages clients to explore their feelings more thoroughly, and speaking with increased rate and volume may help convince them of your credibility or expertise (Cialdini, 1998).

Although people perceive emotions through all sensory modalities, some research suggests that people discern emotions more accurately from auditory than from visual input (Levitt, 1964; M. Snyder, 1974). This finding underscores the importance of vocal qualities in emotional expression and perception. Actors use their entire bodies, including their voices, when portraying various emotions. As an interviewer, your voice quality influences your client's emotional expression.

## Verbal Tracking

It is crucial for interviewers to accurately track what clients say. Although eye contact, body language, and vocal quality are important, they do not, by themselves, represent effective listening. Interviewers demonstrate an ability to track the content of their clients' speech by occasionally repeating key words and phrases. In most cases, clients do not know if you are really hearing what they're saying unless you prove it through accurate verbal tracking.

To use Meier and Davis's (2001) terminology again, verbal tracking involves pacing the client by sticking closely with client speech content (as well as speech volume and tone, as mentioned previously). Verbal tracking involves only restating or summarizing what the client has already said. Verbal tracking does not include your personal or professional opinion about what your client said.

Accurate verbal tracking is easier said than done. At times, clients talk about so many topics, it can be difficult to track them coherently. At other times, you may become distracted by what the client is saying and drift into your own thoughts. For example, a client may mention a range of topics including New York City, abortion, drugs, AIDS, divorce, or other topics about which you may have personal opinions or emotional reactions. To verbally track a client effectively, your internal and external personal reactions must be minimized; your focus must remain on the client, not yourself. This rule is also true when it comes to more advanced verbal tracking techniques, such as clarification, paraphrasing, and summarization.

## Negative Attending Behavior

It has been said that familiarity breeds contempt. When it comes to attending skills, it might be more accurate to say that overuse breeds contempt. It can be disconcerting when someone listens too intensely. Positive attending behaviors, when overused, are obnoxious. Interviewers should avoid overusing the following behaviors:

- *Head nods.* Excessive head nods can be bothersome. After a while, clients may look away from interviewers just to avoid watching their heads bob. One child client stated, "It looked like her head was attached to a wobbly spring instead of a neck."
- *Saying "Uh huh."* This is a very overused ∧ misleading attending behavior. Both novices and professionals can fall into this pattern. While listening to someone for two minutes, they may utter as many as 20 "uh huhs." Our response to excessive "uh huhs" (and the response of many clients) is to simply stop talking to force the person to say something besides "uh huh." *Get rid of saying "... you know?"*
- *Eye contact.* Too much eye contact causes people to feel scrutinized or intimidated. Imagine having a therapist relentlessly stare at you while you're talking about something deeply personal, or while you're crying. Eye contact is crucial, but too much can be overwhelming.
- *Repeating the client's last word.* Some interviewers use a verbal tracking technique that involves repeating a single key word, often the last word, from what the client has said. Overusing this pattern can cause clients to feel overanalyzed, because interviewers reduce 30- or 60-second statements to a single-word response.
- *Mirroring.* Excessive or awkward attempts at mirroring can be damaging. We recall a psychiatrist who used this technique with disturbed psychiatric inpatients. At times, his results were astoundingly successful; at other times, the patients became angry and aggressive because they thought he was mocking them. Similarly, clients sometimes worry that counselors use secret techniques to exert special control over them. They may notice if you're trying to get into a physical position similar to theirs and wonder if you're using a psychological ploy to manipulate them. The result is usually resistance and pursuit. Clients begin moving into new positions, the interviewer notices and changes position to establish synchrony, and the client moves again. If you videotape a session, this is especially entertaining to watch using the fast forward button on your VCR.

Additionally, research indicates that clients perceive the following interviewer behaviors as negative (Cormier & Nurius, 2003; Smith-Hanen, 1977):

- Making infrequent eye contact.
- Turning 45 degrees or more away from the client.
- Leaning back from the waist up.
- Crossing legs away from the client.
- Folding arms across the chest.

As suggested in the previous chapter, it is often difficult to know how you are coming across to others. Consequently, to ensure that you and your colleagues are exhibiting primarily positive rather than negative attending behaviors, you should give and receive constructive feedback to one another (see Putting It in Practice 3.1).

===== **Putting It in Practice 3.1** =====

## Giving Constructive Feedback

Getting and giving feedback regarding attending and listening skills is essential to interviewer development. Specific and concrete feedback regarding eye contact, body language, vocal qualities, and verbal tracking can be obtained through in-class activities, demonstrations, role plays, and audio- or videotape presentations. For example, positive feedback such as: "You looked into your client's eyes with only two or three breaks, and although you fidgeted somewhat with your pencil, it didn't appear to interfere with the interview" is clear and specific (and helpful). General and positive comments (e.g., "Good job!") are pleasant and encouraging, but should be used in combination with more specific feedback; it's important to know what was good about your job.

Sometimes, class activities or role plays don't go well and negative feedback is appropriate. Give negative feedback in a constructive or corrective manner. (This means the feedback shouldn't simply indicate what you did poorly, but also identify what you could do to perform the skill correctly.) For example, constructive negative or corrective feedback might sound like "You kept your eyes downcast most of the time. When you did look up and make eye contact, the interviewee seemed to brighten and become more engaged. So, next time try to maintain your eye contact a little longer."

Getting negative feedback is a sensitive issue because it can be painful to hear that you haven't performed perfectly. In contrast to general positive feedback, general negative comments such as "Terrible job!" should always be avoided. To be constructive, negative feedback should be specific and concrete. Other guidelines for giving negative feedback include:

- Remember, the reason you're in an interviewing class is to improve your interviewing skills. Though hard to hear, constructive feedback is useful for skill development.
- Feedback should never be uniformly negative. Everyone engages in positive *and* negative attending behaviors. If you happen to be the type who easily sees what's wrong, but has trouble offering praise, impose the following rule on yourself: If you cannot think of something positive to say about an interviewer's performance, don't say anything at all.
- It helps to practice giving negative feedback in a positive manner. For example, instead of saying, "Your body was stiff as a board" try saying "You'd be more effective if you relaxed your arms and shoulders more."
- Role players should evaluate themselves first.
- Students should be asked directly after a class interviewing activity whether they would like feedback. If they say no, then no feedback should be given.
- Feedback that is extremely negative is the responsibility of the instructor and should be given during a private, individual supervision session.
- Try to remember the disappointing fact that no one performs perfectly, including the teacher or professor.

## Individual and Cultural Differences

Many individual and cultural differences affect the interview. These differences include, but are not limited to: (a) gender, (b) social class, (c) ethnicity, (d) sexual orientation, (e) age, and (f) physical disabilities (Gilligan, 1982; Gandy, Martin, & Hardy, 1999; Susser & Patterson, 2000). Every client is part of a distinct subculture with associated behavior patterns and social norms (Atkinson & Hackett, 1998). Obviously, attending behaviors that work with young gang members differ from attending behaviors used with geriatric patients. A working knowledge of a wide range of social and cultural norms helps interviewers attend more effectively (see Individual and Cultural Highlight 3.1).

### Individual Differences

If you were to invite 20 people, one by one, into your office for an interview, you would discover that each person was optimally comfortable with slightly different amounts of eye contact, personal space, mirroring, and other attending behaviors. The guidelines discussed previously are based on averages and probabilities. For example, if you interviewed Italian American clients, you might find them, on average, desiring closer seating arrangements than clients with Scandinavian roots. However, this is not the whole story. There also will be times when a *particular* Italian American prefers greater interpersonal distance than a *particular* Scandinavian. If you expect all Italian Americans, all Scandinavians, all African Americans, all women, and so on to be similar, you are stereotyping. Differences between individuals are often greater than the average difference among particular groups, cultural or otherwise. Therefore, although you should be aware of potential differences between members of various groups, you should suspend judgment until you have explored the issue with each individual through observation and by directly discussing these issues.

## MOVING BEYOND ATTENDING

We now move beyond attending and on to other listening responses available to clinical interviewers. The remainder of this chapter is devoted to several interviewer techniques that encourage clients to talk about what is on their minds, not yours.

We would like to provide you with an authoritative guide to every potential interviewer response, complete with a structured format for determining which response should be used at which time during an interview. Unfortunately, or perhaps fortunately, the unique relationship between interviewer and client—and the interviewing process itself—is too complex for any such formula. Differences among clients make it impossible to reliably predict their reactions to various interviewing responses. Some clients react positively to responses we judge as poor or awkward; others react negatively to what might be considered a perfect paraphrase. This section breaks down nondirective interviewing responses into distinct categories, providing general guidelines regarding when and how to use these responses. Effectively applying a particular interviewing response constitutes the artistic side of interviewing, requiring sensitivity and experience as well as other intangibles you cannot absorb from a book. This may seem like bad news but it reflects the true nature of the art.

Not knowing what to say or when to say it can be disconcerting for beginning interviewers, but, truthfully, no one always knows the correct thing to say. For the most part, experienced interviewers have become comfortable with long pauses resulting from not knowing what to say or do next. Meier and Davis (2001) recommend: "When you don't know what to say, say nothing" (p. 11). And Luborsky (1984) elaborates: "Listen . . . with an open receptiveness to what the patient is saying. If you are not sure of what is happening and what your next response should be, listen more and it will come to you" (p. 91). In other words, when you don't know what to say, stick with your basic attending and listening skills.

Margaret Gibbs (1984) expresses the distress many new interviewers experience in her chapter "The Therapist as Imposter" in Claire Brody's book *Women Therapists Working with Women:*

> Once I began my work as a therapist . . . I began to have . . . doubts. Certainly my supervisors seemed to approve of my work, and my patients improved as much as anybody else's did. But what was I actually supposed to be doing? I knew the dynamic, client-centered and behavioral theories, but I continued to read and search for answers. I felt there was something I should know, something my instructors had neglected to tell me, much as cooks are said to withhold one important ingredient of their recipes when they relinquish them. (p. 22)

The missing ingredient Gibbs was seeking could have been experience. Ironically, experience does not make interviewers sure of having the *right* thing to say. Instead, it helps take the edge off the panic associated with not knowing what to say. Experience allows interviewers the confidence required to wait; they know they will eventually think of something useful to say. In addition, experience helps interviewers have more confidence. Nonetheless, part of being an honest professional is to admit and tolerate the fact that sometimes you do not know what to say. Gibbs ends her chapter with the following statements:

> Strategies can cover up, but not resolve, the ambiguities of clinical judgments and interventions. Imposter doubts need to be shared, not suppressed, in the classroom as elsewhere. [There is] evidence to support the idea that uncertainty and humility about the accuracy of our clinical inferences is an aid to increased accuracy. I find this notion enormously comforting. (p. 32)

Knowing what to say, when to say it, and when to be quiet is central to the process of clinical interviewing. Saying "the wrong thing" is a common fear stated by our students.

F. Robinson's (1950) organizational format is used in the following section. We begin with responses that are considered, for the most part, nondirective, and proceed along a continuum toward increasingly directive or therapist-centered responses. Interviewer responses are categorized into three groups:

1. Nondirective listening responses (e.g., silence; see Table 3.1, p. 70).
2. Directive listening responses (e.g., interpretation; see Table 3.2, p. 78).
3. Directive action responses (e.g., advice; see Table 4.2, p. 100).

## NONDIRECTIVE LISTENING RESPONSES

Nondirective listening responses are designed to encourage clients to talk freely and openly about whatever they want. Similar to attending behaviors, these techniques do not overtly direct or lead clients. Instead, they track central client messages by reflecting back to clients what they already said.

Even nondirective responses may influence clients to talk about particular topics. There are at least two reasons for this. First, interviewers may inadvertently, or purposefully, pay closer attention to clients when they discuss certain issues. For example, perhaps an interviewer wants a client to talk about his relationship with his mother. By using eye contact, head nodding, and positive facial expressions whenever the client mentions his mother, the interviewer can direct the client toward "mother talk." Conversely, the interviewer can look uninterested whenever the client shifts topics and discusses something other than his mother. Technically, such an interviewer is using social reinforcement to influence the client's verbal behavior. This selective attending probably occurs frequently in clinical practice. After all, psychoanalytic interviewers are more interested in mother talk, person-centered interviewers are more interested in feeling talk, and behaviorists are more interested in specific, concrete behavioral talk.

Second, clients talk about such a wide range of topics that it is impossible to pay equal attention to every issue a client brings up. Some selection is necessary. For example, imagine a case in which a young woman begins a session by saying:

> "We didn't have much money when I was growing up, and I suppose that frustrated my father. He beat us five kids on a regular basis. Now that I'm grown and have kids of my own, I'm doing okay, but sometimes I feel I need to discipline my kids more . . . harder . . . you know what I mean?"

Pretend you are the interviewer for this case. Which of the many issues this woman brought up would you choose to focus on? And remember, all this—being beaten by her father, being poor, doing okay now, feeling like disciplining her children more severely, and more—was expressed in the session's first 20 seconds.

Which topic did you focus on? Aside from indicating something about your personal values, focusing on any single aspect of this woman's message, selecting only one topic to paraphrase or nod your head to, is a directive listening response. To be truly nondirective, interviewers need to respond equally to every piece of the entire message, which is unrealistic. Therefore, be aware of the powerful influence even nondirective responses have on what clients choose to talk about.

## Silence

In some ways, silence is the most nondirective of all listening responses. Though simple and nondirective, silence is also a powerful interviewer response. It takes time for interviewers and clients to get comfortable with silence. As the following excerpt from Edgar Allan Poe's *Silence: A Fable* suggests, silence can be frightening.

> Hurriedly, he raised his head from his hand, and stood forth upon the rock and listened. But there was no voice throughout the vast illimitable desert, and the characters upon the rock were silence. And the man shuddered and turned his face away, and fled afar off in haste so that I beheld him no more.

Silence can frighten both interviewers and clients. Most people feel awkward about silence in social settings and strive to keep conversations alive. As Lewis Thomas (1974) wrote in *The Lives of the Cell,* "Nature abhors a long silence" (p. 22).

On the other hand, when used appropriately, silence can be soothing. As the Tao Te

Ching states: "Stillness and tranquility set things in order in the universe." Much can be accomplished in stillness and silence. Although the primary function of silence as an interviewer response is to encourage client talk, silence may also allow clients to recover from or reflect on what they have just said. In addition, silence allows the interviewer time to consider and intentionally select a response, rather than rushing into one. However, a word of caution: Interviewers who begin sessions with silence and continue using silence liberally, without explaining the purpose of their silence, run the risk of scaring clients away. This is because when interviewers are silent, great pressure is placed on clients to speak and client anxiety begins to mount.

Silence is a major tool used by psychoanalytic psychotherapists to facilitate free association. Effective psychoanalytic therapists, however, explain the concept of free association to their clients before using it. They explain that psychoanalytic therapy involves primarily the client's free expression, followed by occasional comments or interpretations by the therapist. Explaining therapy or interviewing procedures to clients is always important, but especially so when the interviewer is using potentially anxiety-provoking techniques, such as silence (Luborsky, 1984; Meier & Davis, 2001).

As a beginning interviewer, try experimenting with silence (see Putting It in Practice 3.2). In addition, consider the following guidelines:

- When a role-play client pauses after making a statement or after hearing your paraphrase, let a few seconds pass rather than jump in immediately with further verbal interaction. Given the opportunity, clients can move naturally into very significant material without guidance or urging.
- As you're sitting silently, waiting for your client to resume speaking, tell yourself that this is the client's time to express himself or herself, not your time to prove you can be useful.
- Try not to get into a rut regarding your use of silence. When silence comes, sometimes wait for the client to speak next and other times break the silence yourself.

---

**Putting It in Practice 3.2**

### Getting Comfortable with Silence

Dealing with silences during an interview can be uncomfortable. To help adjust to moments of silence, try some of the following activities:

- If you're watching or listening to an interview (either live or taped), keep track of the length of each silence. Then, pay attention to who breaks the silence. Most importantly, try to determine whether the silence helped the client keep talking about something important or go into a deeper issue or whether the silence was detrimental in some way.
- When a silence comes up during a practice interview, pay attention to your thoughts and feelings. Do you welcome silence, dread silence, or feel neutral about silence?
- Talk with friends, family, or a romantic partner about how he or she feels about silent moments during social conversations. You may find that people have much different feelings about silence. Your goal is to understand how others view silence.

- Avoid using silence if you believe your client is confused, experiencing an acute emotional crisis, or psychotic. Excess silence and the anxiety it provokes tend to exacerbate these conditions.
- If you feel uncomfortable during silent periods, try to relax. Use your attending skills to look expectantly toward clients. This helps them understand that it's their turn to talk.
- If clients appear uncomfortable with silence, you may give them instructions to free associate (i.e., tell them "Just say whatever comes to mind."). Or you may want to use an empathic reflection (e.g., "It's hard to decide what to say next.").
- Remember, sometimes silence is the most therapeutic response available.
- Read the published interview by Carl Rogers (Meador & Rogers, 1984) listed at the end of this chapter. It includes excellent examples of how to handle silence from a person-centered perspective.
- Remember to monitor your body and face while being silent. There is a vast difference between a cold silence and an accepting, warm silence. Much of this difference results from body language.

## Paraphrase or Reflection of Content

The paraphrase is a verbal tracking skill and a cornerstone of effective communication. Its primary purpose is to let clients know you have accurately heard the central meaning of their messages. Secondarily, paraphrases allow clients to hear how someone else perceives them (a clarification function), which can further facilitate expression.

*Paraphrasing* is "the act or process of restating or rewording" (*Random House Unabridged Dictionary,* 1993, p. 1409). In clinical interviewing, the paraphrase is sometimes referred to as a reflection of content (this refers to the fact that paraphrases reflect the content of what clients are saying, but not process or feelings). A paraphrase or reflection of content refers to a statement accurately reflecting or rephrasing what the client has said. The paraphrase does not change, modify, or add to the client's message. A good paraphrase is accurate and brief.

Interviewers often feel awkward when making their first paraphrases; it can feel as if they're restating the obvious. They often simply parrot back to clients what has just been said in a manner that is rigid, stilted, and, at times, offensive. This is unfortunate because the paraphrase, properly used, is a flexible and creative technique that enhances rapport and empathy. As Miller and Rollnick (1991) note, nondirective listening, especially characterized by paraphrasing, is harder than it looks:

> Although a therapist skilled in empathic listening can make it look easy and natural, in fact, this is a demanding counseling style. It requires sharp attention to each new client statement, and a continual generation of hypotheses as to the meaning. Your best guess as to meaning is then reflected back to the client, often adding to the content of what was overtly said. The client responds, and the whole process starts over again. Reflective listening is easy to parody or do poorly, but quite challenging to do well. (p. 26)

Several types of paraphrases are discussed in the following section.

### The Generic Paraphrase

The generic paraphrase simply rephrases, rewords, and reflects what the client just said. Some examples:

**Client 1:** "Yesterday was my day off. I just sat around the house doing nothing. I had some errands to run, but I couldn't seem to make myself get up off the couch and do them."

**Interviewer 1:** "So you had trouble getting going on your day off."

**Client 2:** "I do this with every assignment. I wait till the last minute and then I whip together the paper. I end up doing all-nighters. I don't think the final product is as good as it could be."

**Interviewer 2:** "You see this as a pattern for yourself and think that your procrastination makes it so you don't do as well as you could on your assignments."

Each of these examples of the generic paraphrase is simple and straightforward. The generic paraphrase does not retain everything that was originally said; it rephrases the core of the client's message. It also does not include interviewer opinion, reactions, or commentary, whether positive or negative.

## The Sensory-Based Paraphrase

The neurolinguistic programming (NLP) movement in counseling popularized a concept referred to as *representational systems* (Bandler & Grinder, 1975; Grinder & Bandler, 1976). Representational systems refer to the sensory system—usually visual, auditory, or kinesthetic—that clients prefer to use to experience the world.

If you listen closely to your clients' words, you will notice that some clients rely primarily on visually oriented words (e.g., "I see" or "it looks like"), others on auditory words (e.g., "I hear" or "it sounded like"), and others on kinesthetic words (e.g., "I feel" or "it moved me"). Based on NLP research, when interviewers speak through their client's representational system, empathy, trust, and desire to see the interviewer again are all increased (Brockman, 1980; Hammer, 1983; Sharpley, 1984).

Listening closely for your client's sensory-related words is the key to using sensory-based paraphrases. To sensitize yourself to the three representational systems, we recommend doing an individual or in-class activity in which you generate as many visual, auditory, and kinesthetic words as you can. (Although clients occasionally refer to olfactory and taste experiences, it is rare that clients use these as their primary representational modality.) Examples of sensory-based paraphrases follow, with the sensory words italicized:

**Client 1:** "My goal in therapy is to get to know myself better. I think of therapy as kind of a *mirror* through which I can *see* myself, my strengths, and my weaknesses more *clearly.*"

**Interviewer 1:** "You're here because you want to *see* yourself more *clearly* and believe therapy can really help you with that."

**Client 2:** "I just got *laid off* from my job and I don't know what to do. My job is so important to me. I *feel* lost."

**Interviewer 2:** "Your job has been so important to you, you *feel* adrift without it."

Analyzing the client's spontaneous use of sensory words appears to be the most reliable method for evaluating a client's primary representational system (Sharpley, 1984).

## The Metaphorical Paraphrase

Interviewers can use metaphor or analogy to capture the central message in a client's communication. For instance, often clients come to a professional interviewer because they are feeling stuck, not making progress in terms of personal growth or problem resolution. In such a case, an interviewer might reflect, "So it seems like you're spinning your wheels" or "Dealing with this has been a real uphill battle." Although metaphorical paraphrases might be best suited to kinesthetically oriented clients, many clients respond well to them, perhaps because so much of an experience is captured in so few words. Additional examples follow:

> **Client 1:** "My sister is so picky. We share a room and she's always bugging me about picking up my clothes, straightening up my dresser, and everything else, too. She scrutinizes every move I make and criticizes me every chance she gets."
>
> **Interviewer 1:** "It's like you're in the army and she's your drill sergeant."
>
> **Client 2:** "I'm prepared for some breakdowns along the way."
>
> **Interviewer 2:** "You don't expect it will be smooth sailing." (From C. Rogers, 1961, p. 102)

## Clarification

Several forms of clarification have the same purpose: to make clear for yourself and the client the precise nature of what has been said. The first form of clarification consists of a restatement of what the client said and a closed question, in either order. Rogers was a master at clarification:

> If I'm getting it right . . . what makes it hurt most of all is that when he tells you you're no good, well shucks, that's what you've always felt about yourself. Is that the meaning of what you're saying? (In Meador & Rogers, 1984, p. 167)

The second form of clarification consists of a restatement imbedded in a double question. A double question is an either/or question including two or more choices of response for the client. For example:

- "Do you dislike being called on in class—or is it something else?"
- "Did you get in the argument with your husband before or after you went to the movie?"

Using clarification along with a double question allows interviewers to take more control of what clients say during an interview. In a sense, interviewers try to guess a client's potential response by providing possible choices, similar to the multiple-choice test format.

The third form of clarification is the most basic. It's used when you don't quite hear what a client said and you need to recheck.

- "I'm sorry, I didn't quite hear that. Could you repeat what you said?"
- "I couldn't make out what you said. Did you say you'd be going home after the session?"

There are times during interviews when you do not understand what clients are saying. There are also times when your clients are not sure what they are saying or why they are saying it. Of course, the worst possible scenario is when neither of you has any sense of the meaning or purpose of what's being said. Sometimes, the appropriate response is to wait, as Luborsky (1984) suggests, for understanding to come. However, other times, it is necessary to clarify precisely what clients are talking about. There are also times when clients need to clarify something you've said.

Brammer (1979) provides two general guidelines for clarifying.[a] First, admit your confusion over what the client has said. Second, "try a restatement or ask for clarification, repetition, or illustration" (p. 73). Asking for a specific example can be especially useful because it encourages clients to be concrete and specific rather than abstract and vague.

From the interviewer's perspective, there are two main factors to consider when deciding whether to use clarification. First, if the information appears trivial and unrelated to therapeutic issues, it is best to simply wait for the client to move on to a more productive area. It can be a waste of time to clarify minor details that are only remotely related to interview goals. For example, suppose a client says, "My stepdaughter's grandfather on my wife's side of the family usually has little or no contact with my parents." This presents an excellent opportunity for the interviewer to listen quietly. To attempt a clarification response might result in a lengthy entanglement with distant family relationships. Spontaneous rambling about distant family relations is often a sign that your client is avoiding more important personal issues. If so, do not use a clarification response, or any listening response, because to do so might reinforce this avoidance pattern.

Second, if the information your client is discussing seems important but is not being articulated clearly, you have two choices: Wait briefly to see if the client can independently express himself or herself more clearly, or immediately use a clarification. For example, a client may state:

"I don't know, she was different. She looked at me differently than other women. Others were missing . . . something, you know, the eyes, usually you can tell by the way a woman looks at you, can't you? Then again, maybe it was something else, something about me that I'll understand someday."

An appropriate interviewer clarification might be: "She seemed different; it may have been how she looked at you, or something about yourself you don't totally understand. Is that what you're saying?"

### Nondirective Reflection of Feeling    *let person know you understand how they're feeling*

The primary purpose of nondirective reflection of feeling is to let clients know, through an emotionally oriented paraphrase, that you are tuned in to their emotional state. Nondirective feeling reflections also encourage further emotional expression. Consider the following example of a 15-year-old male talking with an interviewer about his teacher:

**Client:** "That teacher pissed me off big time when she accused me of stealing her watch. I wanted to punch her lights out."
**Interviewer:** "So you were pretty pissed off."
**Client:** "Damn right."

In this example, the interviewer's feeling reflection focuses only on what the client clearly articulated. This is the basic rule for nondirective feeling reflections: Restate or reflect *only* what you clearly hear the client say. Do not probe, interpret, or speculate. Although we might guess at the underlying emotions causing this boy's fury, a nondirective feeling reflection doesn't address these possibilities.

Feelings are, by their very nature, personal. This means any attempt at reflecting feelings is a move toward closeness or intimacy. Some clients who do not want the intimacy associated with a counseling relationship react to feeling reflections by becoming more distant and quiet. Others deny their feelings. You minimize potential negative reactions to feeling reflections by using tentative nondirective reflections.

When offering feeling reflections, interviewers should accurately reflect feeling content and intensity. If you are unsure of what a client is feeling, you may use a tentative reflection. C. Rogers (1951, 1961) would sometimes check with clients after giving a feeling reflection to see if the reflection fit well. Feelings are personal; clients often react negatively when interviewers insist that a particular emotion is present. If you are tentative in your feeling reflection, your client may quickly correct you. For example:

**Client:** "That teacher pissed me off big time when she accused me of stealing her watch. I wanted to punch her lights out."
**Interviewer:** "Seems like you were a little irritated about that. Is that right?"
**Client:** "Irritated, hell, I was pissed."

In this example, the stronger emotional descriptor (pissed) is more appropriate, because the client clearly expressed that he was more than just irritated. Empathy may be adversely affected because the interviewer minimized the intensity of the client's feeling. On the other hand, the adverse effect may be minimized because the interviewer phrased the reflection tentatively (see Putting It in Practice 3.3 to practice your emotional responses to clients).

---

**Putting It in Practice 3.3**

## Enhancing Your Feeling Capacity and Vocabulary

There are many ways to explore and enhance your feeling capacity and vocabulary. Carkhuff (1987) recommends the following activity. Identify a basic emotion, such as anger, fear, happiness, or sadness, and then begin associating to other feelings in response to that emotion. For instance, state, "When I feel sad . . ." and then finish the thought by associating to another feeling and stating it; for example, "I feel cheated." An example of this process follows:

When I feel joy, I feel fulfilled.
When I feel fulfilled, I feel content.
When I feel content, I feel comfortable.
When I feel comfortable, I feel safe.
When I feel safe, I feel calm.
When I feel calm, I feel relaxed.

This feeling association process can help you discover more about your emotional life and help you come up with a wide range of meaningful feeling words. Conduct this exercise individually or in dyads, using each of the 10 primary emotions identified by Izard (1977, 1982):

| | |
|---|---|
| Interest-excitement | Disgust |
| Joy | Contempt |
| Surprise | Fear |
| Distress | Shame |
| Anger | Guilt |

## Summarization

Summarization demonstrates accurate listening, enhances client and interviewer recall of major themes, helps clients focus on important issues, and extracts or refines the meaning behind client messages.

After listening to a client for 20 or 30 minutes, or even after an entire session, it is appropriate and useful to summarize what has been discussed. For example:

> **Interviewer:** "You've said a lot these first 15 minutes, so I thought I'd make sure I'm keeping track of your main concerns. You talked about the conflicts between you and your parents, about how you've felt angry over their neglecting you, and about how it was a relief, but also a big adjustment, to be placed in a foster home. Does that cover the main points of what you've talked about so far?"
>
> **Client:** "Yeah. That about covers it."

Although summarization is conceptually simple, coming up with a summary can be difficult. Memories can quickly fade, leaving us without an accurate or complete recollection of what the client said. Sometimes, because of a desire to be thorough and precise when summarizing, interviewers bite off more than they can chew. For example:

> "Now I want to summarize the four main issues you've discussed today. First, you said your childhood was hard because of your father's authoritarian style. Second, in your current marriage, you find yourself overly critical of your wife's parenting. Third, you described yourself as controlling and perfectionistic, which you think contributes to the ongoing conflict in your marriage. And fourth, uh, fourth [long pause], uh, I forgot what was fourth—but I'm sure it will come to me."

This brings us to the second difficulty in summarizing. Often, a session is full of a variety of topics and themes. There may not be a readily apparent underlying pattern that lends itself to summary. This is especially true at the beginning of therapy. It is difficult to provide a concise summary that captures the essence of what was said without being overly redundant or leaving out a central segment. Therefore, an informal and collaborative approach to summarization can be useful.

There are several advantages to using an informal, interactive, and supportive summary. First, doing so takes pressure off your memory. Second, it places some responsibility on clients to state what *they* think is important. This helps clients recall what they said and helps you know what they think is significant. Third, an interactive approach models a collaborative relationship. In therapy, the counselor is not solely responsible for success. Allowing clients to help decide what's important demonstrates teamwork.

### *Guidelines for Summarizing*

Informal, interactive, and supportive summaries are explained below:

#### Informal

- Instead of saying, "Here is my summary of what you've said," say something like, "Let's make sure I'm keeping up with the main things you've talked about."

- Instead of numbering your points, simply state them one by one. That way, you won't be embarrassed by forgetting a point.

### Interactive

- Pause while summarizing so your client can agree, disagree, or elaborate.
- At the end of a summary, ask if what you've said seems accurate.
- Before you summarize, have your client summarize what he or she felt is important. This way, you obtain your client's views, without tainting them with your opinion. You can always add what you thought was important later.

### Supportive

- In some cases, openly acknowledge that your client has disclosed a large amount of information. For example: "You've said a lot" or "You've covered quite a bit in a short period of time" are reassuring and supportive statements that help clients feel good about what they have said. Of course, you should remain genuine and make these supportive statements only when they are truthful.
- The way you ask a client for a summary should be supportive. Specifically: "I'm interested in what *you* feel has been most important of all you've covered today." Or, "How would you summarize the most important things you've talked about?"

Table 3.1.  **Summary of Nondirective Listening Responses and Their Usual Effects**

| Nondirective Listening Response | Description | Primary Intent/Effect |
|---|---|---|
| Attending behavior | Eye contact, leaning forward, head nods, facial expressions, etc. | Facilitates or inhibits spontaneous client talk. |
| Silence | Absence of verbal activity. | Places pressure on clients to talk. Allows "cooling off" time. Allows interviewer to consider next response. |
| Clarification | Attempted restating of a client's message, preceded or followed by a closed question (e.g., "Do I have that right?"). | Clarifies unclear client statements and verifies the accuracy of what the interviewer heard. |
| Paraphrase | Reflection or rephrasing of the content of what the client said. | Assures clients you hear them accurately and allows them to hear what they said. |
| Sensory-based paraphrase | Paraphrase that uses the client's clearly expressed sensory modalities. | Enhances rapport and empathy. |
| Nondirective reflection of feeling | Restatement or rephrasing of clearly stated emotion. | Enhances clients' experience of empathy and encourages their further emotional expression. |
| Summarization | Brief review of several topics covered during a session. | Enhances recall of session content and ties together or integrates themes covered in a session. |

## THE PULL TO REASSURANCE

Taken together, attending skills and nondirective listening techniques could be considered "nice" behaviors. They involve politely listening to another human being, indicating interest, tuning into feelings, and demonstrating a wide range of caring behaviors.

In addition, if you are listening well, you may also feel a strong pull to say complimentary, reassuring, positive things. However, it is important to know that using compliments or reassurance is not the same as listening nondirectively.

Complimenting someone is an act of self-disclosure. You are expressing *your* taste and *your* approval. Self-disclosure, too, for a clinical interviewer, is a *technique* and should be used in moderation (Pizer, 1997). Reassurance, too, is a *technique*. Clients may behave in ways that beg for reassurance. They want to know if they are good parents, if they did the right thing, if their sadness will lift, and so on. You will feel the pull to reassure them and tell them they are doing just fine.

Premature or global reassurance should not be given to clients. When you reassure, you're assessing a situation and/or a person's coping abilities and declaring that things will improve or come out for the better. Furthermore, empathy and reassurance are not interchangeable. Interviewers should make empathic statements regularly, while reassurance should come in carefully considered, small doses.

## DIRECTIVE LISTENING RESPONSES

Directive listening and action responses are considered directive because they place interviewers in the position of director, choreographer, or expert. To be used effectively, directives require interpersonal and clinical sensitivity. They also require basic knowledge of psychopathology and diagnostic skills.

In some ways, because directive responses are so influential, we should probably wait to discuss them later in this text, after a thorough review of assessment interviewing. Why then, do we include a description of responses such as interpretation, confrontation, and advice giving before we discuss assessment techniques?

To conduct assessment interviews, you must know the complete range of responses available. Assessment interviewing requires both nondirective and directive responses. In addition, unless you have a grasp of all responses available to you, you may use advanced directive techniques inappropriately. Therefore, we present some of the following information *not* so you can master directive or depth psychotherapy skills, but to whet your appetite for more advanced training.

Directive listening responses may be primarily client-centered or they may be primarily interviewer-centered, but they are always used to focus the interview on a particular topic or assessment issue. At their foundation, directive listening responses operate on the assumption that clients need guidance or direction from their therapists.

### Feeling Validation

Reflection of feeling is often confused with a technique referred to as *feeling validation.* Beginning textbooks normally do not distinguish between these two different responses (A. Ivey & Ivey, 1999; Meier & Davis, 2001). Feeling validation occurs when an interviewer acknowledges and approves of a client's stated feelings.

The purpose of feeling validation is to help clients accept their feelings as a natural and normal part of being human. Feeling validation can serve as an ego boost; clients feel supported and more normal because of their interviewer's validating comments. However, this is a controversial issue because some theorists believe that directive and supportive techniques such as feeling validation enhance self-esteem only temporarily, based on the therapist's input rather than real or lasting change in the client. In addition, when therapists liberally use feeling validation, it can foster dependency. As a therapeutic technique, feeling validation contains approval and reassurance, both of which usually produce positive feelings in the recipient. This may be why friends or romantic partners offer each other frequent doses of feeling validation.

All approaches to feeling validation give clients the same message: "Your feelings are acceptable and you have permission to feel them." In fact, sometimes feeling validation gives the message that clients *should* be having particular feelings.

> **Client:** "I've just been so sad since my mother died. I can't seem to stop myself from crying." (Client begins to sob.)
> **Interviewer:** "It's okay for you to be sad about losing your mother. That's perfectly normal. Go ahead and cry if you feel like it."

Notice the preceding interviewer goes beyond feeling reflection to validation of feeling. Obviously, this is not a client-centered or nondirective technique. By openly stating that feeling sad and crying is okay, the interviewer is taking the role of expert and judging whether a client's feelings and behavior are appropriate.

Another way to provide feeling validation is through self-disclosure:

> **Client:** "I get so anxious before tests, you wouldn't believe it! All I can think about is how I'm going to freeze up and forget everything. Then, when I get in there and look at the test, my mind just goes blank."
> **Interviewer:** "You know, sometimes I feel the same way about tests."

In this example, the interviewer uses self-disclosure to demonstrate that he or she has felt similar anxiety. Although using self-disclosure to validate feelings can be reassuring, it is not without risk. In this case, the client may privately wonder if the counselor (who admits to feeling anxiety) can help him or her overcome the anxiety; counselor credibility can be diminished.

Interviewers can also validate or reassure clients by using a concept Yalom (1995) referred to as *universality.*

> **Client:** "I'm always comparing myself to everyone else—and I usually come up short. I wonder if I'll ever really feel completely confident."
> **Interviewer:** "You're being too hard on yourself. Everyone has self-doubts. I don't know anyone who feels a complete sense of confidence."

As illustrated, clients may feel validated when they observe or are informed that nearly everyone else in the world (or universe) feels what they're feeling. Yalom (1995) provides another example:

> Once I reviewed with a patient his 600-hour experience in . . . analysis. . . . When I inquired about his recollection of the most significant event in his therapy, he recalled an incident when he was profoundly distressed about his feelings toward his mother. Despite strong concurrent positive sentiments, he was beset with death wishes for her so that he might inherit a sizable estate. His analyst . . . commented simply, "That seems to be the

way we're built." That artless statement offered considerable relief and furthermore enabled the patient to explore his ambivalence in great depth. (p. 8)

Feeling validation is common in interviewing and counseling. This is partly because people like to have their feelings validated and partly because therapists generally like validating their clients' feelings. In some cases, clients come to therapy primarily because they want to know that that they are normal. Alternatively, some theorists believe that open support, such as feeling validation, reduces client exploration of important issues (i.e., clients figure they must be fine if their therapist says so) and thereby diminishes the likelihood that clients will independently develop positive attitudes toward themselves. Potential effects of feeling validation follow:

- Enhanced rapport.
- Increased or reduced client exploration of the problem or feeling.
- Reduction in client anxiety, at least temporarily.
- Enhanced client self-esteem or feelings of normality (perhaps only temporarily).
- Increased likelihood of client-interviewer dependency.
- Decreased client exploration of important issues.

## Interpretive Reflection of Feeling

Interpretive feeling reflections are feeling-based statements made by interviewers that go beyond the client's obvious emotional expressions. The goal of interpretive feeling reflections is to uncover emotions that clients are only partially aware of. Interpretive feeling reflections may produce insight (i.e., the client becomes aware of something that was previously unconscious or only partially conscious).

Interpretive feeling reflections have been referred to elsewhere as "advanced empathy" (Egan, 1986, p. 212). For example, Egan states:

Basic empathy [nondirective reflection of feeling] gets at relevant surface (not to be confused with superficial) feelings and meanings, while advanced accurate empathy [interpretive reflection of feeling] gets at feelings and meanings that are buried, hidden, or beyond the immediate reach of the client. (p. 213)

Consider, again, the 15-year-old boy who was so angry with his teacher.

**Client:** "That teacher pissed me off big time when she accused me of stealing her watch. I wanted to punch her lights out."
**Interviewer:** "So you were pretty pissed off." (Nondirective feeling reflection.)
**Client:** "Damn right."
**Interviewer:** "You know, I also sense you have some other feelings about what your teacher did. Maybe you were hurt because she didn't trust you." (Interpretive feeling reflection.)

The interviewer's second statement is in pursuit of deeper feelings that the client did not articulate. Interpretive feeling reflections can be threatening to clients because such reflections encourage exploration at a deeper level than the expressed feelings. Interpretive feeling reflections can also significantly strengthen client-interviewer rapport and interviewer credibility.

The reason an interpretive feeling reflection is considered a directive, interviewer-centered response is worth further discussion. You may be wondering why such a response is labeled *interpretive* if it is based on the client's report of personal experience. First, as Egan suggests, the interpretive feeling reflection is based on emotional material "buried" or "hidden" from the client (Egan, 1986, p. 213). When interviewers bring this material to a client's awareness, they are engaging in a directive activity. Second, an interpretive feeling reflection, or Egan's "advanced empathy," assumes that unconscious or out-of-awareness processes are influencing the client's functioning. In making such an assumption, the interviewer is imposing a theoretical construct on the client. Essentially, because an interpretation's goal is to bring unconscious material into consciousness, it is a directive technique (Weiner, 1998). However, as George and Cristiani (1994) suggest, even nondirective feeling reflections can produce this effect: "The classic client-centered technique, reflection of feeling, can be viewed as an interpretation" (p. 162).

Interpretive feeling reflections are powerful techniques that can promote therapeutic breakthroughs. They may also stimulate client defensiveness. As psychoanalytically oriented clinicians emphasize, when it comes to effective interpretations, timing is extremely important (S. Freud, 1940/1949; Weiner, 1998). That's why, in the preceding example, the interviewer initially uses a nondirective feeling reflection and then, only after that reflection has been affirmed, moves to a more probing and interpretive response. Interpretive feeling reflections require a good relationship and previous knowledge of the client as a foundation for effectiveness. In addition, as with nondirective feeling reflections, interpretive feeling reflections should be worded tentatively.

## Interpretation

The purpose of an interpretation is to produce client insight or a more accurate perception of reality. As Fenichel (1945) states, "Interpretation means helping something unconscious to become conscious by naming it at the moment it is striving to break through" (p. 25). When an interviewer provides an interpretation, the interviewer is in essence saying to the client, "This is how I see you and your situation."

### Psychoanalytic or "Classical" Interpretations

According to the psychoanalytic tradition, an interpretation is based on the theoretical assumption that unconscious processes influence behavior. By pointing out unconscious conflicts and patterns, therapists help clients move toward greater self-awareness and higher levels of functioning. This is not to suggest that insight alone produces behavior change. Instead, insight begins moving clients toward more adaptive ways of feeling, thinking, and acting.

There are many forms of classical interpretation, but because it's an advanced skill, we illustrate the technique only briefly here. Consider, one last time, our angry 15-year-old student.

> **Client:** "That teacher pissed me off big time when she accused me of stealing her watch. I wanted to punch her lights out."
> **Interviewer:** "So you were pretty pissed off." (Nondirective feeling reflection.)
> **Client:** "Damn right."
> **Interviewer:** "You know, I also sense you have some other feelings about what your teacher did. Maybe you were hurt because she didn't trust you." (Interpretive feeling reflection.)

**Client:** (Pauses.) "Yeah, well that's a dumb idea . . . it doesn't hurt anymore . . . after a while when no one trusts you, it ain't no big surprise to get accused again of something I didn't do."

**Interviewer:** "So when you respond to your teacher's distrust of you with anger, it's almost like you're reacting to those times when your parents haven't trusted you." (Interpretation.)

In this exchange, the boy gives indirect confirmation of the interpretive feeling reflection's accuracy. He first demeans the interviewer's reflection and then confirms it by noting, "it doesn't hurt anymore." Notice that in this phrase the boy gives the interviewer a signal to search for past traumatic experiences (i.e., the word *anymore* is a reference to the past). This is not surprising. Accurate interpretations often produce "genetic" material (i.e., material from the past). Thus, the interviewer perceives the client's signal and proceeds with a more classical interpretation.

Classical interpretations require knowledge of the client and the client's past and present relationships. In the previous example, the interviewer knows from previous interviews that the boy was sometimes punished by his parents despite the fact that he did not engage in the acts his parents accused him of. The interviewer could have made the interpretation after the boy's first statement, but waited until after the boy responded positively to the first two interventions. This illustrates the importance of timing when using interpretations. As Fenichel (1945) states, "The unprepared patient can in no way connect the words he hears from the analyst with his emotional experiences. Such an 'interpretation' does not interpret at all" (p. 25).

As noted, classical interpretation is an advanced interviewing technique. Much has been written about the technical aspects of psychoanalytic interpretation, what to interpret, when to interpret it, and how to interpret it (Fenichel, 1945; Greenson, 1965, 1967; Weiner, 1998). Reading basic psychoanalytic texts, enrolling in psychoanalytic therapy courses, and obtaining supervision are prerequisites to using classical interpretations. As with interpretive feeling reflections, poorly timed interpretations usually produce resistance and defensiveness.

## Reframing

Other theoretical orientations don't view the effectiveness of interpretation as based on unconscious processes. Instead, interpretation can be seen as an intervention that helps clients view their problems or complaints from another perspective. This approach has been labeled *reframing* by psychotherapists from family systems, solution-oriented, and cognitive orientations (de Shazer, 1985; L. Greenberg & Safran, 1987; Morse, 1997; Watzlawick, Weakland, & Fisch, 1974).

Reframing is used primarily when interviewers believe their clients are viewing the world in a manner that is inaccurate or maladaptive. Consider the following exchange between two members of an outpatient group for delinquent youth and their counselor during a group session:

**Peg:** "He's always bugging me. He insults me. And I think he's a jerk. I want to make a deal to quit picking on each other, but he won't do it."

**Dan:** "She's the problem. Always thinks she's right. Never willing to back down. No way am I gonna make a deal with her. She won't change."

**Counselor:** "I notice you two are sitting next to each other again today."

**Peg:** "So! I'd rather not be next to him."

**Counselor:** "I think you two like each other. You almost always sit next to each other. You're always sparring back and forth. You must really get off on being with each other."

**Others:** "Wow. That's it. We always thought so."

In this example, two teenagers are consistently harassing each other. The interviewer suggests that, rather than mutual irritation and harassment, the two teens are actually expressing their mutual attraction. Although the teens deny the reframe, other group members agree it's possible and begin referring to it in future therapy sessions.

Effective reframing should be based on a reasonable alternative hypothesis. Other examples include:

- To a depressed client: "When you make a mistake, you tend to see it as evidence for failure, but you could also see it as evidence of effort and progress toward eventual success; after all, most successful people experience many failures before persevering and becoming successful."
- To an oppositional young girl: "You think that to say something kind or complimentary to your parents is brown-nosing. I wonder if sometimes saying something positive to your mom or dad might just be an example of your giving them honest feedback" (J. Sommers-Flanagan & Sommers-Flanagan, 1997).
- To a socially anxious client: "When people don't say hello to you, you think they're rejecting you, when it's probably only because they're having a bad day or have something else on their minds."

Reframes may be met initially with denial, but having clients view their interactions or problems in a new way can reduce anxiety, anger, or sadness. Reframes promote flexibility in perceiving or interpreting actions.

## Confrontation

The goal of confrontation is to help clients perceive themselves and reality more clearly. Clients often have a distorted view of others, the world, and themselves. These distortions usually manifest themselves as incongruities or discrepancies. For example, imagine a client with clenched fists and a harsh, angry voice saying, "I wish you wouldn't bring up my ex-wife. I've told you before, that's over! I don't have any feelings toward her. It's all just water under the bridge." Obviously, this client still has strong feelings about his ex-wife. Perhaps the relationship is over and the client wishes he could put it behind him, but his nonverbal behavior—voice tone, body posture, and facial expression—tells the interviewer that he's still emotionally involved with his ex-wife.

Confrontation works best when you have a working relationship with the client and ample evidence to demonstrate the client's emotional or behavioral incongruity or discrepancy. In the preceding example, we wouldn't recommend using confrontation unless there was additional evidence indicating the client's unresolved feelings about his ex-wife. If there was supporting evidence, the following confrontation might be appropriate:

"You mentioned last week that every time you think of your ex-wife and how the relationship ended, you want revenge. And yet today, you're saying you don't have any feelings about her. But judging by your clenched fists, voice tone, and what you said last week about her 'screwing you over,' it seems like you still have very strong feelings about her. Perhaps you *wish* those feelings would go away, but it sure looks like they're still there."

Notice how the interviewer cites evidence to support the confrontation. In this case, the interviewer has decided that the client would be better off admitting to and dealing with his unresolved feelings toward his ex-wife. Therefore, he uses confrontation to help the client see the issue. To increase the likelihood that the client will admit to the discrepancy between his nonverbal behavior and his internal emotions, the confrontation was stated gently and supported by evidence.

Confrontations can range from being very gentle to harsh and aggressive. For example, take the case of a young, newly married man who, 35 minutes into his psychotherapy session, has not yet mentioned his wife (despite the fact that she left two days earlier to return to school about 2,000 miles away). The young man, while discussing a general rise in his anger and frustration, was mildly confronted by his therapist, who observed, "I noticed you haven't mentioned anything about your wife leaving."

In this case, the therapist is using a reflection of content (or lack of content) to gently confront the fact that the client was neglecting to discuss his wife and the relevance of her departure on his mood. The therapist's goal is to get his client to recognize and acknowledge that he was ignoring a possible connection between his negative mood and his wife's recent departure.

Sometimes firmer confrontations may be useful. However, when therapists use more aggressive confrontations, they run the risk of evoking client resistance (Miller & Rollnick, 1991, 2002). Here's an example of a moderately firm confrontation with a substance-abusing client.

**Client:** "Doc, it's not a problem. I drink when I want to, but it doesn't have a big effect on the rest of my life. I like to party. I like to put a few down on the weekends, doesn't everybody?"

**Interviewer:** "Well, you do seem to like to party. But, you've had two DUIs [tickets for driving under the influence], three different jobs, and at least a half dozen fights over the past year. Sounds to me like you've got a major problem with alcohol. If you don't start admitting to it and doing something about it, you're going to continue to have legal trouble, job trouble, and relationship trouble. Do you really think that's no problem?"

Unfortunately, many people believe that confrontations, to be effective, must be harsh and aggressive. Especially in the substance abuse field, there is sometimes a strong belief that confrontations must be an *in-your-face* approach. This is simply not true.

There is, in fact, no persuasive evidence that aggressive confrontational tactics are even helpful, let alone superior or preferable strategies in the treatment of addictive behaviors or other problems. (Miller & Rollnick, 1991, p. 7)

Although stronger or harsher confrontations may sometimes be needed, it is more therapeutic, sensible, and less likely to produce resistance if therapists begin with gentle confrontations, becoming more assertive later.

A final example of an incongruity worthy of confrontation involves a 41-year-old married man who is describing how he picked up a 20-year-old girl over the Internet. The client's statement is followed by three potential interviewer responses, each progressively more confrontational:

**Client:** "I originally met this girl in a chat room. My marriage has been dead for 10 years, so I need to do something for myself. She's only 20, but I'm set up to meet her next week in Dallas and I'm like a nervous Nellie. I've got a friend who's telling me I'm nuts, but I just want some action in my life again."

**Interviewer-1:** "Somehow, you're thinking that having a rendezvous with this young woman, rather than working on things with your wife, might help you feel better."

**Interviewer-2:** "Your plans seem a little risky. It sounds like you're valuing a possible quick sexual encounter with someone you've never met over your 20-year marriage. Have I got that right?"

**Interviewer-3:** "I need to tell you that you're playing out a mid-life fantasy. You've never seen this girl, you don't know if she's really 20, whether she's got AIDS or some other disease, or if she plans to rob you blind. You think getting together with her will help you feel better, but you're just running away from your problems. Sooner or later, getting together with her will only make you feel worse."

A confrontation's effectiveness may be evaluated by examining your client's subsequent response (A. Ivey & Ivey, 1999). For example, a client may blatantly deny the accuracy of your confrontation, partially accept it, or completely accept its accuracy and significance.

True confrontation does not contain an explicit prescription for change. Instead, it implies that action is necessary (but does not specify or prescribe the change). In the next chapter, we review technical responses that explicitly suggest or prescribe action. Table 3.2 summarizes the directive listening responses, while Table 4.1 on page 86 summarizes the directive action responses.

**Table 3.2.   Summary of Directive Listening Responses and Their Usual Effects**

| Directive Listening Response | Description | Primary Intent/Effect |
| --- | --- | --- |
| Interpretive reflection of feeling | Statement indicating what feelings the interviewer believes are underlying the client's thoughts or actions. | May enhance empathy and encourage emotional exploration and insight. |
| Interpretation | Statement indicating what meaning the interviewer believes a client's emotions, thoughts, or actions represent. Often includes references to past experiences. | Encourages reflection and self-observation of clients' emotions, thoughts, and actions. Promotes client insight. |
| Question | Query that directly elicits information from a client. There are many forms of questions. | Elicits information. Enhances interviewer control. May help clients talk or encourage them to reflect on something. |
| Feeling validation | Statement that supports, affirms, approves of, or validates feelings articulated by clients. | Enhances rapport. Temporarily reduces anxiety. May cause the interviewer to be viewed as an expert. |
| Confrontation | Statement that points out or identifies a client incongruity or discrepancy. Ranges from very gentle to very harsh. | Encourages clients to examine themselves and their patterns of thinking, feeling, and behaving. May result in personal change and development. |

## SUMMARY

Attending behavior is primarily nonverbal and consists of culturally appropriate eye contact, body language, vocal qualities, and verbal tracking. Positive attending behaviors open up and facilitate client talk, while negative attending behaviors tend to shut down client communication.

Negative attending behavior consists of a wide range of annoying behaviors, including any positive attending behavior displayed excessively. Considerable cultural and individual differences exist among clients regarding the amount and type of eye contact, body language, vocal qualities, and verbal tracking they prefer. To improve communication and attending skills, beginning interviewers should seek feedback from their peers and supervisors.

Beyond attending behaviors, interviewers employ many different nondirective listening responses—including silence, clarification, paraphrasing, nondirective feeling reflection, and summarization. Each nondirective listening response is designed to facilitate client self-expression. However, even nondirective listening responses influence or direct clients to talk more about some topics than others.

Directive interviewer responses are defined as responses that clearly bring the interviewer's perspective into the session. Interviewers can be too directive, leaving clients feeling as if they have had no control in the interaction. They can also be too nondirective, leaving clients feeling lost and suspecting that the interviewer is evasive or manipulative. Generally, directive interview responses are advanced techniques that encourage clients to change their thinking, feeling, or behavior patterns. Therefore, most directives should be used after an adequate clinical assessment has occurred.

Directive listening responses include interpretive reflection of feeling, interpretation, questioning, feeling validation, and confrontation. These techniques involve the therapist's indicating or pointing out particular issues for clients to focus on during therapy.

## SUGGESTED READINGS AND RESOURCES

Several of the following textbooks and workbooks offer additional information and exercises on attending skills, as well as therapeutic techniques from different theoretical orientations. In addition, some of these readings can enhance your knowledge of and sensitivity to various social and cultural groups.

Bandler, R., & Grinder, J. (1979). *Frogs into princes.* Moab, UT: Real People Press. This is one of the early books on NLP (neurolinguistic programming) and the concept of representational systems.

Cormier, S., & Nurius, P. (2003). *Interviewing strategies for helpers: Fundamental skills and cognitive behavioral interventions* (5th ed.). Monterey, CA: Brooks/Cole. Chapter 4 of this text provides extensive and in-depth information regarding nonverbal behavior.

Gibbs, M. A. (1984). The therapist as imposter. In C. M. Brody (Ed.), *Women therapists working with women: New theory and process of feminist therapy.* New York: Springer. This chapter is a strong appeal to therapists to acknowledge their insecurities and inadequacies. It provides insights into how experienced professionals can and do feel inadequate.

Greenson, R. R. (1967). *The technique and practice of psychoanalysis* (Vol. 1). New York: International Universities Press. This classic work provides extensive ground rules for the use of interpretation.

Meador, B., & Rogers, C. R. (1984). Person-centered therapy. In R. J. Corsini (Ed.), *Current psychotherapies* (3rd ed.). Itasca, IL: Peacock. This chapter contains an excerpt of Rogers's classic interview with the "silent young man."

Miller, J. B. (1986). *Toward a new psychology of women* (2nd ed.). Boston: Beacon Press. This book is about women (and men) and the issues they deal with in contemporary society. It helps articulate the depth and meaning of some difficulties traditionally associated with being female.

Rogers, C. R. (1951). *Client-centered therapy.* Boston: Houghton Mifflin. This text includes Rogers's original discussion of feeling reflection (Chapter 4).

Sue, D. S., Arredondo, P., & McDavis, R. J. (1992). Multicultural counseling competencies and standards: A call to the profession. *Journal of Counseling and Development, 70,* 477–486. Standards and competencies in the area of multicultural issues are outlined for the counseling profession.

Weiner, I. (1998). *Principles of psychotherapy* (2nd ed.). New York: John Wiley & Sons. This is a good general text on psychoanalytically oriented psychotherapy. It provides clear examples and descriptions of interpretation, free association, and other concepts.

Yalom, I. D. (1995). *The theory and practice of group psychotherapy* (5th ed.). New York: Basic Books. Chapters 1 and 2 discuss therapeutic factors in group psychotherapy. These factors are extremely relevant to individual psychotherapy and help illustrate the importance of specific responses, such as feeling validation.

# Chapter 4

# *DIRECTIVES: QUESTIONS AND ACTION SKILLS*

*Grown-ups love figures. When you tell them that you have made a new friend, they never ask you any questions about essential matters. They never say to you, "What does his voice sound like? What games does he love best? Does he collect butterflies?" Instead, they demand: "How old is he? How many brothers has he? How much does he weigh? How much money does his father make?" Only from these figures do they think they have learned anything about him.*

—Antoine de Saint-Exupéry, *The Little Prince*

---

**CHAPTER OBJECTIVES**

Clinical interviewers must move beyond listening and assess clients through the skillful use of questions. The interview is not an investigation, but, at times, the interviewer takes the role of investigator. In addition, interviewers sometimes encourage clients to take specific actions—actions the interviewer deems adaptive or healthy. In this chapter, we analyze a wide range of questions and directive action responses often used by clinical interviewers. After reading this chapter, you will know:

- The many types of questions available to interviewers, how to use them, and their usual effects (and side effects).
- The benefits and liabilities of using questions with clients.
- How asking certain questions can be inappropriate and how asking other questions can be unethical.
- General guidelines for using questions in an interview.
- How and why clinical interviewers use a range of directive action responses, including explanation, suggestion, advice, agreement, disagreement, urging, approval, and disapproval.

---

Imagine digging a hole without a shovel or building a house without a hammer. For many interviewers, conducting an interview without using questions constitutes an analogous problem: How can you be expected to complete a task without using your most basic tool?

Despite the central role of questions for interviewing, we have managed to avoid discussing them until this chapter. The reason for this is similar to having a carpenter consider building a house without a hammer. Our purpose has been to stimulate your creativity and to help you understand the depth, breadth, and application of your other listening and communication tools. If you can develop your complete range of interviewing skills, it may help you avoid depending too much on questions to conduct interviews.

Questions are an incredibly diverse and flexible interviewer tool; they can be used to stimulate client talk, to restrict it, to facilitate rapport, to show interest in your clients, to show disinterest, to gather information, to pressure clients, and to ignore the client's viewpoint. As you proceed through the section on using questions and directive action responses, reflect on how it feels to freely use what many of you will consider your most basic tool.

## USING QUESTIONS

When you ask a question, in any context, you take control of the conversation. Questions, by definition, are directive and are an integral part of human communication. In the context of clinical interviewing, questions constitute a technique and deserve our scrutiny. Asking questions, especially if you are interested in particular information, can be hard to resist. Unfortunately, as in the case of *The Little Prince,* there is also no guarantee that the questions you ask (and their corresponding answers) are of any interest whatsoever to the person being questioned.

### Types of Questions

Interviewers have many types of questions at their disposal. It is important to differentiate among them because different types of questions tend to produce different client responses and response patterns. The most common questions used by interviewers are open, closed, swing, indirect or implied, and projective.

*Open Questions*
Open questions are designed to facilitate verbal output. By definition, open questions require more than a single-word response; they cannot be answered with a simple yes or no. Ordinarily, open questions begin with the word *How* or *What.* Writers sometimes classify questions that begin with *Where, When, Why,* and/or *Who* as open questions, but such questions are really only partially open because they don't facilitate talk nearly as well as *How* and *What* questions (Cormier & Nurius, 2003; Hutchins & Cole, 1997). The following hypothetical dialogue uses questions sometimes classified as open:

> **Interviewer:** "When did you first begin having panic attacks?"
> **Client:** "In 1996, I believe."
> **Interviewer:** "Where were you when you had your first panic attack?"
> **Client:** "I was just getting on the subway in New York City."
> **Interviewer:** "What happened?"
> **Client:** "When I stepped inside the train, my heart began to pound. I thought I would die. I just held onto the metal post next to my seat as hard as I could because I was afraid I would fall over and be humiliated. I felt dizzy and nauseated. Then I got off the train at my stop and I've never been back on the subway again."
> **Interviewer:** "Who was with you?"
> **Client:** "No one."

**Interviewer:** "Why haven't you tried to ride the subway again?"

**Client:** "Because I'm afraid I'll have another panic attack."

**Interviewer:** "How are you handling the fact that your fear of panic attacks is so restrictive for you?"

**Client:** "Well, frankly, not so good. I've been slowly getting more and more scared to go out. I'm afraid that soon I'll be too scared to leave my house."

As you can see, open questions vary in their degree of openness. They do not uniformly facilitate depth and breadth of talk from clients. Although questions beginning with *What* or *How* usually elicit the most elaborate responses from clients, such is not always the case. More often, it is the way a particular *What* or *How* question is phrased that produces very specific or very wide-ranging client responses. For example, "What time did you get home?" and "How are you feeling?" are usually answered very succinctly. The openness of a particular question should be judged primarily by the response it usually elicits.

Questions beginning with *Why* are unique in that they commonly elicit defensive explanations. Meier and Davis (2001) state, "Questions, particularly 'why' questions, put clients on the defensive and ask them to explain their behavior" (p. 23). *Why* questions frequently produce one of two responses. First, some clients respond with *"Because!"* and then proceed to explain, sometimes through very detailed and intellectual responses, why they are thinking or acting or feeling in a particular manner. Second, some clients defend themselves with "Why not?" or, because they feel attacked, they seek reassurance by confronting their therapist with "Is there anything wrong with that?" This illustrates why clinicians usually minimize *Why* questions—they exacerbate defensiveness and intellectualization, and diminish rapport. On the other hand, in cases where rapport is good and you want the client to speculate or intellectualize regarding a particular aspect of his or her life, *Why* questions may be appropriate and useful in helping your client take a closer, deeper look at certain patterns or motivations.

### Closed Questions

Closed questions can be answered with a yes or no response (Hutchins & Cole, 1997). Although some people classify them as open, questions that begin with *Who, Where,* or *When* direct clients toward very specific information; therefore, we believe they generally should be considered closed questions (see Putting It in Practice 4.1).

Closed questions restrict verbalization and lead clients toward more specific responses than open questions. They can serve as a technique for reducing or controlling how much clients talk. Restricting verbal output is useful when interviewing clients who are excessively talkative. Also, getting clients to describe their experiences in a particular way can be helpful when conducting diagnostic interviews (e.g., in the preceding example about a panic attack on the New York subway, a diagnostic interviewer may ask, "Did you feel lightheaded or dizzy?" to confirm or disconfirm the presence of symptoms associated with panic attacks).

Sometimes, interviewers inadvertently or intentionally transform an open question into a closed question with a tag query. For example, we often hear students formulate questions such as, "What was it like for you to confront your father after all these years—was it gratifying?"

As you can see, transforming open questions into closed questions greatly limits how much a client can elaborate when giving a response. Unless clients faced with such questions are exceptionally expressive or assertive, they focus solely on whether they

---

**Putting It in Practice 4.1**

## Open and Closed Questions

The four sets of questions that follow are designed to obtain information pertaining to the same topic. Imagine how you might answer these questions, and then compare your imagined responses.

1. *(Open)* "How are you feeling about being in psychotherapy?"
   *(Closed)* "Are you feeling okay about being in psychotherapy?"
2. *(Open)* "What happened next, after you walked onto the subway and you felt your heart begin to pound?"
   *(Closed)* "Did you feel lightheaded or dizzy after you walked onto the subway?"
3. *(Open)* "What was it like for you to confront your father after having been angry with him for so many years?"
   *(Closed)* "Was it gratifying for you to confront your father after having been angry with him for so many years?"
4. *(Open)* "How do you feel?"
   *(Closed)* "Do you feel angry?"

Notice and discuss with other classmates the differences in how you (and clients) are affected by open versus closed questioning.

---

felt gratification when confronting their father; they may or may not elaborate on feelings of fear, relief, resentment, or anything else they may have experienced.

Closed questions usually begin with words such as *Do, Does, Did, Is, Was,* or *Are.* They are very useful if you want to solicit specific information. Traditionally, closed questions are used more toward the interview's end, when rapport is already established, time is short, and efficient questions and short responses are needed (Morrison, 1994).

If you begin an interview with frequent nondirective responses, but later change styles to obtain more specific information through closed questions, it is wise to inform the client of this shift in strategy. For example, you might state:

"Okay, we have about 15 minutes left and there are a few things I want to make sure I've covered, so I'm going to start asking you very specific questions."

### Swing Questions

Swing questions can be answered with a yes or no, but are designed to produce a more elaborate discussion of feelings, thoughts, or issues (Shea, 1998). In a sense, swing questions inquire as to whether the client wants to respond. Such questions usually begin with *Could,* or *Would, Can,* or *Will.* For example:

"Could you talk about how it was when you first discovered you had AIDS?"
"Would you describe how you think your parents might react to finding out you're gay?"
"Can you tell me more about that?"
"Will you tell me what happened in the argument between you and your husband last night?"

Ivey (1993) considers swing questions the most open of all questions: "*Could* [italics added] questions are considered maximally open and contain some of the advantages of closed questions in that the client is free to say 'No, I don't want to talk about that.' *Could* [italics added] questions reflect less control and command than others" (p. 56).

For swing questions to function effectively, you should observe two basic rules. First, avoid using swing questions unless adequate rapport has been established (Shea, 1998). If rapport is not adequately established, a swing question may backfire and function as a closed question (i.e., the client responds with a shy or resistant yes or no, and rapport may be damaged). Second, avoid using swing questions with most children and adolescents. This is because children and adolescents often interpret swing questions concretely and may respond oppositionally (J. Sommers-Flanagan & Sommers-Flanagan, 1997). For example, if you ask young clients "Would you like to tell me about how you felt when your dad left?" they frequently respond with "No!," which is obviously uncomfortable and unhelpful.

## Indirect or Implied Questions

Indirect or implied questions often begin with *I wonder* or *You must* or *It must* (Benjamin, 1981, p. 75). They are used when interviewers are curious about what clients are thinking or feeling, but don't want to pressure clients to respond. Following are some examples of indirect or implied questions:

"I wonder how you're feeling about your upcoming wedding."
"I wonder what your plans are after graduation."
"I wonder if you've given any thought to searching for a job."
"You must have some thoughts or feelings about your parents' divorce."
"It must be hard for you to cope with the loss of your health."

Indirect questions, when overused, can seem sneaky or manipulative. You should use them only occasionally and usually when adequate rapport has developed.

## Projective Questions

Projective questions help clients identify, articulate, and explore and clarify unconscious or unclear conflicts, values, thoughts, and feelings. Projective questions begin with some form of *What if* and invite client speculation. Often, projective questions are used to trigger mental imagery and help clients explore thoughts, feelings, and behaviors they might have if they were in a particular situation. For example:

"What would you do if you were given one million dollars, no strings attached?"
"If you had three wishes, what would you wish for?"
"If you needed help or were really frightened, or even if you were just totally out of money and needed some, who would you turn to right now?" (J. Sommers-Flanagan & Sommers-Flanagan, 1998, p. 193)
"What if you could go back and change how you acted during that party (or other significant life event); what would you do differently?"

Projective questions are also used for evaluating client values and judgment. For example, an interviewer can analyze a response to the question "What would you do with one million dollars?" to indirectly glimpse a client's values and self-control. The million-dollar question also can be used to evaluate client decision-making or judgment. Projective questions are often included in mental status examinations (see Chapter 7).

## Benefits and Liabilities of Questions

Interviewers have different feelings about using questions. Some of our student interviewers have commented:

> "I felt more powerful as an interviewee."
>
> "I felt more in control."
>
> "I felt more pressure."
>
> "It was hard to think of questions while I was trying to listen to the client, and it was hard to listen to the client while I was thinking of questions I might ask."
>
> "I seemed to have less patience. I had an impulse to cut in and ask questions all the time."
>
> "I felt less pressure. I really liked asking questions!"

Obviously, asking questions produces reactions—in interviewers as well as clients. It is important to sort out these reactions. Some are unique to each individual, while others are more standard or universal. Unfortunately, it is often difficult to balance our own needs to ask—or not ask—questions, with clients' needs to be asked—or not be asked—questions.

Asking questions commonly produces several positive results. Open questions can lead clients to discuss their thoughts and feelings in more depth. Closed questions can help interviewers pinpoint specific information that would otherwise be difficult to access. When interviewers assume an authoritative role and control the interview with questions, some clients feel relieved. Questions can also help clarify or specify what clients are trying to talk about. Questions are excellent tools for eliciting specific, concrete examples of client behavior. Skillful questioning is essential to diagnostic interviewing (see Table 4.1).

Using questions can also produce negative results. Questioning emphasizes the interviewer's interests and values, not the client's. Consequently, clients may react to questioning by feeling their viewpoint is unimportant. Of course, effective interviewers can reduce this risk by asking the client sensitive questions, such as: "What have we not yet discussed that you feel is important?" Questioning also sets up the interviewer as an

**Table 4.1.   Question Classification**

| Word Question Begins With | Type of Question | Usual Client Responses |
|---|---|---|
| What | Open | Factual and descriptive information |
| How | Open | Process or sequential information |
| Why | Partially open | Explanations and defensiveness |
| Where | Minimally open | Information pertaining to location |
| When | Minimally open | Information pertaining to time |
| Who | Minimally open | Information pertaining to a person |
| Do/Did | Closed | Specific information |
| Could/Would/Can/Will | Swing | Diverse info, sometimes rejected |
| I wonder/You must | Indirect | Exploration of thoughts and feelings |
| What if | Projective | Information on judgment and values |

expert who is responsible for asking the right questions and, sometimes, for coming up with the right answers. Liberal questioning highlights power, responsibility, and authority differentials inherent in interviewing situations.

Questioning can reduce client spontaneity and may make clients feel defensive, especially if they are asked several questions in a row. Clients may sit back passively, waiting for the interviewer to ask the right question. This produces a paradox: Interviewers usually begin asking questions because they want information, but sometimes asking too many questions decreases client verbal initiative, increases defensiveness, and results in less information being obtained. Excessive questioning may also foster dependency; clients begin relying too heavily on the interviewer for questions and answers to important problems in their lives. Again, we should note that more directive therapeutic approaches generally advocate the use of direct questions and place the therapist more in the expert role. This is a reasonable perspective, as long as it is consistent with the interviewer's theoretical orientation and is done with full knowledge of the potential liabilities. Benjamin (1981) has commented on excessive use of questions:

> Yes, I have many reservations about the use of questions in the interview. I feel certain that we ask too many questions, often meaningless ones. We ask questions that confuse the interviewee, that interrupt him. We ask questions the interviewee cannot possibly answer. We even ask questions we don't want the answers to, and consequently, we do not hear the answers when forthcoming. (p. 71)

Some clients prefer to be asked many questions because questions provide clear guidelines regarding what to say. In contrast, less structured or less directive techniques may produce anxiety or frustration because clients are unsure of how to proceed. Although questions are used primarily to gather information, they are also helpful in providing interviewers with control over an interview's course and direction.

## Interviewer Curiosity and Professional Ethics

It is normal for interviewers to have urges to ask clients inappropriate questions. Most counselors sometimes feel the desire to ask clients questions just to satisfy their own curiosity. For example, if a client mentions he or she grew up in the Portland, Oregon, area and the interviewer is from there, he or she may feel an impulse to ask: "Where did you go to high school?" or "Did you ever go dancing at the Top of the Cosmo restaurant?" Although asking these questions may help with evaluating social status or academic background, the questions are more likely designed exclusively to satisfy the interviewer's curiosity. Additionally, such questions may give the interview a social, rather than therapeutic, flavor. Furthermore, giving in to curiosity questioning may devolve into excess self-disclosure ("Yeah, I remember one night at the Cosmo when I had a couple of drinks and . . ."), which might be interpreted as the beginnings of a friendship-type, mutual relationship rather than a professional relationship. It is important to remember that everything you do, including self-disclosure, should be to further the client's welfare (Pizer, 1997).

Ethical issues may arise if interviewers follow their impulses and ask clients inappropriate questions. An ethical dilemma popularized by A. Lazarus (1994) focused on whether it is acceptable, at the end of a therapy hour, for a therapist to ask his or her client for a ride somewhere (provided the client is going that direction anyway). Our position is that, in nearly every case, mental health professionals should get their personal needs met outside the therapeutic relationship, even supposedly innocuous ones such as catching a ride. It is possible to be too rigid in your application of this principle. However, we generally avoid boundary violations because they may lead to more frequent inappropriate impulses and eventual ethical violations (R. Sommers-Flanagan, Elliot, & Sommers-Flanagan, 1998).

## Guidelines in Using Questions

Both clients and interviewers sometimes have strong reactions to questions. To optimize your use of questions, keep in mind the following five guidelines:

1. Prepare your clients for questions.
2. Do not use questions as your predominant listening or action response.
3. Make your questions relevant to client concerns.
4. Use questions to elicit concrete behavioral examples.
5. Approach sensitive areas cautiously.

### *Prepare Your Clients for Questions*

A simple technique that reduces negative fallout from questioning is to forewarn and prepare your client for intensive questioning. This often helps clients feel less defensive and more cooperative. You can forewarn clients by saying:

> "I need some specific information from you. So, for a while, I'll be asking you some questions to help me get that information. Some of the questions may seem odd or may not make much sense to you, but I promise, there's a reason behind my questions."

### *Do Not Use Questions as Your Predominant Listening or Action Response*

Questions should always be used in combination with other listening responses, especially nondirective listening responses. Be sure to follow your client's response to your query, at least occasionally, with a listening response:

> **Interviewer:** "What happened when you first stepped onto the subway?"
> **Client:** "When I stepped inside the train, I felt my heart begin to pound. I thought I was going to die. I just held onto the metal post as hard as I could because I was afraid I would fall over and be humiliated. Then I got off the train at my stop and I've never been back on the subway again."
> **Interviewer:** "So that was a pretty frightening experience for you. You were doing about everything you could to stay in control. Was anyone with you when you went through this panicky experience?"

Unless a variety of sensitive listening responses are used in combination with repeated questions, clients are likely to feel bombarded or interrogated (Benjamin, 1981, 1987; Cormier & Nurius, 2003).

### *Make Your Questions Relevant to Client Concerns*

Clients are more likely to view you as competent and credible if you focus squarely on their major concerns. Therefore, to use questions skillfully, aim your queries directly at what the client believes is important.

It may be hard for clients to understand the purpose of certain diagnostic or mental status questions. For example, when interviewing a depressed client, eating patterns, sleeping patterns, concentration ability, sexual interest, and so on should be closely evaluated. The following questions would be relevant:

"How has your appetite been?"
"Have you been sleeping through the night?"
"Have you had trouble concentrating?"
"Do you find yourself interested in sex lately?"

Imagine how a depressed client who is irritable, psychologically naïve, and who believes, somewhat accurately, that her bad mood is related to 10 years of emotional abuse from her husband might perceive such a series of questions. She might think, "I couldn't believe that counselor! What do my appetite, sex life, and concentration have to do with why I came to see her?" Unless clients can see the relevance of their counselor's questions, the questions can decrease rapport and thus reduce the client's interest in therapy.

## Use Questions to Elicit Concrete Behavioral Examples

Perhaps the best use of questions is to obtain clear, concrete life examples from clients. Instead of relying on abstract client descriptions, questions can be used to obtain specific behavioral examples:

**Client:** "I have so much trouble with social situations. I guess I'm just an anxious and insecure person."
**Interviewer:** "Could you give me an example of a recent social situation when you felt anxious and thought you were insecure?"
**Client:** "Yeah, let me think. Well, there was the party at the frat the other night. Everyone else seemed to be having a great time and I just felt left out. I'm sure no one wanted to talk with me."

In this exchange, although the interviewer asks a swing question to obtain specific information, the client remains vague. Repeated open and closed questions may be needed to help clients be more specific and concrete in describing their anxiety. For example:

"What exactly was happening when you felt anxious and insecure at the party?"
"Who was standing near you when you had these feelings?"
"What thoughts were going through your mind?"
"What ways would you rather have acted in this situation if you could do it over?"

Moursund (1992) provides a helpful suggestion for obtaining additional information when tracking a client's experience: "If there are major gaps in the client's story, ask for information to fill them; do so with open-ended questions. Say 'What did you do next?' rather than 'Did you talk to her about it?'" (p. 23).

## Approach Sensitive Areas Cautiously

Be especially careful when questioning sensitive areas. As Wolberg (1995) notes, it is important *not* to question new clients in sensitive areas (e.g., appearance, status, sexual difficulties, failures). Wolberg suggests instead that clients be allowed to talk freely

========== Putting It in Practice 4.2 ==========

## Types of Interviewer Questions: A Review

Without looking back through the chapter, respond to the following queries:

1. Give two examples of an open question.
2. Give three examples of a closed question.
3. Give an example of a swing question.
4. Give an example of an indirect question.
5. Give an example of a projective question.

After you are clear on the particular types of questions available to you during an interview, try the following practice activities:

1. Find a partner and practice using the various types of questions.
2. Sit down, relax, and imagine how and when you might use the different types of questions. Visualize yourself asking questions in an interview setting.
3. Practice asking different types of questions into a video- or audiotape recorder.

about sensitive topics, but if blocking occurs, questioning should be avoided until the relationship is better established; early in therapy, relationship building is a higher priority than information gathering.

Despite Wolberg's (1995) generally good advice, sometimes the therapeutic relationship must take a back seat to information gathering. This is especially true when conducting an intake interview, when a client is in crisis, or when the setting demands a speedy assessment. For example, if a client is suicidal or homicidal, gathering assessment data for competent clinical decision-making is top priority (J. Sommers-Flanagan & Sommers-Flanagan, 1995a). Similarly, if you are a designated intake worker and you won't be seeing the client for counseling, information gathering is probably more important than relationship building. However, make this clear to your client by saying something like:

"This interview is just for assessment purposes. I'll be gathering information about you to pass on to your counselor. So if it seems like I'm firing a lot of questions your way, that's probably because I am." (See Putting It in Practice 4.2 for a review of types of questions.)

## DIRECTIVE ACTION RESPONSES

Directive action responses encourage clients to change the way they think, feel, or act. They are essentially persuasion techniques, pushing clients toward specific change. Directives are used when interviewers believe, based on clinical judgment and/or the client's personal welfare, that change should occur in the client's life, attitudes, or behavior. Such responses require that interviewers take responsibility for determining what client changes might be desirable. This is true even when interviewers and clients work collaboratively, because even then interviewers must decide what advice to offer and when to offer it. Of course, clients decide whether to apply interviewers' opinions, suggestions, or advice.

Directive action responses require that interviewers evaluate *what* changes a client should make to improve his or her life. Many textbooks and graduate programs in counseling and psychology encourage the application of techniques or directives that foster client change (Cormier & Nurius, 2003; Egan, 1998; George & Cristiani, 1994; Hutchins & Cole, 1997; Okun, 1997). Although it is true that directive techniques are effective methods of producing client change, our position is similar to L. Seligman's (1996); that is, interviewers should be well-trained in evaluation and assessment techniques before applying technical interventions. The following descriptions are provided primarily to help you differentiate between these types of responses and other, less directive techniques. Beginning interviewers should use these tech-niques cautiously and with supervision.

The directive action responses described in this section are organized in order of intensity, from milder to stronger persuasive techniques.

## Explanation (Providing Information That Influences Behavior)

An *explanation* is a descriptive statement used to make something plain or understandable. In an interview context, an explanation often describes one of the following:

The process of counseling.

The meaning or implications of a particular symptom.

How to implement a specific piece of advice or therapeutic strategy.

Clients usually ask their therapists questions because they need or want some specific information. Client questions about therapy frequently fall into the following three categories:

1. Questions about therapy process: How long will it take for me to feel better?
2. Questions about their normality or sanity: Is it normal for me to feel this way?
3. Questions about how to make personal changes: How do I change the way I think, or behave, or feel?

The first, and perhaps most important, use of explanation is for role induction or psychotherapy socialization. *Role induction* consists of informing or educating clients about what to expect in therapy, especially regarding the respective roles of therapist and client. Role induction is needed because many clients have little or no information about what a clinical interview, or counseling, entails. Research on role induction has indicated, not surprisingly, that clients benefit from knowing what to expect and how to act in therapy (Luborsky, 1984; Mayerson, 1984; M. Nelson & Neufeldt, 1996).

Interviewing should not be a mysterious process, and almost all clinical practitioners periodically stop and explain a little bit about core counseling concepts to their clients. Imagine that a client tells you, toward the end of your first session, about her emerging feelings of hopelessness:

"I'm not sure if I should tell you this, but I just keep thinking that none of these things we're talking about will ever change. It's nothing personal, but I think I'll never change."

This statement includes several interesting issues. First, when clients say, "I don't know if I should talk about this" or "I'm not sure what I'm supposed to say," it often means some explanation (or role induction) is needed. When clients are uncertain about the counseling process, it is your job to reduce the confusion.

Second, when clients do not know if they should talk about something, they should be encouraged to discuss it, at least so interviewer and client can collaboratively decide whether the information is important. Discussing issues together enhances the collaborative relationship.

Third, although the client is suggesting otherwise, his or her feelings may well be related to the interviewer—the client's perceptions of the interviewer's competence or because his or her appearance or personality style reminds the client of someone else. If so, the client needs to know that he or she can express concerns, whether those concerns are based on reality or imagination. These concerns may be signs of transference and should not be ignored (neither should they be interpreted, but clients can benefit from talking openly about their feelings about therapy and about the therapist).

Fourth, when clients attend their first counseling sessions, they often feel worse because they are focusing on and discussing uncomfortable problems. Consequently, explaining to clients that they may feel hopeless, mixed up, or angry while discussing their problems can prevent premature therapy dropouts.

The following explanations might help if a client has strong negative feelings about being interviewed:

- "If you're unsure about whether you should talk about something in here, I want you just to go right ahead and talk about it as much as you can. That way, at least we can decide together whether it's important."
- "Sometimes, people develop strong feelings about their counselors or about counseling. Usually, these feelings are important to talk about, even if they're negative."
- "You know, it's not all that unusual to have negative feelings during counseling. Many people feel worse before they feel better. That's just part of what people experience when they face their problems head on."

A second type of explanation is needed when clients are experiencing symptoms, but are puzzled about what the symptoms mean. For example, clients with anxiety disorders often believe they are "going crazy" or "losing their mind" or "dying" (Barlow & Craske, 1994; Wells, 1997). They believe they may have a psychotic disorder and that they will undoubtedly end up institutionalized. In reality, the prognosis for most anxiety disorders is positive. This should be explained to the client because symptom explanations, even diagnosis, can be very reassuring for clients. For example:

"I know you think there's something wrong with your mind, because your symptoms are very frightening. But based on your personal history, family history, and the symptoms you have, it's safe to tell you that you're not going crazy. The problems you're experiencing are not unusual. They respond very well to counseling."

The third type of explanation involves giving clients information about how to apply a particular therapy technique. An example follows:

**Client:** "I don't know what causes my anxiety. It comes out of nowhere. Is there anything I can do to get more in control over these feelings?"

**Interviewer:**  "The first step to controlling anxiety usually involves identifying the thoughts or situations that cause you to feel anxious. I'd like you to try the following experiment. Keep a log of your anxiety level. You can use a pocket-sized notebook to record when you feel anxious. Write down how anxious you feel on a scale of 0 to 100, 0 being not anxious at all and 100 being so anxious you think you're going to die. Then, right next to your anxiety rating, list the thoughts you're thinking and the situation you're in. Bring your anxiety log to the next session and we can start figuring out what's causing your anxiety."

In this example, a cognitive-behavioral therapist has given instructions to initiate anxiety monitoring. As a matter of course, when providing instructions, you should always ask the client if he or she has any questions to make sure your instructions are understood (i.e., "Do you have any questions about how to monitor your anxiety?").

The explanation an interviewer gives is dictated, in part, by his or her theoretical orientation. Specifically, behavior therapists explain to their clients the importance of behavior and self-monitoring; cognitive therapists explain how thoughts influence or cause behavior and emotions; person-centered therapists explain how sessions should consist of whatever clients feel is important; solution-oriented therapists explain how important and helpful it is to talk about successes; and psychoanalytic therapists explain to their clients the importance of "saying whatever comes to mind." Whether interviewers are describing free association or explaining how to engage in guided imagery, they are still using explanation.

## Suggestion

*Suggestion* isn't usually discussed in introductory interviewing texts (Egan, 2002; Hutchins & Cole, 1997). This may be because suggestion is traditionally associated with psychoanalytic or hypnotic approaches (Erickson, Rossi, & Rossi, 1976; Kihlstrom, 1985; J. Watkins, 1992). It may also be because some authorities define suggestion as "a mild form of advice" and discuss it in the context of advice giving (Benjamin, 1981, p. 134).

Although sometimes interchangeable, suggestion and advice are two distinct and different interviewer responses. Specifically, to *suggest* means to "bring before a person's mind indirectly or without plain expression," whereas to *advise* is "to give counsel to; offer an opinion or suggestion worth following" (*Random House Unabridged Dictionary,* 1993, p. 187). Advice is a more directive approach than suggestion.

A suggestion is an interviewer statement that directly or indirectly suggests or predicts a particular phenomenon will occur in a client's life. Suggestion is designed to move clients consciously or unconsciously toward engaging in a particular behavior, changing their thinking patterns, or experiencing a specific emotion.

Suggestions are often given when clients are in a hypnotic trance, but they may also be given when clients are fully alert and awake (J. Watkins, 1992). For example:

**Client:**  "I have never been able to stand up to my mother. It's like I'm afraid of her. She's always had her act together. She's stronger than I am."
**Interviewer:**  "If you look closely at your interactions with her this next week, you may discover ways in which you're stronger than she."

Another suggestion procedure occurs when the interviewer suggests that the client will have a dream about a particular issue. This example is classic in the sense that psychoanalytic therapists use suggestions to influence unconscious processes:

**Client:** "This decision is really getting to me. I have two job offers but don't know which one to take. I'm frozen. I've analyzed the pros and cons for days and just swing back and forth. One minute I want one job and the next minute I'm thinking of why that job is totally wrong for me."

**Interviewer:** "If you relax and think about the conflict as clearly as possible in your mind before you drop off to sleep tonight, perhaps you'll have a dream to clarify your feelings about this decision."

In this example, suggestion is mixed with advice. The interviewer advises the client to relax and clearly think about the conflict before falling asleep and suggests a dream will subsequently occur.

We've found that suggestive techniques can be especially helpful when working with difficult young clients. For example, young clients are enthusiastically interested in "hypnosis" when, in contrast, they are opposed to "relaxation" (J. Sommers-Flanagan & Sommers-Flanagan, 1996). In addition, gentle and encouraging suggestions with delinquent young clients may have a positive influence (J. Sommers-Flanagan, 1998). We use the following suggestion technique when discussing behavioral alternatives with young clients:

**Client:** "That punk is so lame. He deserved to have me beat him up."

**Interviewer:** "Maybe so. But you can do better than resorting to violence in the future. I *know* you can do better than that."

Young clients sometimes view this technique as a vote of confidence in their problem-solving abilities. From an Adlerian (A. Adler, 1931) perspective, this form of suggestion is viewed as a method for encouraging clients.

Suggestion should be used with caution. Occasionally, it can be viewed as a sneaky or manipulative strategy. Additionally, sometimes suggestion backfires and evokes opposition. For example, each suggestion used in examples from this section could backfire, producing the following results:

The woman continues to insist that her mother is stronger.

The client does not recall his dreams or is unable to make any connections between his dreams and his decision-making process. (This might be viewed as resistance by psychoanalytically oriented therapists.)

The delinquent boy insists that physical violence is his best behavioral option.

## Giving Advice

All advice essentially contains the message, "Here's what I think you should do." *Giving advice* is very much an interviewer-centered activity; it casts interviewers in the expert role.

It is important to avoid advice giving early in the interview process because giving advice is easy, common, and sometimes coolly received. Usually, friends and relatives freely give advice to one another, sometimes effectively, other times less so. You may wonder, if advice is readily available outside therapy, why would interviewers bother using it?

The answer to this question is simple: People desire advice—especially expert advice—and sometimes advice is a helpful therapeutic change technique (Haley, 1973).

Nonetheless, advice remains controversial; many interviewers use it, and others passionately avoid it (Benjamin, 1981; C. Rogers, 1957).

In many cases, clients try to get quick advice from their interviewers during their first session. However, premature problem solving or advice giving in a clinical interview is usually ineffective (Egan, 2002; Meier & Davis, 2001). Interviewers should thoroughly explore a specific issue with a client before trying to solve the problem or render advice. A good basic rule is to find out everything the client has already tried before jumping in with prescriptive advice.

Sometimes it is difficult to keep yourself from giving advice. Imagine yourself with a client who tells you:

"I'm pregnant and I don't know what to do. I just found out two days ago. No one knows. What should I do?"

You may have good advice for this young woman. In fact, you may have gone through a similar experience or known someone who struggled with an unplanned pregnancy. The woman in this scenario may also desperately *need* constructive advice (as well as basic information). However, all this is speculation, because based on what she has said, we still do not even know if she needs information or advice. All we know is she says she "doesn't know what to do." If she discovered she was pregnant two days ago, she's probably spent nearly 48 hours thinking about the options available to her. At this point, telling her what she should do would likely be ineffective and inappropriate.

Giving premature advice shuts down further problem solution exploration. We recommend starting nondirectively:

"So you haven't told anyone about the pregnancy. And if I understand you correctly, you're feeling that maybe you should be taking some particular action, but you're not sure what."

You can always get more directive and provide advice later.

Some clients will push you hard for advice and keep asking, "But what do you think I should do?" In many cases, you should use an explanation and open-ended question when clients pressure you for advice. For example:

"Before we talk about what you should do, let's talk about what you've been thinking and feeling about your situation. I may have some good advice for you, but first, tell me what you've thought about and felt since discovering you're pregnant."

Or, in this case, simply an open-ended question might be appropriate: "What options have you thought of already?"

Clients are typically more complex, thoughtful, and full of constructive solutions than we think they are (and typically more resourceful than *they* think they are). It is an injustice to provide advice before exploring how they have tried solving their own problems. Solution-oriented interviewers emphasize client skills and resources by asking questions like, "How did you manage to change things around?" or "What's the longest you've gone without being in trouble with the law? How did you do that?" (Bertolino, 1999, pp. 34–35)

Providing redundant advice (i.e., advice to take some action that others have previously suggested or to take an action that the client has already unsuccessfully tried) can damage your credibility. To avoid providing redundant advice, ask clients what advice they've already received from friends, family, and past counselors. However, despite its liabilities, sometimes advice is both needed and helpful. In the words of Miller and Rollnick (1991), "Well-tempered and well-timed advice to change can make a difference" (p. 20; see also Putting It in Practice 4.3).

## Agreement-Disagreement

A common directive action response used by beginning interviewers is *agreement*. Agreement occurs when an interviewer makes a statement indicating harmony with the client's opinion. Agreement is rewarding to interviewer and client, partly because, as studies from social and clinical psychology have shown, people like to be with others who have attitudes similar to their own (Hatfield & Walster, 1981; Kurdek & Smith, 1987; Yalom, 1995).

As with advice giving, you should explore why you feel like agreeing with your client. Why do you want clients to know you agree with them? Is agreement being used therapeutically, or are you agreeing because it feels good to let someone else know your opinions are similar? Are you agreeing with clients to affirm their viewpoint, or yours?

Using agreement has several potential effects. First, agreement can enhance rapport. Second, if your clients think you are a credible authority, agreement can affirm the correctness of their opinion (i.e., "If my therapist agrees with me, I must be right."). Third, agreement puts you in the expert role, and your opinion is sought in the future.

---

**Putting It in Practice 4.3**

## A Little Advice on Giving Advice

As you might guess, we have some advice about advice giving. Specifically, you should become aware of when and why you want to give a client advice. Review and contemplate the following questions.

When you feel like giving advice, is it . . .

1. just to be helpful?
2. to prove you're a competent therapist?
3. because you've had the same problem and so you think you know how the client can be helped?
4. because you think you have better ideas than your client will ever come up with?
5. because you think your client will never come up with any constructive ideas?

Your responses to these questions can help determine whether your advice giving motives are pure or not. As you may have guessed, we're not strong advocates of giving advice. On the other hand, we also believe that advice, when well-timed and received from the proper person, can be tremendously powerful. When it comes to giving advice, our advice to you is: (a) be aware of why you're giving it, (b) wait for the appropriate time to deliver it, (c) avoid giving advice in a moralistic or pedantic manner, and (d) avoid giving redundant advice (i.e., advice that the client has already received from someone else).

Fourth, agreement can reduce client exploration (i.e., "Why explore my beliefs any longer; after all, my therapist agrees with me.").

Wherever there is agreement, there can also be disagreement. It is simple, rewarding, and somewhat natural to express when you are in agreement with someone else. On the other hand, disagreement is often socially unacceptable or socially undesirable. People sometimes muffle their disagreement, either because they are unassertive or because they fear conflict or rejection.

In a clinical interview, however, interviewers are in a position of power and authority. Consequently, interviewers sometimes lose their inhibition and disagree openly with clients. Depending on the issue, the result can be devastating to clients, disruptive to therapy, and may involve abuse of power and authority. Imagine, for example, a client and therapist having the following interaction about U.S. foreign policy not long after the September 11, 2001, terrorist attacks:

**Client:** "I am so angry about what happened in New York. I think we need a quick and decisive military action. We need to bomb Afghanistan to its knees."

**Interviewer:** "I'm uncomfortable with what you're saying. You're focusing solely on retaliation and I don't think that's very constructive."

**Client:** "Well, those Arabs started it and I think we need to finish it."

**Interviewer:** "Do you use this same philosophy in your personal relationships? Maybe you need to look a little closer at the implications of what you're saying."

As you can see from this interaction, when emotionally laden political and social issues are raised, it is possible for an interviewer to lose his or her therapeutic focus and deteriorate into sociopolitical positioning. In this case, the interviewer uses disagreement and disapproval to express his or her political-social agenda and leads the interaction into a destructive arena. Further, the therapist subsequently begins to link the client's political views to his or her personal life in a premature and inappropriate way. This sort of approach can become a clear abuse of interviewer power and status.

Disagreement may also be subtle. Sometimes, silence, lack of head nodding, or therapist neutrality is interpreted as disagreement. It is important to monitor your reactions to clients so you know if you tend to nonverbally and inadvertently communicate disagreement (or disapproval) to clients.

The purpose of disagreement is to change client opinion. The problem with disagreement is that countering one opinion with another opinion may deteriorate into a personal argument, resulting in increased defensiveness by interviewer and client. Therefore, interviewers generally should not use personal disagreement as a basis for their therapeutic intervention. The cost is too high, and the potential benefit can be achieved through other means. Two basic guidelines apply when you feel compelled to disagree with clients:

- If you have an opinion different from a client regarding a philosophical issue (e.g., abortion, mixed-race marriage, sexual practices), remember it's not your job to change your client's opinion; it's your job to help him or her with maladaptive thoughts, feelings, and/or behaviors.
- If, in your professional judgment, the client's belief or opinion is maladaptive (e.g., is causing stress, is ineffective), then you may choose to confront the client and provide him or her with factual information designed to facilitate client change toward more adaptive beliefs. (In such a case, you provide information or explanation rather than disagreement.)

A good example of when an interviewer should employ explanation instead of disagreement is in the area of child rearing. Clients often use ineffective or inappropriate child-rearing techniques and then support such techniques by citing their opinion or experience. Interviewers should avoid bluntly rushing in and telling clients that their opinion is "wrong." Instead, clients should be encouraged to examine whether they are consistently accomplishing their discipline goals by using a particular strategy:

**Client:** "I know some people say spanking isn't good. Well, I was spanked when I was young and I turned out fine."

**Interviewer:** "So, you feel like being spanked as a child didn't have any negative affect on you."

**Client:** "Right. I'm doing okay."

**Interviewer:** "It's true that many parents spank and many parents don't. Maybe, instead of looking at whether you or I think spanking is okay, we should look at your goals for parenting your son. Then, we can talk about what strategies, including spanking, might best help you accomplish your parenting goals."

In this case, empirical evidence indicates that the behavior discussed (spanking) may produce undesirable consequences (Bauman & Friedman, 1998; Sheline, Skipper, & Broadhead, 1994; Straus, Sugarman, & Giles-Sims, 1997). Additionally, numerous professional groups (e.g., the American Psychological Association, American Academy of Pediatrics) recommend that parents develop alternatives to physical punishment for managing children (American Academy of Pediatrics, 1998; Hyman, 1997). Therefore, eventually, the interviewer may discuss with the client the potential undesirable consequences of physical punishment. Generally, this discussion should focus on the client's child-rearing goals and objectives, rather than whether the interviewer does or doesn't "believe in spanking." An exception to this guideline occurs when a therapist suspects the client is physically abusing a child. However, even in cases when child abuse is suspected and reported to the department of family services, the decision is based on violation of a legal standard, rather than therapist-client philosophical disagreements.

## Urging

*Urging* is a step beyond advice giving. It involves pressuring or pleading with clients to take a specific action. When interviewers urge clients to take a specific action, they are using the power of their expert or director role.

Urging is not common during clinical interviews, but there are situations when urging is appropriate. These situations involve primarily crisis (e.g., when the client is in danger or dangerous). For example, in cases involving battered women, often the woman needs to be urged to take her children and move to a battered women's shelter for safety. Similarly, in child abuse cases, if you are interviewing the abuser, you may urge him to report himself to the local agency responsible for protecting children.

In noncrisis situations, urging is even less common. One noncrisis situation where urging may be appropriate is in the treatment of anxiety disorders. This is because clients with anxiety disorders tend to reinforce their fears by avoiding potentially anxiety-producing situations. They become more and more incapacitated by their fearful expectations and avoidance behaviors. A major component of treatment involves graduated exposure to previously anxiety- or fear-producing situations. Not surprisingly, people suffering from anxiety disorders often need their therapists to urge them to face their fears (McCarthy & Foa, 1990; Plaud & Eifert, 1998).

## Approval-Disapproval

*Approval* refers to an interviewer's sanction of client thoughts, feelings, or behavior. To give your approval is to render a favorable judgment. To use approval and disapproval as interviewing responses, interviewers must have the knowledge, expertise, and sensitivity necessary for rendering judgments on their clients' ideas and behavior. Approval and disapproval are sometimes avoided (or used) because they place significant power in the interviewer's hands. Many interviewers prefer that clients judge, accept, and approve of their own thoughts, feelings, and behavior rather than rely on another person's external evaluation.

The concept of approval-disapproval is similar to agreement-disagreement. An interviewer's inclination to agree or disagree with a client, however, generally comes from a desire for social harmony. Approval-disapproval is a step further. When approving or disapproving of client behavior, interviewers take on greater moral authority.

Many clients seek approval from their therapists. In this regard, clients are vulnerable; they need or want a professional's stamp of approval. As interviewers, we must ask whether we should accept the responsibility, power, and control that needy and vulnerable clients want to give us. In some ways, choosing to bestow approval or disapproval on clients is similar to playing God. Who are we to decide which feelings, thoughts, or behaviors are good or bad?

Clients who seek their interviewers' approval may be feeling temporarily insecure or suffering from longstanding needs for approval. Strong needs for approval may stem from feeling rejected and disapproved of as a child. Giving approval can be a powerful therapeutic technique. Interviewer approval can enhance rapport and increase client self-esteem. It also fosters dependent relationships. When a client's search for approval is rewarded, the client is likely to resume a search for approval when or if the insecure feelings begin again.

In some cases, it is difficult to avoid feeling disapproval toward clients. It is especially difficult to maintain a sense of professional neutrality when your client is talking about child abuse, wife battering, rape, murderous thoughts and impulses, deviant sexual practices, and so on. Keep in mind the following facts:

- Clients who engage in deviant or abusive behavior have been disapproved of before, usually by people who mean a great deal to them and sometimes by society. Nonetheless, they have not stopped engaging in deviant or abusive behavior. This suggests that disapproval is ineffective in changing their behavior.
- Your disapproval only alienates you from someone who needs your help to change.
- By maintaining objectivity and neutrality, you are not implicitly approving of your client's behavior. There are other responses besides disapproval (e.g., explanation and confrontation) that show your client that you believe change is needed.
- If you cannot listen to your client's descriptions of his or her behavior without disapproval, refer the client to another qualified professional.
- Disapproval is associated with reduced rapport, feelings of rejection, and early termination of counseling.

Similar to agreement and disagreement, approval and disapproval can be communicated subtly to clients. For example, responding with the word *okay* or *right* can be interpreted by clients as approval—even when you may simply be using these words as a verbal tracking response. Be aware that your verbal and nonverbal behavior may communicate subtle messages of approval or disapproval.

Table 4.2. Summary of Directive Action Responses and Their Usual Effects

| Directive Action Response | Description | Primary Intent/Effect |
|---|---|---|
| Explanation | Statement providing factual information, usually about the interview process, client problem, or implementation of a treatment strategy. | Clarifies client misconceptions. Helps client attain maximal benefit from counseling. |
| Suggestion | Interviewer statement that directly or indirectly suggests or predicts that a particular phenomenon will occur. | May help clients consciously or unconsciously move toward engaging in a particular behavior, thinking a specific thought, or experiencing a particular emotion. |
| Advice | Recommendation given to the client by the interviewer. A prescription to act, think, or feel in a specific manner. | Provides the client with ideas regarding new ways to act, think, or feel. If given prematurely, can be ineffective and can damage interviewer credibility. |
| Agreement-Disagreement | Statement indicating harmony or disharmony of opinion. | Agreement may affirm or reassure a client, enhance rapport, or shut down exploration of thoughts and feelings. Disagreement can produce conflict and stimulate arguments or defensiveness. |
| Urging | Technique of pressuring or pleading with a client to engage in specific actions or to consider specific issues. | May produce the desired change or may backfire and stimulate resistance. May be considered offensive by some clients. |
| Approval-Disapproval | Favorable or unfavorable judgment of the thoughts, feelings, or behavior of a client. | Approval may enhance rapport and foster client dependency. Disapproval may reduce rapport and produce client feelings of rejection. |

Some interviewer responses not discussed here, such as scolding and rejection, are even more interviewer-centered than approval and disapproval (see Benjamin, 1981). Others, such as humor and self-disclosure, are difficult to place along a continuum of interviewer responses or are discussed elsewhere in this text. Table 4.2 includes a summary of directive action responses described in this section.

## SUMMARY

Questions possibly constitute the most basic interviewer tool. They consist of an exceptionally versatile range of listening and action responses. As such, they may be used to facilitate or detract from the clinical interview process.

Many types of questions are available to interviewers, ranging from maximally open (*what* or *how*), minimally open (*where, when,* and *who*), to closed (can be answered with yes or no) questions. Swing questions, beginning with the words *could, would, can,* or *will,* require adequate rapport but often yield in-depth responses. Indirect questions, beginning with *I wonder* or *you must,* are implied questions that allow a client to respond or not. Projective questions usually begin with *what if* and invite client speculation.

To maximize the effectiveness of questions, interviewers should adhere to several basic guidelines, including (a) preparing clients for liberal question use, (b) mixing questions with less directive interviewer responses, (c) using questions relevant to client problems, (d) using questions to elicit concrete behavioral information, and (e) approaching sensitive areas cautiously.

Directive action responses encourage client action. They are based on the assumption that a particular client, for his or her personal welfare, should engage in a particular behavior. Directive action responses include explanation, suggestion, advice, agreement-disagreement, urging, and approval-disapproval. Each of these techniques provides clients with guidelines toward specific action. Beginning interviewers are advised to explore their motives before using directive action responses.

## SUGGESTED READINGS AND RESOURCES

Several of the following books offer additional information and exercises on using questions, directive action skills, and therapeutic techniques from different theoretical orientations.

Benjamin, A. (1987). *The helping interview* (3rd ed.). Boston: Houghton-Mifflin. Chapter 5 of Benjamin's classic work is devoted to a discussion and analysis of the uses and abuses of questions.

Bertolino, B. (1999). *Therapy with troubled teenagers.* New York: John Wiley & Sons. In this book, Bertolino describes and provides numerous examples of strength-based, solution-oriented approaches to moving young clients toward positive action.

de Shazer, S. (1985). *Keys to solution in brief therapy.* New York: W. W. Norton. This is one of the first clear and concise books written on solution-oriented therapy. The author provides many examples of using active and directive interviewing approaches.

Egan, G. (2002). *The skilled helper* (7th ed.). Egan's now classic textbook has a strong emphasis on action-oriented interviewing skills.

Glasser, W. (2000). *Counseling with choice theory.* New York: HarperCollins. In this book, William Glasser, the originator of choice theory and reality therapy, describes several cases during which he uses active and directive choice theory interviewing approaches.

# Chapter 5

# *RELATIONSHIP VARIABLES AND CLINICAL INTERVIEWING*

> *One brief way of describing the change which has taken place in me is to say that in my early professional years I was asking the question, How can I treat, or care, or change this person? Now, I would phrase the question in this way: How can I provide a relationship which this person may use for . . . personal growth?*
> —Carl Rogers, *On Becoming a Person*

---

### CHAPTER OBJECTIVES

Most clinicians and researchers agree that it is crucial for clinical interviewers to establish a positive therapeutic relationship with clients. In this chapter, we examine the nature of a helping relationship from the perspective of several different theoretical orientations. After reading this chapter, you will know:

- The "core conditions" of congruence, unconditional positive regard, and accurate empathy as defined by Carl Rogers.
- The relationship among and misconceptions about Rogers's core conditions.
- Psychoanalytic and interpersonal variables that often affect the relationship between interviewer and client, including transference, countertransference, identification, internalization, resistance, and the working alliance.
- How behavioral and social psychology relationship variables, including interviewer expertness, attractiveness, and trustworthiness, can be integrated into a clinical interview.
- How feminist relationship factors of mutuality and empowerment can be employed in an interviewing situation.

---

In his counseling work, Carl Rogers became disillusioned with traditional psychoanalytic and behavioral methods of personality and behavior change. Instead, he began to focus on a "certain type of relationship" (1961, p. 33) that seemed to facilitate personal development. Rogers came to view this relationship as all-important to the success of counseling, psychotherapy, teaching, and even international peacekeeping (1962, 1969, 1977, 1983). He boldly claimed that the psychotherapeutic relationship he envisioned was necessary *and* sufficient for positive personal development.

In the years since Rogers's early publications (i.e., *Counseling and Psychotherapy,* 1942, and *Client-Centered Therapy,* 1951), research has addressed the importance of relationship factors in counseling and psychotherapy. The overall conclusion is that a warm, personable, and confiding relationship is a significant therapeutic factor common to virtually all forms of counseling and psychotherapy (Frank & Frank, 1991; Glasser, 2000; Hubble, Duncan, & Miller, 1999; Wright & Davis, 1994). Most clinicians heartily agree with half of Rogers's claims about therapy (Mearns, 1997). That is, a good psychotherapeutic relationship is considered a necessary but not always sufficient ingredient for positive client personal development or change.

This chapter focuses on core relationship conditions from a variety of theoretical perspectives. We begin by examining the core relationship conditions that Rogers considered crucial to therapeutic success and then review therapeutic relationship variables commonly associated with psychoanalytic, cognitive-behavioral and social psychology, and feminist approaches to therapy.

## CARL ROGERS'S CORE CONDITIONS

Carl Rogers (1942) believed that establishing a therapeutic relationship constituted the essence and totality of what is therapeutic about counseling. Rogers's three core conditions are:

- Congruence.
- Unconditional positive regard.
- Accurate empathy.

In Rogers's (1961) own words:

> Thus, the relationship which I have found helpful is characterized by a sort of transparency on my part, in which my real feelings are evident; by an acceptance of this other person as a separate person with value in his own right; and by a deep empathic understanding which enables me to see his private world through his eyes. When these conditions are achieved, I become a companion to my client, accompanying him in the frightening search for himself, which he now feels free to undertake. (p. 34)

### Congruence

*Congruence* means that a person's thoughts, feelings, and behavior match. There are no discrepancies; congruent interviewers think, feel, and behave in a consistent and integrated manner. Congruent interviewers are described as genuine, authentic, and comfortable in their interactions with clients.

Congruence implies spontaneity and honesty. Rogers (1961) was clear that congruence requires expression of "various feelings and attitudes which exist in me" (p. 33). He also emphasized that congruent expression is important even if it consists of attitudes, thoughts, or feelings that do not, on the surface, appear conducive to a good relationship.

#### Implications of Congruence

When discussing congruence in clinical interviewing, students often wonder how this concept plays out in a typical interview. Typical questions about congruence include:

> Does congruence mean I can say what I really think about the client right to his or her face?

If I feel sexually attracted to a client, should I be "congruent" and tell him or her?

If I feel like touching a client, should I go ahead and do so? Am I being ingenuine if I restrain myself?

What if I don't like a client or something a client does? Am I being incongruent if I don't tell him or her?

These are important and sometimes controversial questions. You can certainly be consistent and integrated without being excessively transparent; sometimes, the cost of too much expressed internal reaction outweighs the benefit. For example, from the psychoanalytic perspective, Luborsky (1984) states:

> In trying to gain a good measure of trust and rapport, therapists typically experience a natural temptation to impart to the patient information about themselves. . . . This temptation generally should be resisted since, on balance, it provides fewer benefits than it does potential long term problems. (p. 68)

Carl Rogers would agree that the congruent counselor is dedicated primarily to the client's welfare. To take an action or make a disclosure that might detract from the client's potential growth would therefore be incongruent.

To evaluate and use congruence, you should view it from Carl Rogers's perspective. When counseling, Rogers became deeply absorbed with his clients. He strove to completely understand his clients, from their points of view, which is precisely why he named his approach "client-centered" and later "person-centered." This focus greatly reduced his need to judge or express negative feelings toward clients. Moreover, Rogers (1958) clearly stated that the aim of client-centered therapy was not for interviewers to talk about their own feelings:

> Certainly the aim is not for the therapist to express or talk about his own feelings, but primarily that he should not be deceiving the client as to himself. At times he may need to talk about some of his own feelings (either to the client, or to a colleague or superior) if they are standing in the way. (pp. 133–134)

This statement illustrates how Rogers believed good judgment should be used before using self-disclosure with clients. Often, discussing your feelings with peers or supervisors is more appropriate than discussing feelings directly with your client.

For Rogers, being truly present and committed to listening to and helping clients was the most important attribute the interviewer offered. Rogers was a remarkable individual who was almost always genuinely interested in listening to whatever his clients were saying; he was truly committed to his clients' personal growth and development. Quite amazingly, even after decades of counseling, he reported only rarely feeling anger or irritation toward his clients (C. Rogers, 1972).

## Tempering Your Congruence

Gazda, Asbury, Balzer, Childers, and Walters (1984) provide excellent advice about how to determine when or if you should be spontaneously expressive in an interview. Although Gazda et al. are referring to the use of touch in counseling, their advice is sound with respect to most spontaneous interviewer behaviors: "Whom is it for—me, the other person, or to impress those who observe?" (p. 111). In other words, interviewers should explore motives underlying potentially spontaneous behaviors.

With regard to touch, we take a stance that might be even more conservative than

Gazda and his associates. We believe that if you are going to touch a client, you need to be sure you are doing so purely for the client's benefit and not for your own gratification. In addition, you need to be sure your touch will not feel invasive or overbearing and that it will not be misinterpreted. If you have any doubts, you should not touch your client.

In his book *The Road Less Traveled,* M. Scott Peck (1978) outlines a controversial view on sexual relations with clients, a view in which expressive action is tempered by clinical judgment and a personal and professional commitment to client growth:

> Were I ever to have a case in which I concluded after careful and judicious consideration that my patient's spiritual growth would be substantially furthered by our having sexual relations, I would proceed to have them. In fifteen years of practice, however, I have not yet had such a case, and I find it difficult to imagine that such a case could really exist. (p. 176)

We have never come across a case in which an interviewer or psychotherapist had sexual relations with a client based on completely unselfish motives. In fact, sexual relations between therapist and client are always inappropriate, unacceptable, and unethical; therapist-client sex results in trauma and victimization (Sonne & Pope, 1991). We agree with Pope's (1990) terminology for sexual relations between therapists and clients: *sexual abuse of clients.* When such terminology is used, it becomes obvious: Sexual abuse of clients can never be a therapeutic endeavor.

It is not unusual for therapists to occasionally feel sexually attracted to their clients. In fact, as Welfel (2002) states: "Sexual attraction to clients is an almost universal phenomenon among therapists, but most do not act on that attraction and handle their reactions in a responsible manner" (p. 133).

If you feel sexual attraction toward clients, it is unacceptable for you to act on that attraction, either by touching your client sexually or by speaking of your attraction to the client. To speak of your attraction burdens your client with the knowledge of your attraction. When you experience sexual attraction to a client, seek supervisory and collegial input and assistance.

Although congruence suggests spontaneous expression, adhering to the following guidelines will help you temper your spontaneity with good clinical judgment:

- Examine your motives. Are you expressing yourself solely for your client's benefit?
- Consider if what you want to say or do is therapeutic. Are there any possibilities that your client will respond in a negative or unpredictable manner to your expression?
- Congruence does not mean that you say whatever comes to mind. It means that whenever you do choose to speak, you do so with honesty and integrity.

Feminist therapists strongly advocate congruence, or authenticity, in interviewer-client relations. Brody (1984) describes the range of responses that an authentic interviewer might use:

> To be involved, to use myself as a variable in the process, entails using, from time to time, mimicry, provocation, joking, annoyance, analogies, or brief lectures. It also means utilizing my own and others' physical behavior, sensations, emotional states, and reactions to me and others, and sharing a variety of intuitive responses. This is being authentic. (p. 17)

Brody advocates using a wide range of sophisticated and advanced therapeutic strategies, but she is also an experienced clinician. Authentic or congruent approaches to interviewing are best if combined with good clinical judgment, which is obtained, in part, through clinical experience.

A final example from Peck (1978) illustrates the struggle between psychoanalytic and person-centered or feminist perspectives when it comes to congruence:

> After a year of this [therapy], she [the client] asked me in the middle of a session, "Do you think I'm a bit of a shit?"
>
> "You seem to be asking me to tell you what I think of you," I replied, brilliantly stalling for time.
>
> That was exactly what she wanted, she said. But what did I do now? What magical words or techniques or postures could help me? I could say, "Why do you ask that?" or "What are your fantasies about what I think of you?" or "What's important, Marcia, is not what I think of you but what you think of yourself." Yet I had an overpowering feeling that these gambits were cop-outs, and that after a whole year of seeing me three times a week the least Marcia was entitled to was an honest answer from me as to what I thought of her. (pp. 170–171)

At some point, you will be faced with similar questions, and you will need to decide how to respond. Do you deny your client a human and congruent response for the sake of preserving neutrality, professionalism, and technical correctness? Or, do you forsake professional and technical neutrality and respond to your client as "just" another human being? Interviewers with psychoanalytic training tend to stay with professional neutrality, whereas person-centered, existential, and feminist interviewers choose more open, humanistic approaches. This does not mean therapists from these theoretical orientations always and immediately answer direct client questions. Most questions requiring therapist self-disclosure, judgment, or advice should be discussed and explored before answered (or immediately afterwards), no matter what the counseling orientation (see Putting It in Practice 5.1 for further discussions on self-disclosure).

## Unconditional Positive Regard

Carl Rogers (1961) defines *unconditional positive regard* as: ". . . a warm regard for him *[sic]* as a person of unconditional self-worth—of value no matter what his condition, his behavior, or his feelings" (p. 34). Unconditional positive regard suggests warmth, caring, respect, and a nonjudgmental attitude.

No one knows clients better than they know themselves. Therefore, even as interviewers, we are not in a good position to judge clients. Usually, all we know is a thin slice or sample of their lives and behavior; consequently, our judgments are based on inadequate information. We have not lived with our clients, we have not observed them at great length, and we cannot directly know their internal motives, thoughts, or feelings. Even if it were possible to have complete information on clients, rendering judgment on good or bad qualities of clients' thoughts, feelings, or behavior would be inappropriate.

The term *unconditional positive regard* suggests more than a neutral acceptance of clients. Rogers (1961) stated, "the safety of being liked and prized as a person seems a highly important element in a helping relationship" (p. 34). Rogers is referring to positive or affectionate feelings interviewers need to have for their clients to feel safe enough to explore their self-doubts, insecurities, and weaknesses. Research shows that therapy is more effective when therapists have positive feelings toward their clients (Moras & Strupp, 1982; Strupp & Hadley, 1979).

======= **Putting It in Practice 5.1** =======

## The Pros and Cons of Self-Disclosure

Clients will ask you personal questions. It's only a matter of how many personal questions you get asked. In addition, from time to time you'll feel the urge to disclose something about yourself—both appropriately and inappropriately—to a client. Consequently, the big questions to ask right now include:

- Is there anything basically wrong about self-disclosing personal information to clients?
- Are there any benefits associated with therapist self-disclosure?
- How much disclosure is too much?
- Is it possible that refusing to disclose anything about myself might damage my relationship with my client?

As with most therapy issues, therapists have widely differing opinions about self-disclosure, depending on their theoretical orientation, personality style, positive and negative personal experiences, and personal preferences. Here are a few distinct viewpoints.

Julia Segal, a counselor in Britain, is strongly opposed to self-disclosure. She summarizes her views in a book chapter titled "Against Self Disclosure." She states:

> There are many reasons for counsellors not to disclose information about themselves. Discussion of the counsellor's experience takes the focus off the client. It can be a means of avoiding serious and painful issues, both for the client and for the counsellor. In particular, it can prevent confrontation of issues about the client's belief in the counsellor's competence and the difficulties of two people being different from each other. There is really no predicting what any disclosure will mean to a client, and it may simply confuse the issues and increase the client's protectiveness toward the counsellor. It also removes the possibility of uncovering and examining the client's assumptions about the counsellor, some of which may be false but very illuminating. Lastly, I maintain, it is important for the counsellor to retain privacy and clear boundaries in the relationship in order to be free to use . . . empathy in the full service of the client. (Segal, 1993, p. 14)

In somewhat surprising contrast, a psychoanalytic writer recently articulated the benefits of "Playing one's cards face up in analysis" (Renik, 1999, p. 521). Previously, Renik (1995) wrote:

> Self-disclosure for the purposes of self-explanation facilitates the analysis of transference by establishing an atmosphere of authentic candor. Of course, therapeutic benefits are most extensive and enduring when based upon expansion of the patient's self-awareness. (p. 466)

If you find it hard to figure out whether and how much to self-disclose to clients, join the club. Both the empirical research and clinical anecdotes suggest that self-disclosure can be either facilitative or nonfacilitative of therapy (Stricker & Fisher, 1990).

In the end, whether and how much you self-disclose to clients is totally up to you. We tend to encourage a little therapist spontaneity from time to time—as long as you plan for it.

An important question for interviewers is: "How can I express or demonstrate unconditional positive regard toward my clients?" It's tempting to try expressing positive feelings directly to clients, either by touching or making statements such as "I like (or love) you," "I care about you," "I will accept you unconditionally," or "I won't judge you in here."

Expressing unconditional positive regard directly to clients is usually ineffective— or even dangerous. First, direct expressions of regard may be interpreted as phony or inappropriately intimate. Second, direct expressions of affection may imply that you want a friendship or loving relationship with your client. Third, even professional interviewers sometimes have negative feelings toward their clients. If you claim "unconditional acceptance," you are promising the impossible, because you cannot (and will not) always like your clients.

The question remains: How do you express positive regard, acceptance, and respect to clients indirectly? Here are some ideas: First, by keeping appointments, by asking how your clients like to be addressed and then remembering to address them that way, and by listening sensitively and compassionately, you establish a relationship characterized by affection and respect. Second, by allowing clients freedom to discuss themselves in their natural manner, you communicate respect and acceptance. Third, by demonstrating that you hear and remember specific parts of a client's story, you communicate respect. This usually involves using paraphrases, summaries, and sometimes interpretations. Fourth, by responding with compassion or empathy to clients' emotional pain and intellectual conflicts, you express concern and acceptance. This is what Othmer and Othmer (1994) mean when they say that finding the suffering and showing compassion are rapport-building strategies. Fifth, clinical experience and research both indicate that clients are sensitive to an interviewer's intentions. Thus, by clearly making an effort to accept and respect your clients, you are communicating a message that may be more powerful than any therapy technique (Strupp & Binder, 1984; Wright & Davis, 1994).

In the following example, the interviewer sensitively uses a feeling-oriented summary along with a gentle interpretation to express unconditional positive regard:

"Earlier, you mentioned feeling hurt when a woman you care about rejected you. Now you're talking about your mother and how you felt she abandoned you to take care of your father and his alcoholism. It seems like there might be a connection or pattern there."

Although this interviewer comment is designed to facilitate insight into relationship patterns (Luborsky, 1984), it also lets your client know how closely you are listening. As a result, your client may feel honored and respected, and the relationship may take on a greater intimacy. Remembering what your client says requires deliberate attentiveness. Using intellect, intuition, and empathy to mirror the client's inner world communicates a deep respect that is the very essence of unconditional positive regard.

## Accurate Empathy

Empathy is a popular concept in clinical interviewing, counseling, and psychotherapy. Empathy is vital to initial rapport and, according to some schools of thought, crucial to eventual psychotherapeutic change (Kohut, 1984; C. Rogers, 1951; see Table 5.1). Unfortunately, empathy is as complex as it is popular. Take, for example, the definition of empathy in *Webster's Dictionary:*

**Table 5.1.   Empathy and Other Theoretical Orientations**

Writers and clinicians of various theoretical orientations and professional perspectives have emphasized the importance of empathy in interviewing, counseling, and psychotherapy. Below is a brief sampling from some prominent writers and clinicians.

*Psychoanalytic Psychotherapy:* "Empathy is the operation that defines the field of psychoanalysis. No psychology of complex mental states is conceivable without the employment of empathy" (Kohut, 1984, pp. 174–175).

*Psychiatric Interviewing:* "When the patient reveals his suffering, tell him that you understand, show your empathy, and express your compassion" (Othmer & Othmer, 1994, p. 27).

*Feminist Theory:* "We have a long tradition of trying to dispense with, or at least to control or neutralize, emotionality, rather than valuing, embracing, and cultivating its contributing strengths. . . . However attained, these qualities bespeak a basic ability that is very valuable. It can hardly be denied that emotions are essential aspects of human life" (J. Miller, 1986/1997, pp. 38–39).

*Behavior Therapy:* "Any behavior therapist who maintains that principles of learning and social influence are all one needs to know in order to bring about behavior change is out of contact with clinical reality. . . . The truly skillful behavior therapist is one who can both conceptualize problems behaviorally and make the necessary translations so that he interacts in a warm and empathic manner with his client" (Goldfried & Davison, 1976, pp. 55–56).

*Marriage Counseling:* "A major design of the treatment is to enable each spouse to receive empathic understanding when he or she communicates with the therapist, and for the task of the spouse who is listening to be defined as an attempt to put aside his or her complaints and empathically enter the world of the other" (Lansky, 1986, p. 562).

*Counseling Difficult Adolescents:* "If you find yourself having a hard time connecting with a challenging youth, quit talking and start listening. Remember, meaningful relationships develop from warm, friendly, accepting, and nonjudgmental attitudes conveyed through active, empathic listening (Richardson, 2001, pp. 55–56).

---

The action of understanding, being aware of, being sensitive to, and vicariously experiencing the feelings, thoughts, and experience of another of either the past or present without having the feelings, thoughts, and experience fully communicated in an objectively explicit manner. (1985, p. 407)

According to this definition, empathy requires inference. Because we cannot know "in an objectively explicit manner" the feelings, thoughts, and experience of another, we must use our intellect and our emotional responses to infer what this other person might be feeling, thinking, and experiencing. Consequently, empathy is both an intellectual and affective process.

Although Webster's definition may seem complex, even more in-depth efforts have been made to define the empathic process. For example, Buie (1981) describes four components of empathy:

1. Cognitive or intellectual understanding of the client.
2. Low-intensity feelings, memories, and associations experienced by the interviewer in response to client communications.
3. Imaginative imitation empathy (similar to Carkhuff's [1987] empathy question; see the following section).

4. Affective contagion or a resonating with clients' emotional expressions (J. Watkins, 1978).

Empathy is a complex affective-cognitive-experiential concept that continues to stimulate analysis and research (Duan, 2000; Tamburrino, Lynch, Nagel, & Mangen, 1993).

Carkhuff (1987) refers to the intellectual part of empathy as "asking the empathy question" (p. 100). "By answering the empathy question we try to understand the feelings expressed by our helpee. We summarize the clues to the helpee's feelings and then answer the question, How would I feel if I were Tom and saying these things?" (p. 101).

Asking the empathy question is useful for enhancing empathic sensitivity. However, it also oversimplifies the empathic process in at least two ways. First, it assumes that the interviewer (or helper) has an accurately calibrated affective barometer within, allowing for objective readings of client emotional states. The fact is, clients and therapists may have had such different personal experiences that the empathy question produces completely inaccurate results; just because *you* would feel a particular way if you were in the client's shoes doesn't mean the client feels the same way. As Pietrofesa and associates state, "Some skeptics suggest that an empathic response is a projection" (Pietrofesa, Hoffman, & Splete, 1984, p. 238). If interviewers rely solely on Carkhuff's empathy question, they may project their own feelings onto clients. For example, consider what might happen if an interviewer tends to view events pessimistically, while her client usually uses denial or repression to put on a happy face. The following exchange might occur:

**Client:** "I don't know why my dad wants us to come to therapy now. We've never been able to communicate. It doesn't even bother me any more. I've accepted it. I wish he would."

**Interviewer:** "It must make you angry to have a father who can't communicate effectively with you."

**Client:** "Not at all. I'm letting go of my relationships with my parents. Really, I don't let it bother me."

In this case, thinking about how it would feel to never communicate effectively with her own father may make the interviewer feel angry or sad. However, her comment is a projection, based on her own feelings, not on the client's. Accurate empathic responding stays close to client word content and nonverbal messages. If this client had previously expressed anger or was currently looking upset or angry (e.g., by staring downward, tightening her body, and talking in tense voice tones), the interviewer might choose to reflect anger. However, instead the interviewer's comment is an inaccurate feeling reflection and, as such, is rejected by the client. The interviewer could have stayed more closely with what her client expressed by focusing on key words. For example:

"Coming into therapy now doesn't make much sense to you. Maybe you used to have some feelings about your lack of communication with your dad, but it sounds like you feel pretty numb about the whole situation now."

This second response is more accurate. It touches on how the client felt before, what she presently thinks, as well as the numbed affective response. There may be unresolved sadness, anger, or disappointment, but for the interviewer to connect with these buried feelings requires an interpretation, which would need to be supported with clear evidence before it could be experienced by the client as empathic. Recall from Chapter 3 that interpretations and interpretive feeling reflections must be supported by adequate evidence to be effective.

Instead of focusing solely on what you would feel if you were in your client's shoes, it is more effective to also reflect intellectually on how other clients (or other people you know) might feel and think in response to this particular experience. Carl Rogers (1961) emphasized that feeling reflections should be stated tentatively so the client feels able to freely accept or dismiss them. Keep in mind the defensive style of your clients. If they are using defense mechanisms such as rationalization or denial, you need to first acknowledge, in an empathic manner, their defensive thinking. For example:

> **Client:** "I don't know why my dad wants us to come to therapy now. We've never been able to communicate. It doesn't even bother me any more. I've accepted it. I wish he would."
>
> **Interviewer:** "Coming into therapy now doesn't make much sense to you. Maybe you used to have some feelings about your lack of communication with your dad, but it sounds like you feel pretty numb about the whole situation now."
>
> **Client:** "Yeah, I guess so. I think I'm letting go of my relationships with my parents. Really, I don't let it bother me."
>
> **Interviewer:** "Maybe one of the ways you're protecting yourself from how you felt about your lack of communication with your dad is to distance yourself from your parents. Otherwise, it could still bother you, I suppose."
>
> **Client:** "I, yeah. I guess if I let myself get close to my parents again, my dad's lame communication style would bug me again."

Obviously, this client still has feelings about her father's poor communication. *Accurate* empathy allows the client to begin admitting her feelings.

A second way in which Carkhuff's (1987) empathy question is simplistic is that it treats empathy as if it had to do *only* with accurately reflecting client feelings. Certainly, accurate feeling reflection is an important part of empathy, but, as Rogers (1961), Webster's (1985), and others (Buie, 1981; Duan, 2000; Margulies, 1984) indicate, empathy also involves *thinking* and *experiencing* with clients. This is why empathic acknowledgment of clients' defensive styles is important to empathic responding. Clients protect themselves from emotional pain through defense mechanisms (i.e., largely unconscious patterns of distorting reality that are ego-protective; A. Freud, 1946). Consequently, to be maximally empathic, interviewers need to address not only feelings, but also the way clients shield themselves from feelings. As Sigmund Freud (1921/1955) suggested, empathy "plays the largest part in our understanding of what is inherently foreign to our ego" (p. 108).

Accurate empathy is usually based on a combination of at least the following four strategies:

1. Acknowledging and reflecting surface or buried feelings as clients express them through verbal and nonverbal messages. This may include matching representational systems, mirroring, paraphrasing, reflection of feeling, interpretation, and other responses (see Chapter 3).
2. Noticing how clients are thinking about, coping with, and defending against their emotional pain.
3. Coming up with an answer to Carkhuff's empathy question, How would I feel if I were in the client's shoes?

4. Demonstrating that you're interested in discussing important issues and trying to comprehend, through a variety of listening and attending techniques, how clients are experiencing these issues.

## The Effects of Empathy

Obviously, empathy enhances rapport. Empathy also has many other positive effects. First, empathy helps clients explore personal issues more freely. When clients feel understood, they are also more open and willing to talk about their concerns in detail; empathy elicits information (Egan, 2002).

Second, as Carl Rogers (1961) emphasized, empathy, combined with unconditional positive regard, allows clients to explore themselves more completely than they would otherwise: "It is only as I see them (your feelings and thoughts) as you see them, and accept them and you, that you feel really free to explore all the hidden nooks and frightening crannies of your inner and often buried experience" (p. 34). Rogers is claiming that accurate empathy helps clients become aware of previously unconscious material. He is also claiming that accurately empathic responses, similar to accurate interpretations, result in increased client self-awareness.

Third, empathy enhances the working alliance (Greenson, 1967). Empathic responding helps clients believe the interviewer is on their side, a perception that also considerably increases trust and motivation (Krumboltz & Thoresen, 1976).

Fourth, research has shown that empathy is related to positive treatment outcome (see Duan, Rose, & Kraatz, 2002). In fact, some authors go so far as to suggest that empathy is the basis for all effective therapeutic interventions: "Because empathy is the basis for understanding, one can conclude that there is no effective intervention without empathy and all effective interventions have to be empathic" (Duan et al., 2002, p. 209).

## Misguided Empathic Attempts

Just because you want to express empathy to your clients does not mean you will be successful in communicating empathy. Often, early interviews are filled with self-disclosures and other attempts to let clients know they are understood. Classic empathic statements that beginning interviewers often use, but should avoid, include the following (J. Sommers-Flanagan & Sommers-Flanagan, 1989):

1. "I know how you feel" or "I understand."
   In response to such a statement, clients may wonder, "How could she know how I feel; she's only known me for 15 minutes," or they may reason, "If she really knew how I felt, or had been through what I've been through, she'd be getting therapy, not being a therapist."
2. "I've been through the same type of thing."
   Clients may respond with skepticism or ask you to elaborate on your experience. Suddenly the roles are reversed: The interviewer is being interviewed.
3. "Oh my God, that must have been terrible."
   Clients who have experienced trauma sometimes are uncertain about how traumatic their experiences really were. Therefore, to hear a professional exclaim that what they lived through and coped with was "terrible" can be too negative. The important point here is whether you are leading or tracking the client's emotional experience. If the client is giving you a clear indication that he or she senses the "terribleness" of his or her experiences, reflecting that the experiences "must have been terrible" is empathic. However, a better empathic response would re-

move the judgment of "must have" and get rid of the "Oh my God" (i.e., "Sounds like you felt terrible about what happened.").

4. "Gee, you poor thing" or "That's awful. You must be a strong person to have made it through that."

Again, these statements contain judgments and offer sympathy. The client may feel complimented but may subsequently feel reluctant about sharing other emotions or weaknesses, for fear of further judgments by the expert. Or, once clients are rewarded for looking strong, they may choose to present all their material in the same light.

Clients often have ambivalent feelings about their experiences. For example, take the following interviewer-client interaction:

**Interviewer:** "Can you think of a time when you felt unfairly treated? Perhaps punished when you didn't deserve it?"

**Client:** "No, not really. (15-second pause) Well, I guess there was this one time. I was supposed to clean the house for my mother while she was gone. It wasn't done when she got back, and she broke a broom over my back."

**Interviewer:** "She broke a broom over your back?" (stated with a slight inflection, indicating interviewer disapproval or surprise with the mother's behavior)

**Client:** "Yeah. I probably deserved it, though. The house wasn't cleaned like she had asked."

In this situation, the client is experiencing mixed feelings about her mother. On the one hand, the mother treats her unfairly, and on the other hand, the client feels guilty because she was a bad girl who did not follow her mother's directions. The interviewer is trying to convey empathy through voice tone and inflection. This technique is appropriately chosen because focusing too strongly on the client's guilt or indignation and anger would prematurely shut down exploration of the client's ambivalent feelings. Despite the interviewer's tentative and minimal expression of empathy, the client defends her mother's punitive actions. This suggests that the client had already accepted (by age 11, and still accepted in this session, at age 42) her mother's negative evaluation of her. From a person-centered or psychoanalytic perspective, a stronger supportive statement such as "That's ridiculous, mothers should never break brooms over their daughters' backs" may have closed off any exploration of the client's victim guilt about the incident.

From a nondirective perspective, minimally empathic, nondirective responses that communicate empathy through voice tone, facial expression, and feeling reflection are usually more advantageous than open support and sympathy. There is always time for open support later, after the client has explored both sides of the issue.

## The Relationship among Rogers's Core Conditions

Rogers believed that the desire to judge clients or respond to them out of his own need was greatly reduced through empathy. He found that the interrelatedness of empathy, unconditional positive regard, and congruence modified the spontaneity associated with congruence. Accurate empathy also diminishes the tendency to judge clients and thus enhances unconditional positive regard. Empathy, unconditional positive regard, and congruence are not competing individual constructs. (In statistical terms, they are not orthogonal.) Instead, they form a single triarchic construct; they complement one another.

## PSYCHOANALYTIC AND INTERPERSONAL RELATIONSHIP VARIABLES

The following interviewing relationship variables are derived from psychoanalytic, object relations, and interpersonal theoretical perspectives.

### Transference

Sigmund Freud (1940/1949) defined *transference* as a process that occurs when "the patient sees in his analyst the return—the reincarnation—of some important figure out of his childhood or past, and consequently transfers on to him feelings and reactions that undoubtedly applied to this model" (p. 66). Subsequently, Sullivan (1970) defined a similar process that he referred to as *parataxic distortion:* "The real characteristics of the other fellow at that time may be of negligible importance to the interpersonal situation. This we call parataxic distortion" (p. 25).

Transference is characterized by inappropriateness; the client responds to the interviewer by acting, thinking, or feeling in an inappropriate manner. S. Freud (1912/1958) stated that transference "exceeds anything that could be justified on sensible or rational grounds" (p. 100). Sometimes, but not always, intense and obvious transference issues can come to the surface early in an interview or early in the therapeutic process. For example, an angry, confused young man had an especially negative reaction to his female counselor. He became verbally violent during an initial screening interview, stating repeatedly, "Women. You [expletives deleted] women can't understand where I'm coming from. No way. Women just don't get me. Like you. You don't get me." Because the counselor had not behaved in a manner that warranted such a strong reaction, it is likely this client was displacing "feelings, attitudes, and behaviors" based on previous interactions he had experienced with females (Gelso & Hayes, 1998, p. 51).

More commonly, like many relationship variables, transference is abstract, vague, and elusive. To notice it, you have to pay attention to idiosyncratic transactions clients initiate with you; for example, clients respond to you in ways that are more emotional than the situation warrants, they make assumptions about you that have little basis in reality, and they express unfounded and unrealistic expectations regarding you or therapy.

A fairly common old map on new terrain is the client's unspoken belief that you, too, will evaluate him, find him lacking, and reject him. An example is a client who expressed evaluation anxiety regarding her performance on a psychological test and cognitive-behavioral homework assignment. She stated tentatively, "You know, some of those things the test says about me don't seem accurate. I must have done something wrong when I took the test." This comment is revealing because when clients are provided with inaccurate psychological test feedback, they often begin questioning the test's validity, rather than their own performance. Similarly, she stated, "I did the assignment, but I'm not sure I had the right idea." Again, she made this statement when, in fact, she turned in a very thorough homework assignment. She did exactly as instructed, but her self-doubt was triggered because she viewed her therapist as an authority figure who might evaluate her negatively. Her expectation of criticism suggests, based on the psychoanalytic perspective, that she had been harshly, and perhaps inappropriately, criticized before. In this sense, her reaction is similar to the child who flinches when approached by an adult whose arm is extended. The child flinches because of previous physical abuse; the flinch may be an automatic and unconscious response. Similarly, clients who have been exposed to excessive criticism have an automatic and unconscious tendency to prepare themselves (or flinch) when exposed to evaluative situations. This is an example of transference.

Transference reactions may become self-fulfilling prophecies. The client, expecting rejection, negative evaluation, or lack of empathy scans for those possibilities. Therefore, every subtle rejection, every frown, and every missed empathic opportunity is interpreted by the client, who is an expert at detecting these transgressions, as fulfilling her unconscious assumptions of how people treat her. The client may then begin responding negatively to these small but magnified errors by harshly rejecting the interviewer's paraphrases or feeling reflections. Soon the interviewer is thinking, "I don't know what it is about her, but she's getting under my skin." If the interviewer fails to notice this pattern, this misplaced map, the client may eventually succeed in eliciting a negative evaluation of herself.

As S. Freud (1940/1949) stated, "Transference is ambivalent" (p. 66). Transference may manifest itself in positive (e.g., affectionate, liking, or loving) or negative (hostile, rejecting, or cold) attitudes, feelings, or behaviors. Each can be a productive area to work through with the client as therapy progresses. However, during initial stages, the wisest course for interviewers is to be astute observers, noticing responses and behaviors that seem to come from old terrain and past relationships in the client's life, but not commenting on these patterns.

It is tempting to attribute overly positive, warm, or complimentary attitudes as being legitimate responses by the client, while attributing hostile, rejecting, cold attitudes to a defect in the client's character. Neither attribution should be made early in therapy. Instead, interviewers use their knowledge of transference responses to sharpen their observational skills and remain accepting and neutral whether transference responses are positive or negative.

Interpretation of transference early in the therapeutic relationship should be avoided. Adequate rapport and a working relationship should always precede interpretation (Meissner, 1991). Further, transference interpretation requires advanced skills and firm theoretical grounding that should be obtained from specialized texts and professional supervision (Weiner, 1998). A generally accepted rule is to notice but ignore mildly positive transference reactions, dealing first with negative transference. Of course, interpretation of both positive and negative transference should be delayed until evidence for the inappropriateness of these reactions becomes clear and more easily interpreted.

Simply being aware that a client might be exhibiting transference reactions provides important information. A statement of hostility or warmth from the client can provide an opportunity to explore the client's problem areas more deeply. The interviewer can simply respond by asking, "When are some times you've felt similar feelings in the past?" This question neatly deflects the comment back to the client and reduces the chances that the interviewer might respond defensively or accusingly by stating, "Well, you make me nervous, too" or "Sounds like that's an old problem from your past." After all, if clients are really exhibiting transference, it pertains more to them and their history than it does to their real relationship with you. Furthermore, through gentle questioning you can explore significant past relationships.

Transference gives interviewers a special opportunity to glimpse not only the client's past relationships, but also his or her contemporary relationships. Research suggests that the core conflictual relationship theme (CCRT) observed in therapy is highly similar to contemporary relationship patterns observed outside therapy (Fried, Crits-Christoph, & Luborsky, 1990; Kivlighan, 2002). Overall, psychoanalytic, interpersonal, and even behavioral clinicians have commented on the advantage of working with transference reactions (Goldfried & Davison, 1994; Sullivan, 1970). Fenichel (1945) states, "The transference offers the analyst a unique opportunity to observe directly the past of his patient and thereby to understand the development of his conflicts" (p. 30).

Psychoanalytically oriented interviewers usually refrain from self-disclosure because talking about their own real feelings muddies the transference. When pressed by clients for a congruent or genuine response, psychoanalytic-oriented interviewers usually take shelter behind the professional relationship. For example:

> **Client:** "I like being with you so much that I wish we could get together outside therapy. I wish we could go out to lunch and do the kinds of things that friends do."
>
> **Interviewer:** "I want you to know how important it is for us to maintain our professional relationship. Even if I wanted to have a friendship with you, I wouldn't, because to do so could have a negative effect on our work together."

The psychoanalytic response is much cooler and more distant than the person-centered or feminist response in similar situations. Although person-centered and feminist interviewers maintain professional client-therapist boundaries, they might be more warm and open:

> **Client:** "I like being with you so much that I wish we could get together outside therapy. I wish we could go out to lunch and do the kinds of things that friends do."
>
> **Interviewer:** "Yeah, I can really relate to that because I enjoy our time together too. And in some ways, spending time together outside therapy would be nice for me too. But counseling is a special kind of relationship. Each of us has a role, or a job to do, and if we added in other roles, like being friends, it could get in the way of the work you're doing here. Does that make sense to you?"

Whether positive or negative, take your clients' reactions to you with a grain of salt. If you take your clients' emotional reactions to you too personally, you will probably experience strong emotional reactions. Strong or disproportionate emotional reactions to clients constitute countertransference.

## Countertransference

*Countertransference* is similar to transference, except it happens to interviewers rather than clients. Countertransference, like transference, stems from conflicts, attitudes, and motives not consciously experienced. Countertransference also consists of emotional, attitudinal, and behavioral responses that are inappropriate in terms of their intensity, frequency, and duration. It is important and helpful for professional interviewers to become aware of their own countertransference patterns (Beitman, 1983; Szajnberg, Moilanen, Kanerva, & Tolf, 1996; see Putting It in Practice 5.2).

Although countertransference is similar to transference, there are several important differences. Originally, S. Freud (1940/1949) identified countertransference as a reac-

---

**Putting It in Practice 5.2**

## Coping with Countertransference

*Countertransference* is defined as therapist emotional and behavioral reactions to clients. As an example, imagine an interviewer who lost his mother to cancer when he was a child. His father's grief was very severe. As a consequence, little emotional support was available when the interviewer was a child. The situation eventually improved, his father recovered, and the interviewer's conscious memory consists of a general sense that losing his mother was very difficult. Now, years later, he's a graduate student, conducting his first interviews. Things are fine until a very depressed middle-aged man comes in because he recently lost his wife. What reactions might you expect from the interviewer? What reactions might catch him by surprise?

Countertransference reactions may be more or less conscious, more or less out of the therapist's awareness. These reactions, if unmanaged, can have a negative effect on therapy. The following guidelines are provided to assist you in coping with countertransference reactions:

- Recognize that countertransference reactions are normal and inevitable. If you experience strong emotional reactions, persistent thoughts, and behavioral impulses toward a client, it does not mean you are a "sick" person or a "bad" interviewer.
- If you have strong reactions to a client, consult a colleague or supervisor.
- Do some additional reading about countertransference. It is especially useful to obtain reading materials pertaining to the particular type of client you're working with (e.g., eating disorder clients, depressed clients, antisocial clients).
- If your feelings, thoughts, and impulses remain despite efforts to deal with them, two options may be appropriate: Refer your client to another therapist, or obtain personal psychotherapy to work through the issues that have been aroused in you.

---

tion to client transference. This is certainly the case sometimes. On occasion, clients treat their interviewers with such open hostility or admiration that interviewers find themselves caught up in the transference and behave in ways that are very unusual for them. For example, at a psychiatric hospital, a patient once unleashed an unforgettable accusation against her therapist:

> "You are the coldest, most computer-like person I've ever met. You're like a robot! I talk and you just sit there, nodding your head like some machine. I bet if I cut open your arms, I'd find wires, not veins!"

Certainly, this accusation might be considered pure transference. Perhaps the client was responding to her therapist in this manner because, in the past, she experienced males as emotionally unavailable. On the other hand, as the saying goes, it takes two to tango. As interviewers, we need to look at our own contributions to the therapist-client dance.

Taking a hard look at his reactions to this particular patient, the therapist consulted with colleagues and a supervisor, engaged in self-reflection, and came to several conclusions about his behavior with her. First, he admitted to behaving cooler and less emotionally than he generally did with clients. Second, he was frightened of her demands for emotional intimacy. Consequently, he responded by protecting himself by becoming more inhibited and robotic. Third, his supervisor reassured him that countertransference reactions to severely disturbed patients are not unusual. The therapist took solace in the fact that he was not the first clinician to experience countertransference; he also worked to respond to the client more therapeutically, rather than reacting with his own fears of intimacy.

Interviewers respond to transference reactions in unique ways that elicit, in turn, unique responses from each client. In the preceding example, important men in her past had been emotionally unavailable to the client. Her outrage toward emotionally unavailable men often drew emotional (and sometimes physical) counterattacks from men with whom she had relationships. Her therapist's continued withdrawal into emotional neutrality was unusual for her (and him), and so she kept up a raging attack, possibly in an effort to obtain some type of reaction from him. In turn, he kept constricting his reactions to her, out of fears of intimacy and losing control.

Many theorists go beyond Freud's definition of countertransference and define it more broadly as "any unconscious attitude or behavior on the part of the therapist which is prompted by the needs of the therapist rather than by the needs of the client" (Pipes & Davenport, 1999, p. 161). In other words, countertransference may begin with the interviewer's (rather than the client's) unconscious agenda.

Freud originally considered transference an impediment to psychotherapy, but later modified his position, suggesting that the analysis of transference, conducted properly, is a crucial therapeutic tool. In contrast, Freud always considered countertransference to be an impediment to psychotherapy. That is, he thought good psychoanalysts should deal with their own inner conflicts through analysis; their high levels of self-awareness would then reduce the likelihood of their experiencing countertransference reactions. "Recognize this counter-transference . . . and overcome it" because "no psychoanalyst goes further than his own complexes and internal resistances permit" (S. Freud, 1910/1957, p. 145). In fact, research has shown that therapists reputed as excellent are also rated as having better self-awareness and less countertransference potential than therapists considered average (Van Wagoner, Gelso, Hayes, & Diemer, 1991).

Many contemporary psychoanalysts and object relations theorists have broken with Freud's negative view of countertransference and believe there is much to be gained from an interviewer's countertransference reactions (Beitman, 1983; Weiner, 1998). For example, if a client provokes strong and unusual feelings of fear, disappointment, or sexual attraction, it may be worthwhile to scrutinize yourself to determine if your emotional response is from your own personal issues. Only after scrutinizing yourself can you assume that your client's behavior is an indicator of the client's usual effect on people outside psychotherapy.

Countertransference reactions can teach us about ourselves and our underlying conflicts. They are a source of information about ourselves and our clients. Although it may be a hindrance and make it difficult to distinguish our own issues from those of clients', countertransference can facilitate the therapeutic process.

Clinicians from various theoretical orientations acknowledge the reality of countertransference. Goldfried and Davison ( 1976), the authors of *Clinical Behavior Therapy*, offer the following advice: "The therapist should continually observe his own behavior and emotional reactions, and question what the client may have done to bring about such reactions" (p. 58). Similarly, Beitman (1983) suggests that technique-oriented counselors may fall prey to countertransference. He believes that "any technique may be used in the service of avoidance of countertransference awareness" (p. 83). In other words, clinicians may repetitively apply a particular therapeutic technique to their clients (e.g., progressive muscle relaxation, mental imagery, or thought stopping) without realizing they are applying the techniques to address their own needs, rather than the needs of their clients (see Putting It in Practice 5.2 and Individual and Cultural Highlight 5.1).

## Identification and Internalization

*Identification* and *internalization* are terms that come primarily from psychoanalytic and object relations theory. However, concepts that share very similar meanings can be found in other schools of thought, a fact that underscores the importance of identification and internalization and their central role in therapeutic relationship development and treatment outcome. For example, behaviorists emphasize the importance of modeling in behavior therapy (Bandura, 1969; Raue, Goldfried, & Barkham, 1997). According to social learning theory, we adopt many specific behavior patterns because we've watched others perform such behavior previously (i.e., we have seen the behavior modeled). Furthermore, as D. Myers (1989) states, "We more often imitate those we respect and admire, those we perceive as similar to ourselves, and those we perceive as successful" (p. 251). Obviously, parents are important models to children, but interviewers and psychotherapists may also teach clients new behavior patterns through explicit, as well as subtle, modeling procedures.

Psychoanalytic and object relations theorists use the concepts of identification and internalization to describe what learning theorists consider modeling (G. Adler, 1996; Eagle, 1984; J. Greenberg & Mitchell, 1983). Specifically, individuals identify with others whom they love, respect, or view as similar. Through this identification process, individuals come to incorporate or internalize unique and specific ways in which that loved or respected person thinks, acts, and feels. In a sense, identification and internalization result in the formation of identity; we become like those we have been near but also like those whom we love, respect, or view as similar to ourselves.

Identification is enhanced when clients feel understood by their interviewer or therapist at points where their values run deepest or their distress is most poignant. If identification is achieved, superficial dissimilarities do not detract from the therapy relationship. In other words, empathy enhances identification and reduces the importance of surface differences. Clients can say internally, "I can identify with this person. Even though we are different in some ways, she understands where I'm coming from." More importantly, clients can also think, "Because she understands and has heard the worst of my fears, and she still is hopeful, maybe she can help me resolve my problems." If differences between you and a given client are large and central, identification may be difficult or impossible.

For instance, one client wanted to work on deeply troubling issues she had because she had chosen not to marry, which is unacceptable in her family. She carefully selected a middle-aged female therapist, thinking she would find the basic understanding that she needed to work on her feelings. Unfortunately, after a very few sessions, the therapist interpreted the woman's no-marriage decision as adolescent rebellion. There were some basic differences between the therapist's worldview and the client's, which made rapport, empathy, and eventual identification very unlikely.

Identification is the precursor to internalization. Object relations theorists hypothesize that as we develop, we internalize components of various caretakers and others in

═══ INDIVIDUAL AND CULTURAL HIGHLIGHT 5.1 ═══

## Coping with Cultural Countertransference

Pitfalls of countertransference are lurking everywhere. Imagine that you're a Vietnam War vet and therapist, and a Southeast Asian client comes to you for therapy. Unless you've done your personal work previously, you're likely to have a few reactions and issues to work through.

Countertransference is omnipresent (and tricky) because it can be triggered by so many different variables. Not only can you succumb to a client who behaves in ways similar to your domineering sister, but you can also overreact to clients who sound whiney or who are particularly handsome or particularly homely. Countertransference does not discriminate: We all can and will be affected by it.

As an example, the renowned group psychotherapist Irvin Yalom (1989) writes eloquently about his negative countertransference toward an obese client:

> Of course, I am not alone in my bias. Cultural reinforcement is everywhere. Who ever has a kind word for the fat lady? But my contempt surpasses all cultural norms. Early in my career, I worked in a maximum security prison where the *least* heinous offense committed by any of my patients was a simple, single murder. Yet I had little difficulty accepting those patients, attempting to understand them, and finding ways to be supportive.
>
> But when I see a fat lady eat, I move down a couple of rungs on the ladder of human understanding. I want to tear the food away. To push her face into the ice cream. "Stop stuffing yourself! Haven't you had enough, for Chrissakes?" I'd like to wire her jaws shut!
>
> Poor Betty—thank God, thank God—knew none of this as she innocently continued her course toward my chair, slowly lowered her body, arranged her folds and, with her feet not quite reaching the floor, looked up at me expectantly.

Your client's cultural background (or physical appearance) may trigger inappropriate countertransference reactions. These reactions may range from traditional discrimination ("I shouldn't expect much educational ambition from my American Indian or African American clients") to guilt and pity ("I need to be especially nice to minority clients because they've been so mistreated over the years") to competition ("Women and minorities are taking all the best jobs in psychology and now I'm stuck working with this militant Sri Lankan woman who's filing a sexual harassment suit against her employer").

There are many examples of cultural countertransference in the research literature. For example, a recent study showed that hospital staff in the United Kingdom are more likely to restrain patients from other races than they are to restrain patients from their own race (S. Lee et al., 2001). Similarly, mental health professionals from the United States have been found to overdiagnose psychotic disorders in patients of African American descent (M. Zuckerman, 2000).

As you read this section, you may find yourself wondering: "What's the difference between countertransference and racism?" That's an excellent question. What do you think the differences (and similarities) might be?

---

**Putting It in Practice 5.3**

## Identification and Internalization:
## Viewing Yourself as a Role Model

Although identification and internalization are concepts that emerge primarily in ongoing psychotherapy relationships, these concepts do have some practical relevance for beginning interviewers. We recommend that you explore the types of relationships and interpersonal behaviors you believe are important to the process of identification and internalization.

1. Think about yourself and whom you have chosen to emulate. Do you have conscious awareness of specific people whom you view as role models?
2. Why have you chosen those particular people?
3. What traits of your role models do you find most desirable?
4. Think about yourself and which traits and behaviors you have that clients might consciously or unconsciously adopt.
5. How do you feel about the fact that clients may be modeling themselves after you?

---

our early environment. These internalizations serve as the basis for how we feel about ourselves and how we interact with others (G. Adler, 1996; Fairbairn, 1952; Kernberg, 1976; Kohut, 1972, 1977; J. Watkins & Watkins, 1997). If we internalize "bad objects" (i.e., abusive parents, neglectful caretakers, vengeful siblings), we may experience disturbing self-perceptions and interpersonal relationships. Psychotherapy involves a relationship that can replace maladaptive or bad internalizations with more adaptive or good internalizations, derived from a relatively healthy psychotherapist. Strupp (1983) states: "[I have] stressed the importance of the patient's identification with the therapist, which occurs in all forms of psychotherapy. Since the internalization of 'bad objects' has made the patient 'ill,' therapy succeeds to the extent that the therapist becomes internalized as a 'good object'" (p. 481).

As Strupp (1983) points out, "Since the patient tends to remain loyal to early objects of his childhood, defending these internalizations against modification, therapy inevitably becomes a struggle" (p. 481). Therefore, identification and internalization processes are especially relevant in long-term psychotherapy cases, when interviewer-client contact is extensive. For clients to give up their loyalties to early childhood objects and develop new loyalties to more adaptive objects, longer term therapy may be required (see Putting It in Practice 5.3).

### Resistance

At times, we are at odds with our clients. We want them to talk about their life history, and they want to talk about their last trip to the mall, the Olympic games, or some other matter that seems distant or irrelevant. If clients are avoiding important topics, yet at the same time wanting the benefits of therapy, it is likely that resistance is occurring.

Some of the best examples of resistance come from the medical world. We avoid the dentist even though our tooth aches because we do not want to face the pain involved in drilling or extracting a tooth. We have physical aches, pains, lumps, bumps, or other symptoms, but we don't go to the physician. Perhaps we fear discovery of a disease, perhaps we fear the potential costs or treatment procedures (e.g., medicine, traction, surgery), or perhaps we simply don't recognize the severity of our symptoms. Whatever the case, we are engaging in resistance. Children provide excellent examples of resistance. They resist shots and bad-tasting medicine, even though they want to start feeling better.

Change is never easy. People need to proceed at their own pace and to feel safe as they take each step. Resistance often develops when change feels too difficult or too fast. Clients slow down, shut down, retreat, engage in meaningless chatter, cry incessantly, don't cry at all, or just drop out of therapy.

Like defense mechanisms, resistance is learned early in life and applied when feelings of fear or anxiety are present. Therefore, it is not easily overcome. A person must first recognize that resistance is occurring and then begin looking for why it has developed.

*Recognizing Resistance*

Recognizing behaviors that represent resistance is both simple and complex. It's simple because almost any behavior can represent resistance. Resistance may entail talking too little or too much. It can be manifest by focusing only on the present or by dwelling too much on the past. Recognizing resistance is complex for the same reason: Almost any specific behavior pattern, if engaged in excessively, can constitute resistance.

Weiner (1998) identifies five common forms of resistant behavior: "(a) reducing the amount of time spent in the treatment; (b) restricting the amount or range of conversation; (c) isolating the therapy from real life; (d) acting out; and (e) flight into health" (p. 178). *Reducing time spent in treatment* may consist of arriving late, leaving early, missing appointments, or terminating therapy prematurely. *Restricting conversation in therapy* occurs when clients avoid talking about or refuse to talk about certain topics. One young man we worked with adamantly refused to discuss any aspect of his past; this blatantly resistant behavior was extremely difficult to work through. *Isolating therapy from real life* occurs when clients deny or minimize the relevance therapy has for their lives (Wilkes, Belsher, Rush, & Frank, 1994). Examples of resistant *acting out* may involve client activities such as leaving a therapy session abruptly, calling the therapist at home, or behaving in a sexually or aggressive impulsive manner as a distraction from deeper issues. Finally, *flight into health* refers to times when clients suddenly and abruptly pronounce themselves healed. Of course, once *cured,* clients have no need for therapy or to explore personal issues.

*Managing Resistance*

With clients who are immediately resistant to counseling, slightly paradoxical, but caring, statements can help. For example, an interviewer might mention that it is quite common for people to feel frightened or reluctant about discussing personal topics and, therefore, it certainly is not necessary to take such a risk right away. This approach encourages oppositional clients to prove you wrong, and they may begin talking about more personal material. At the same time, clients realize that you understand how hard it is for them and may believe their reluctant feelings are normal. This belief, in turn, may reduce anxiety and thereby reduce resistance. A word of caution: Most paradoxical techniques are risky and require supervision.

Another method for dealing with resistance involves talking about the resistance itself, rather than trying to probe more deeply into underlying conflicts or anxieties (which often only exacerbates resistance). Psychoanalytic psychotherapists refer to this as *interpretation of defense.* For our purposes, it's sufficient to describe this process as "noticing" the resistance. For example, if resistance is manifest through discussion of irrelevant or inane topics, you may say, "I notice when we begin talking about how your relationship to your spouse might be making you more depressed, you usually begin talking about television shows, how this office is decorated, international issues, and anything but your relationship with your spouse." Sometimes, simply noticing resistance patterns, similar to a confrontation, encourages clients to examine their behavior and begin making constructive changes.

A third method for dealing with resistance involves discussing what makes resistance necessary. This approach is sometimes easier for clients, because you're backing away from the difficult issue itself. To use this technique, you could say, "Obviously, you don't want to talk about your father's death. So instead, let's just talk briefly about what makes it so hard to talk about." Or, you might engage the client by using a slightly projective technique: "What might happen if you did start talking about your father's death?" Clients may respond to such strategies by discounting the importance of the topic (e.g., "My father died two years ago; it isn't a big deal now."). Or, they may acknowledge that "talking about my dad's death makes me feel sad, and I don't want to feel that right now."

Sometimes, the most prudent approach is to avoid dealing with resistance during initial interviews. Especially if you are going to have further contact with a particular client, it may be best to simply make a mental note of when the client seems reluctant or resistant. You can always address it later.

One final point on resistance: Resistance should not be considered "bad" client behavior. In fact, research suggests that client resistance is an opportunity and that resistance, when worked through, becomes associated with positive treatment outcome (Mahalik, 2002). Additionally, we believe resistance emanates from the very center of a person and is part of the force that gives people stability and predictability in their interactions with others. Without resistance, we would change with each passing whim, ever at the mercy of those around us. Resistance exists because change and pain are often frightening and more difficult to face than retaining our old ways of being, even when the old ways are maladaptive. Finally, with culturally or developmentally different clients, resistance may actually be caused when the therapist refuses to make culturally or developmentally sensitive modifications in his or her approach (J. Sommers-Flanagan & Sommers-Flanagan, 1997).

## Working Alliance

Psychoanalytically oriented clinicians believe therapy involves the simultaneous development of three different relationships between therapist and client. These three relationships are (a) the transference relationship, (b) the real (human) relationship, and (c) the working alliance or therapeutic relationship.

The term *working alliance* was originally discussed by psychoanalytic theorists and refers to an explicit or implicit professional contract between client and interviewer (Greenson, 1965; Zetzel, 1956). More recently, the working (or therapeutic) alliance has become one of the most frequently studied concepts in counseling and psychotherapy (Constantino, Castonguay, & Schut, 2002). In summarizing the research literature, Constantino and associates offer this conclusion:

> Based on the current state of our empirical knowledge, it seems reasonable to say that regardless of the treatment approach (psychodynamic, cognitive-behavioral, gestalt, interpersonal, eclectic, drug counseling, or management), the length of therapy, the type of

problems presented by clients (depression, bereavement, anxiety, substance abuse, and so on), and the type of change aimed at (specific target complaints, symptom reduction, interpersonal functioning, general functioning, intrapsychic change and so on), therapists should make deliberate and systematic efforts to establish and maintain a good therapeutic alliance. (pp. 111–112)

Strupp (1983), among others, has pointed out that a client's ability to establish a therapeutic or working alliance is predictive of his or her potential to grow and change as a function of psychotherapy. In other words, if clients cannot or will not engage in a working alliance with an interviewer, there is little hope for change. Conversely, the more completely clients enter into such a relationship, the greater their chances for positive change (Krupnick et al., 1996; Raue, Castonguay, & Goldfried, 1993). Many researchers and theorists agree that, ironically, people's abilities to enter into productive relationships are determined in large part by the quality of their early interpersonal relations (Mallinckrodt, 1991). Therefore, unfortunately, those most in need of a curative relationship may be those least able to enter into one (Strupp, 1983).

Ainsworth's (1989) and Bowlby's (1969, 1988) work on attachment has been applied to components of the psychotherapy process. Specifically, as infants explore and learn from their environment, they venture away from their caretakers for short periods, returning from time to time for reassurance of safety, security, making sure they have not been abandoned by their caretakers. This venturing and returning is one mark of a secure, healthy attachment. Similar to a caretaker, a therapist provides a safe base from which clients can explore and to which they can return. In optimal situations, all of the relationship factors discussed in this chapter come into play to help interviewers serve as a safe base to which clients can return for comfort, support, and security.

## RELATIONSHIP VARIABLES AND BEHAVIORAL AND SOCIAL PSYCHOLOGY

Social and behavioral psychology has contributed significantly to our understanding of interviewer-client relationships. In particular, Stanley Strong (1968) identified three characteristics that make it more likely that clients will accept suggestions and recommendations put forth by their interviewers. These characteristics are expertness, attractiveness, and trustworthiness.

### Expertness (Credibility)

As Othmer and Othmer (1994) claim, empathy and compassion are important, but effective interviewers must also show expertise and establish authority. In other words, no matter how understanding and respectful you are of your client, at some point you must demonstrate that you're competent. Behaviorists generally refer to this as establishing credibility. Goldfried and Davison (1976) state, "The principle underlying this utilization technique is that it reinforces the client's perception of the . . . [therapist's] credibility" (p. 62). Clients generally want their interviewers to be competent and credible.

There are many ways that therapists can *look* credible, including:

- Displaying your credentials (e.g., certificates, licenses, diplomas) on office walls.
- Keeping shelves of professional books and journals in the office.

- Having an office arrangement conducive to open dialogue.
- Being professionally groomed and attired.

Specific interviewer *behaviors* also communicate expertise, credibility, and authority. Othmer and Othmer (1994) identify three strategies for showing expertise. First, they suggest that interviewers help clients put their problems in perspective. For example, you may reassure your clients that their problems, although unique, are similar to problems other clients have had that were successfully treated. Second, they recommend that interviewers show knowledge by communicating to clients a familiarity with their particular disorder. This strategy often involves naming the client's disorder (e.g., panic disorder, obsessive-compulsive disorder, dysthymia). Third, they note that interviewers need to deal effectively with their clients' distrust. For example, when clients express distrust by questioning your credentials, you should manage such challenges effectively.

Finally, when it comes to expertness, Cormier and Nurius (2003) express an appropriate warning: "Expertness is not in any way the same as being dogmatic, authoritarian, or one up. Expert helpers are those perceived as confident, attentive, and, because of background and behavior, capable of helping the client resolve problems and work toward goals" (p. 50).

## Attractiveness

With therapists, as with love, beauty is in the eye of the beholder. However, there are some standard features that most people view as attractive. Because of its subjective nature and the fact that self-awareness is an important attribute of effective clinical interviewers, we refer you to the activity included in Individual and Cultural Highlight 5.2. This activity helps you explore behaviors and characteristics you might find attractive if you went to a professional interviewer. Note that when we speak of what is attractive, we are referring not only to physical appearance but also to behaviors, attitudes, and personality traits.

## Trustworthiness

*Trust* is defined as "reliance on the integrity, strength, ability, surety, etc., of a person or thing; confidence" (Random House, 1993, p. 2031). Establishing trust is crucial to effective interviewing. S. Strong (1968) emphasized the importance of interviewers being perceived as trustworthy by their clients, finding that when interviewers are perceived as trustworthy, clients are more likely to believe what they say and follow their recommendations or advice.

It is not appropriate to express trustworthiness directly in an interview. Saying "trust me" to clients may be interpreted as a signal that they should be wary about trusting. As is the case with empathy and unconditional positive regard, trustworthiness is an interviewer characteristic that is best implied; clients infer it from interviewer behavior.

Perceptions of interviewer trustworthiness begin with initial client-interviewer contacts. These contacts may be over the telephone or during an initial greeting in the waiting room. The following interviewer behaviors are associated with trust:

- Initial introductions that are courteous, gentle, and respectful.
- Clear and direct explanations of confidentiality and its limits.

---

=== INDIVIDUAL AND CULTURAL HIGHLIGHT 5.2 ===

## Defining Interviewer Attractiveness

Attractiveness is an elusive concept, but being aware of our own values and of how we appear to others is invaluable in interviewer development. Reflect on the following questions:

1.  How you would like your interviewer to look? Would your ideal interviewer be male or female? How would he or she dress? What type of facial expressions would you like to see? Lots of smiles? Do you want an expressive interviewer? One with open body posture? A more serious demeanor? Imagine all sorts of details (e.g., use of makeup, type of shoes, length of hair).
2.  Now, think about what racial or ethnic or other individual characteristics you would like your interviewer to have? Do you want someone whose skin color is the same as yours? Do you want someone whose accent is just like yours? Would you wonder, if you had a counselor with an ethnic background different from your own, if that person could really understand you? How about your counselor's age or sexual orientation; would those characteristics matter to you?
3.  What types of technical interviewing responses would your attractive interviewer make? Would he or she use plenty of feeling reflections or be more directive (e.g., using plenty of confrontations or explanations)? Would he or she use lots of eye contact and "uh-huhs," or express attentiveness some other way?
4.  How would an attractive interviewer respond to your feelings? For example, if you started crying in a session, how would you like him or her to act and what would you like him or her to say?
5.  In your opinion, would an attractive interviewer touch you, self-disclose, call you by your first name, or stay more distant and focus on analyzing your thoughts and feelings during the session?

Ask these same questions of a fellow student or a friend or family member. Although you may find initially that you and your friends or family don't seem to have specific criteria for what constitutes interviewer attractiveness, after discussion, people usually discover that they have stronger opinions than they originally thought. Be sure to ask fellow students of racial/ethnic backgrounds, ages, and sexual orientations different from yours about their ideally attractive therapist.

---

- Acknowledgment of difficulties associated with coming to a professional therapist (e.g., Othmer and Othmer's [1994] "putting the patient at ease").
- Manifestations of congruence, unconditional positive regard, and empathy.
- Punctuality and general professional behavior.

With clients who are very resistant to counseling (e.g., involuntary clients), it is often helpful to state outright that the client may have trouble trusting the therapist. For example:

"I can see you're not happy to be here. That's often the case when people are forced to attend counseling. So, right from the beginning, I want you to know I don't expect you to trust me or like being here. However, because we'll be working together, it's up to you to decide how much trust to put in me and in this counseling. Also, I might add, just because you're required to be here doesn't mean you're required to have a bad time."

Throughout counseling relationships, clients periodically test their interviewers (Fong & Cox, 1983; Horowitz et al., 1984). In a sense, clients "set up" their interviewers to determine whether they are trustworthy. For example, children who have been sexually abused often immediately behave seductively when they meet an interviewer; they may sit in your lap, rub up against you, or tell you they love you. Left alone with an interviewer for the first time, some abused children even ask the interviewer to undress. These behaviors can be viewed as blatant tests of interviewer trustworthiness (i.e., the behaviors ask, "Are you going to abuse me, too?"). It is important for therapists to recognize tests of trust and to respond, when possible, in ways that enhance the trust relationship.

## FEMINIST RELATIONSHIP VARIABLES

Feminist theory and psychotherapy emphasize the importance of establishing an egalitarian relationship between client and interviewer (L. Brown & Brodsky, 1992; Warwick, 1999). The type of egalitarian relationship preferred by feminist interviewers is one characterized by mutuality and empowerment.

### Mutuality

*Mutuality* refers to a sharing process; it means that power, decision making, goal selection, and learning are shared. Although various psychotherapy orientations (especially person-centered) consider treatment a mutual process wherein clients and therapists are open and human with one another, nowhere are egalitarian values and the concept of mutuality emphasized more than in feminist theory and therapy (Birch & Miller, 2000; Nutt, Hampton, Folks, & Johnson, 1990).

The following example illustrates this concept:

### CASE EXAMPLE

*Betty, a 25-year-old graduate student, comes in for an initial interview. The interviewer's supervisor has urged the interviewer to stay neutral and to resist any urge toward self-disclosure. The interviewer says, "Tell me about what brings you in at this time." Betty begins crying almost immediately and says, "My mother is dying of cancer. She lives two hundred miles away but wants me there all the time. I'm finishing my PhD in chemistry and my dissertation chair is going on sabbatical in three months. I have two undergraduate courses to teach, and my husband just told me he's thinking of leaving me. I don't know what to do. I don't know how to prioritize. I feel like I'm disappearing. There's hardly anything left of me. I'm afraid. I feel like a failure being in therapy, but . . ." Betty cries a while longer.*

*The interviewer feels the overwhelming sadness, fear, and confusion of these situations. She is tempted to cry herself. She works hard, internally, to think of something appropriately neutral to say. After just a slight pause, in a kind voice, she says, "All of these things leave you feeling diminished, afraid, perhaps like you're losing a sense of who you are. Being in therapy adds to the sense of defeat." Betty says, "Yes, my mother always said therapists were for weak folks. Her term was* addle-brained. *My husband refuses to see anyone. He thinks if I stay home and drop this education thing, we could be happy together again. Sometimes I feel that even my dissertation chair would be happier if I just gave it up."*

*The interviewer responds, "The important people in your life somehow want you to do things differently than you are doing."*

Although the preceding interactions are acceptable, if both Betty and the interviewer stay with this modality, Betty would finish knowing very little about her therapist and she would feel, generally, that the therapist was the provider of insight, and she, Betty, was the provider of problems.

In a more mutuality-oriented interaction, when the interviewer feels overwhelming sadness, fear, and confusion, she might say, "Wow, Betty. Those are some *very* difficult situations. Just hearing about all that makes me feel a little bit of what you must be feeling—sad and overwhelmed." Betty might then say, "Yes. I feel both. It's nice to have you glimpse that. See, my mom says counseling is a waste of time. My husband thinks I'm too busy outside the home . . . and I even get the same message from my dissertation chair." The interviewer might then say, "Yeah. It's hard to decide to get into therapy, or to even keep going when those close to you disapprove of your choices."

The differences in responses may not seem huge, but the underlying framework of the interviewer-client relationship being built in mutuality-oriented therapies contrasts sharply with traditional frameworks. The client is not excluded from the interviewer's emotional reactions. She is not given the message that she is the bearer of problems and the interviewer is the bearer of insights or cures. Instead, the groundwork is laid for a relationship that includes honest self-disclosure on the interviewer's part and that may, later in therapy, even include times when the client observes and comments on patterns in the interviewer's behavior. In a mutuality-oriented relationship, interviewers and therapists are ready to respond to such offers from clients in a genuine manner that neither merely reflects client statements nor interprets them as coming from client pathological needs (L. Brown, 1994).

When interviewers engage in mutuality, they usually do so for the ultimate purpose of empowering clients. Their clients see therapy as a working relationship in which they are equal members rather than subordinates. Although mutuality does not entirely alter the fact that a certain amount of authority must rest with the counselor (Buck, 1999), the feminist interviewer actively works to teach clients to respond to authority with a sense of personal worth and with their own personal authority. Feminist therapists believe that respectful, reciprocal interactions can result in a growing sense of personal power in clients.

## Empowerment

Most therapies have as underlying goals the development, growth, and health of clients. However, therapies vary in the routes they take to reach these goals; and, therefore, different approaches inevitably leave clients with different beliefs as to how they "got better." The interviewer who begins therapy with an emphasis on authenticity and mutuality usually hopes that clients attribute their gains, growth, and life improvements to their own efforts and to the strength and potential residing within them. Rather than set up relationship rules that separate client from therapist along the lines of dependency/neediness versus authority/expertise, the interviewer interested in empowerment affirms that both participants in the therapy process are human and therefore more similar than different.

Interviewers have skills and knowledge that clients may not have; in feminist therapy, these skills are viewed as tools clients can avail themselves of to help themselves grow. Clients understand that there are no magical formulas and no authority figures to instruct them, to be obeyed, or to offer mysterious insights previously unavailable. Instead, interviewers interact in ways that validate their clients' life experiences and attempts at solving their own problems. Interviewers recognize that often, people come to therapy in part because of the pressures, discrimination, and mistreatment we all experience in varying degrees as we interact in society. These experiences of disenfranchisement are acknowledged for what they are rather than interpreted as something intrapsychically askew in the client.

Beginning in 1911, Alfred Adler established himself as an early feminist theorist and spoke articulately about issues associated with empowerment:

> All our institutions, our traditional attitudes, our laws, our morals, our customs, give evidence of the fact that they are determined and maintained by privileged males for the glory of male domination. (Adler, 1927, p. 123)

Adler's assertion points out a key issue in feminist theory. That is, pathological conditions among women are often constructed and sustained by social-political factors (Olson, 2000). Consequently, the concept of empowerment for a feminist involves consciousness-raising among oppressed groups (especially women) and encourages them to stand up and claim their personal power.

Initially, incorporating mutuality, authenticity, and empowerment into the interviewing relationship may be threatening to interviewers. Doing so is an advanced skill. It requires knowing how to be authentic without burdening the client, and it requires being able to welcome and enhance a sense of mutuality while maintaining enough control so that hope for change via therapy is not lost. Finally, it requires having the patience and wisdom to allow clients to find their own way, thus empowering them, rather than issuing edicts on how to become empowered.

## INTEGRATING RELATIONSHIP VARIABLES

The relationship variables discussed in this chapter are not an exhaustive list. You may have noticed that we did not discuss relationship variables derived from many different therapeutic approaches including gestalt, choice theory (reality therapy), solution-oriented, cognitive, and others. Instead, due to space limitations we focused primarily on theoretical perspectives that emphasize relationship variables as curative factors in counseling and psychotherapy.

Because the variables discussed are advocated by different schools of thought, it should not be surprising that some of the variables contradict one another. For example, although mutuality and expertness are not exact opposites, greater interviewer expertness is usually associated with less interviewer-client mutuality.

The purpose of this chapter is to enhance your awareness of important relationship variables, rather than convince you that a single type of therapeutic relationship is preferred. We believe person-centered, feminist, solution-oriented, and cognitive-behavioral-oriented interviewers should all be sensitive to potential transference, countertransference, and other reactions within sessions. Similarly, psychoanalytic interviewers enhance their effectiveness if they are attentive to issues involving congruence, empathy, and empowerment.

## SUMMARY

The early work of Carl Rogers (1942, 1951, 1961) articulated the importance of relationship variables in psychotherapy. Similarly, clinical interviewing is characterized, to some degree, by the formation of a special type of relationship between interviewer and client.

Rogers identified three core conditions he believed were necessary and sufficient for personal growth and development to occur: congruence, unconditional positive regard, and accurate empathy. Congruence is synonymous with genuineness or authenticity and generally means the interviewer is open and real with clients. However, it is inappropriate for interviewers to be completely congruent or authentic with clients all of the time because the purpose of counseling is to facilitate the client's (and not the therapist's) growth. Similar to congruence, unconditional positive regard and accurate empathy are complex relationship variables that, for the most part, must be communicated indirectly to clients.

Several relationship variables derived from interpersonal and psychoanalytic theories influence the clinical interview process. These include, but are not limited to, transference, countertransference, identification, internalization, resistance, and the working alliance. Further reading and supervised clinical experience is needed before interviewers should be expected to understand and effectively manage these particular relationship variables. Beginning interviewers should strive to recognize and discuss situations where these factors appear to be affecting the therapeutic process.

Behavioral and social psychologists also have examined interviewing processes and identified several variables associated with effective interviewing and counseling. Specifically, interviewers viewed as credible experts who are personally and professionally attractive and trustworthy are generally more influential therapists. Interviewers can appear and behave in ways that lead clients to view them as highly expert, attractive, and trustworthy.

Finally, feminist theorists and psychotherapists emphasize the importance of establishing egalitarian relationships between interviewers and clients, incorporating the concepts of mutuality and empowerment. They believe open, mutual relationships facilitate therapeutic processes and help empower clients to be their own advocates and to attribute their growth to the power that resides in themselves. Feminists generally consider social oppression to be a large contributor to client psychopathology and work to empower clients to stand up and claim their personal power.

The relationship variables described in this chapter are both diverse and similar. It is a challenge for interviewers of all theoretical orientations to do their best to integrate these divergent relationship factors into the clinical interview.

## SUGGESTED READINGS AND RESOURCES

Fong, M. L., & Cox, B. G. (1983). Trust as an underlying dynamic in the counseling process: How clients test trust. *Personnel and Guidance Journal, 62,* 163–166. This article lists and describes six common ways that clients test their counselors' trust.

Greenson, R. R. (1965). The working alliance and the transference neurosis. *Psychoanalytic Quarterly, 34,* 155–181. This article presents Greenson's classic discussion of the working alliance.

Miller, J. B. (1986). *Toward a new psychology of women* (2nd ed.). Boston: Beacon. Jean Baker Miller's classic discussion of the psychology of women is crucial reading for interviewers interested in the feminist perspective.

Olson, M. E. (2000). *Feminism, community, and communication.* Binghamton, NY: Haworth Press. This edited volume contains nine essays and an interview with a family therapist trainer. It emphasizes the social construction of identity and examines the contribution of the dominant U.S. culture.

Rogers, C. R. (1961). *On becoming a person.* Boston: Houghton-Mifflin. This text contains much of Rogers's thinking regarding congruence, unconditional positive regard, and empathy.

Wilkinson, S., & Kitzinger, C. (Eds.). (1996). *Representing the other: A feminism and psychology reader.* London: Sage. This book explores when and how we should represent members of groups to which we ourselves do not belong. Discussions include when and how to represent diverse groups such as children, prostitutes, gay men with HIV/AIDS, and infertile women.

Worell, J. & Johnson, N. G. (Eds.). (1997). *Shaping the future of feminist psychology: Education, research, and practice.* Washington, DC: American Psychological Association. This edited volume provides an in-depth review of feminist perspectives on research, supervision, assessment, and training in feminist therapy.

# PART THREE

# STRUCTURING AND ASSESSMENT

# Chapter 6

# *AN OVERVIEW OF THE INTERVIEW PROCESS*

*It is good to have an end to journey toward; but it is the journey that matters, in the end.*
—Ursula K. Le Guin, *The Left Hand of Darkness*

---

### CHAPTER OBJECTIVES

Every interview has a flow or pattern. Even when interviewers decide to be completely nondirective and let the client free associate during an entire session, there is a beginning, a middle, and an end to the interview process. In this chapter, we examine the structure of a typical clinical interview; we take a close look at how interviews typically begin, proceed, and end, and how you can smoothly integrate many essential activities into a single clinical hour. After reading this chapter, you will know:

- Common structural models—or ways to describe what happens during the course of a clinical interview—identified in the literature.
- How to handle the introduction stage of an interview, including phone contact, initial meetings, rapport development, putting clients at ease, using small talk, and providing clients with information about what to expect during an interview.
- How to handle the interview's opening stage, including your opening statements and the client's opening response.
- How to handle information-gathering and assessment tasks associated with the body stage of an interview.
- General methods for evaluating client psychopathology.
- How to handle the closing stage of an interview, including how to reassure and support clients; how to summarize crucial issues and themes; how to instill hope in, guide, and empower clients; and how to tie up loose ends before ending a session.
- How to handle the termination stage of an interview, including time boundaries, guiding termination, and dealing with feelings about the end of the session.

---

The clinical interview cannot and should not be an interaction that runs along a prescribed path from point A to point B. True, we can dissect the interview into components, and, in fact, we do so in this book; but in the end, each interview involves at least two unique human beings, interacting with and responding to each other. This guarantees that no two interviews are ever the same.

Learning to conduct an effective interview shares many commonalities with learning other new skills, such as dancing or driving an automobile. This is particularly true when it comes to structural components of an interview. Most beginning interviewers rigidly conform to taking the proper step at the proper time. For example, as an interviewer, you may find yourself thinking, "I need to establish rapport here. . . . Now it is time to elicit information. . . . Time to prepare for closing." In contrast, experienced interviewers gather information, maintain rapport, and begin dealing with closure all at the same time. But they didn't begin their careers with such an ability (Tracey, Hays, Malone, & Herman, 1988).

Human interactions are guided by spoken and unspoken rules that depend on variables such as setting, purpose, individual differences, and cultural differences. For the most part, humans are not conscious of sequences involved as they negotiate their way through the day. We do not sit down and analyze each step; we just move smoothly through the routines of getting to work or going to the laundromat or attending a surprise party. When meeting someone, we generally know when to say what and when to stand or sit or offer a hand for a handshake. But this ease, established after much repetition, did not always exist. For everything from laundromat behavior to social interaction, we have learned effective, efficient steps through observation, trial and error, feedback, and specific instructions.

This chapter clarifies the rhythm and unspoken rules of the clinical interview. Our purpose is to provide a road map for conducting interviews so that you are more comfortable with the continuity of this unique 50-minute hour. If you know and feel comfortable with these rules, you expend less energy contemplating what is next and more energy on understanding, evaluating, and helping your clients.

Although the interviewing structure presented here primarily illustrates how typical assessment interviews proceed, it also has implications pertaining to psychotherapy or counseling sessions. Therapy sessions proceed in a similar manner. The major difference is that the *body* of a therapy interview naturally involves the application of therapy interventions, rather than information gathering (see the next section).

## STRUCTURAL MODELS

Just as many professional and social interactions have a normal, implicit sequence, ritual, or set of phases, so does the clinical interview. Shea (1998) identifies these phases as:

1. The introduction.
2. The opening.
3. The body.
4. The closing.
5. The termination.

Shea's five-part format is helpful partly because it enlarges on the more common "beginning, middle, and end" schema sometimes referred to in training texts (Benjamin, 1987). Shea's model also remains generic and atheoretical; it may be applied to virtually all interviewing situations. This chapter outlines and discusses tasks and potential pitfalls associated with each interview phase.

In adopting Shea's (1998) format, we are not implying that his format is universally endorsed by all clinical interviewers. Other models are worth mentioning. For example,

Foley and Sharf (1981) identify five sequential interviewer duties or activities common to an interview:

1. Putting the patient at ease.
2. Eliciting information.
3. Maintaining control.
4. Maintaining rapport.
5. Bringing closure.

Like all models in the literature, Foley and Sharf's model has many similarities to Shea's model.

One of the more descriptive stage approaches to interview structure has been described by A. Ivey & Ivey (1999), who also identifies five stages or components in a typical clinical interview:

1. Establishing rapport and structuring.
2. Gathering information, defining the problem, and identifying assets.
3. Determining outcomes (setting goals).
4. Exploring alternatives and confronting client incongruities.
5. Encouraging generalization of ideas and skills to situations outside therapy.

As you compare the models presented, you probably notice similarity but not complete uniformity among them. In part, this reflects the fact that interviewers and clients vary in their approaches and responses to clinical interviews; each has an individual sense of timing and propriety.

The astute interviewer initially allows clients to set the pace as much as possible because observing this process yields valuable information to the interviewer. Being allowed to set the pace also provides clients with a sense of control and safety; they do not feel rushed from stage to stage. Ideally, interviewers guide clients gently forward through the interview, allowing them to rush through or linger on a given point. The interviewer is responsible for managing the essential elements of a good interview, seeing that it does not run overtime, and ensuring it covers what is necessary, given the setting and expectations. However, the less overtly and rigidly this responsibility is exercised, the better. Be organized and attentive to interview structure while remaining flexible.

## THE INTRODUCTION

Shea (1998) defines the introduction phase as follows: "The introduction begins when the clinician and the patient first see one another. It ends when the clinician feels comfortable enough to begin an inquiry into the reasons the patient has sought help" (p. 58). The introduction phase of an interview involves mainly "putting the patient at ease" (see Foley & Sharf, 1981; Othmer & Othmer, 1994; Chapter 4 of this text) or, as Shea words it, "decreasing the patient's anxiety" (p. 58).

### Telephone Contact

In some situations, the introduction phase actually begins before you see the client. You may set up your initial appointment with the client by telephone. Whether you do this yourself or a receptionist makes the call, be aware that the therapeutic relationship begins with the initial contact. The phone call, the paperwork, and the clarity and warmth with which clients are greeted can put them at ease or confuse and intimidate.

Interviewers vary greatly in how they inform clients of financial arrangements, session lengths, and intake procedures. Some leave these duties to trained office personnel. Some provide the information in written form. Others go over it verbally with the client before the first session. Still others give this information during the interview. The important point is that first contact, whether via mail, phone, questionnaire, or in person, directly affects your relationship with clients.

The following brief transcript illustrates a typical initial telephone contact:

**Interviewer:** "Hello, I'm trying to reach Bob Johnson."

**Client:** "That's me."

**Interviewer:** "Bob, this is Chelsea Brown. I'm a therapist at the University Counseling Center. I understand you might be interested in counseling, and I'm calling to see if you'd like to set up an appointment."

**Client:** "Yeah, that's right. I filled out a questionnaire, so I guess that's where you got my number."

**Interviewer:** "Right. If you're still interested in coming for counseling, we should set up a time to meet. Do you have particular days and times that work best for you?"

**Client:** "I guess Tuesday or Thursday afternoons look best . . . after 2 P.M., but before 6 P.M."

**Interviewer:** "How about this Thursday, the 24th, at 4 P.M.?"

**Client:** "Sounds fine to me."

**Interviewer:** "I guess since you were in the counseling center to fill out a questionnaire, you know how to find the center."

**Client:** "Yep. So, do I just go to the same building?"

**Interviewer:** "Yes. Just be sure to check in with the receptionist when you arrive. In fact, you might want to come a few minutes early. The receptionist will give you a few forms to fill out and that way you can finish them before we start meeting at 4. Is that okay?"

**Client:** "Sure, no problem."

**Interviewer:** "Okay, then, I guess we're all set. I'll look forward to meeting you on Thursday, the 24th, at 4 P.M."

**Client:** "Okay, see you then."

Note several points in this dialogue. First, scheduling the initial appointment is a collaborative activity—hopefully the first of many—that occurs between interviewer and client. This activity begins the working alliance. It can be very difficult to schedule an appointment with some clients, perhaps because of the common problem of finding a meeting time for two busy people or perhaps because of client rigidity, resistance, or ambivalence about coming for counseling. The preceding dialogue illustrates a simple, straightforward scheduling experience. Such is not always the case. It is important to be very clear about your available times for meeting with clients before initiating the phone call.

Second, the interviewer clearly identifies herself, her status (i.e., therapist), and her place of employment. Depending on the situation, you may want to be even clearer about these facts. For example, when students in our upper-level interviewing courses contact volunteers, the students say something like, "I'm a student in Psych 455, and I received your name and number from Dr. Baxter."

Third, the interviewer checks to make sure the client knows how to get to the interview location. If you are calling a new client and there is a possibility the client does not know how to reach the interviewing office, you should prepare clear directions before making the call. Some agencies even provide a map.

Fourth, the interviewer asks the potential client what days and times would be best for him. If your schedule is particularly busy, you may want to first identify days and times when you have openings. Whatever the case, it is not necessary to disclose specific information about why you cannot meet at a particular time. For example, do not say, "Oh, I can't meet then because I have to pick up my daughter from school" or "I'm in class then." Such disclosures are unnecessary and provide too much personal information for an initial telephone contact. Especially at first, it is better to say little to clients about your personal background.

Fifth, the interviewer closes by repeating the appointment time and noting that she is looking forward to meeting the client. She also clarifies exactly what the client should do when arriving at the center (i.e., check in with the receptionist). Avoid saying things like, "Check in with the receptionist and I'll be right out to meet you," because you do not know when the client will arrive. If he arrives 25 minutes early, you are stuck—either you meet him 25 minutes early or you end up not following through with what you said over the telephone.

Overall, be well prepared when making initial telephone contact with potential clients. You may want to practice telephone conversations in class or with a supportive friend or family member. If you have done your homework, you will be more able to focus on how clients present themselves and on the task of working together to schedule an appointment.

## Initial Face-to-Face Meeting

Privacy is important to consider when first meeting clients. Most clinics and agencies have public waiting rooms with seating for more than one person at a time. It is more difficult to keep a client's identity anonymous in these settings than in the surroundings maintained by single clinicians in private practice. Therefore, it is incumbent on interviewers who work in relatively public settings to consider how they can best respect their clients' privacy. A favorite option involves having the receptionist point out or describe a new client so you can walk up and say the client's name in a quiet, friendly voice, not easily overheard by others in the room. Then smile and introduce yourself. In such a scenario, you can quickly assess whether the client might welcome a handshake; if so, offer a hand and simply say, "Come back this way," and lead the client to the private consulting office.

Many issues are associated with first impressions. You need to be aware of how much hinges on first impressions and how much information you gain by being especially observant of your client's behavior during the first few moments of your meeting. It is likely that clients will be nervous, although some may be excited, some may be angry, and some might appear quite nonchalant, as if they could not care less about seeing a therapist.

Assuming your new client is nervous, you have an excellent opportunity to observe how he or she expresses nervousness. Is he or she quiet? Loud? Smoking or clinging to a coffee cup? Chewing his or her nails or lip? Formal, informal, talkative, withdrawn, pale, or flushed? These are observations you can use to begin to form your composite impression of the client. The initial meeting may give you a sense of how your client deals with anxiety and stress.

As you observe your client's behavior, your client is simultaneously sizing up you and the situation. To increase the consistency of client perceptions, some professionals always follow an introductory ritual that includes some or all of the following:

1. Shaking hands.
2. Offering something to drink.
3. Chatting about the weather or another neutral subject as they go to the private interviewing room.

A standard greeting ritual can be comforting and can free you to be more observant. Standardization strengthens your ability to make inferences from your observations (see Putting It in Practice 6.1). You can design your greeting ritual to reflect a warm, welcoming, professional image. Not every interviewer uses a standardized ritual, how- ever. Many interviewers never establish an exact routine; they like to size up clients in- dividually and offer whatever seems to be called for. Sometimes, this is a firm hand- shake and/or comforting social banter. On other occasions, less contact and less informal verbal exchange seem wiser.

This leads to the issue of how to address your clients. The first rule in addressing clients is to go with the "base rates" (i.e., the known norm for the group of which the client is a part). For example, when you're meeting with a middle-aged or older male, it is a safe bet that he will be comfortable being addressed as "Mr." Later, when you sit down in the room with your client, if you are not sure whether you have addressed him in a proper manner, ask how he prefers to be addressed.

Other groups have less clear base rates. For example, women over 30 may strongly prefer being referred to as "Ms." rather than "Mrs." or vice versa, so it is difficult to know in advance which to try. "Ms." may offend fewer women under 40 than "Mrs.," but you may choose to go with the woman's entire name: "Are you Susan Smith?" If you sense you have used the wrong strategy, check with your client and correct yourself and apologize ("Would you prefer I call you Mrs. Smith? Okay. Sorry about that. I wasn't sure how you wanted to be greeted."). The effort to address clients as they want to be addressed communicates respect and acceptance.

The second rule of addressing clients is: When in doubt, choose the least potentially offensive or more formal alternative. Addressing a woman over 40 by first and last name is an example of a least offensive alternative. Another example, this time with re- gard to shaking hands, is to wait until the client either reaches out for your hand or simply stands up and begins moving toward your office. Waiting for the client to reach forward helps avoid trying to shake hands with people who prefer not to.

## Establishing Rapport

*Rapport* is a generic relationship variable. Interviewers of all theoretical orientations acknowledge the importance of having good rapport with clients. However, rapport has probably been popularized more by behavioral, humanistic, and feminist clinicians than by psychoanalytically oriented psychotherapists. Positive *rapport* is defined as ". . . connection, especially harmonious or sympathetic relation" (Random House, 1993, p. 1601).

=== **Putting It in Practice 6.1** ===

## Standardized Introductions

In some ways, it's best to use a standardized introduction procedure with all clients, because the more consistent you are, the more certain you can be that individual differences in how clients present themselves reflect actual differences in personality styles. If you vary your introduction routine based on your mood or other factors, client reactions may vary, based on differences in your approach to them. In other words, differences in their reactions to you may represent something about you, rather than something about them. Standardization is a part of good psychological science. If you have a standard approach, you increase the reliability, and possibly the validity, of your observations.

On the other hand, as an interviewer, you do not want to be mechanistic or ingenuine in your approach to clients. A strictly standardized approach probably comes across to clients as ingenuine or distant. Similarly, it's important to respond not only to each client's unique individual characteristics, but also to typical differences found in social or cultural groups. For example, the same introductory approach would usually not be equally effective with male adolescents and female senior citizens. Individuals in these two groups usually have significantly different styles of relating to others. To assume you can treat them identically during the introduction phase of an interview is a mistake. Keep in mind that the introductory phase is crucial to establishing rapport with clients. Excessive standardization may adversely affect rapport. When dealing with different individuals in the introductory phase of an interview, you should follow two general guidelines:

• Go with the base rates.
• Choose the least offensive alternative.

Some beginning interviewers are put off by the fact that standardization and routine are part of the interviewing process. After all, we're dealing with unique individuals, and shouldn't we give each one a unique and human response? Our answer to that question is no and yes. No, it is not necessary to give each client a unique or different response just for the sake of avoiding ritual or consistency. And yes, we should give each client a human response.

For example, we usually begin first sessions with a description of the limits of confidentiality and a discussion of how an initial interview is sometimes uncomfortable because it involves two strangers getting to know each other. Although this is part of a standardized introduction, we sincerely mean what we're saying every time; we genuinely want each client to understand the concept of confidentiality and its limits. Simply because we say virtually the same statement to hundreds of clients does not mean we're operating on auto-pilot.

A balance between standardization and flexibility is best. Be consistent and yet genuine. Deviate from your standard routine when it seems clinically appropriate and not just when the mood strikes you.

Effective interviewers take specific steps to establish good rapport with their clients. Many technical responses discussed in Chapter 3 are associated with developing rapport (e.g., paraphrase, reflection of feeling, and feeling validation). Othmer and Othmer (1994) outline six strategies for developing good rapport:

1. Put the patient and yourself at ease.
2. Find the suffering; show compassion.
3. Assess insight; become an ally.
4. Show expertise.
5. Establish authority.
6. Balance the roles.

## Common Client Fears

Clients have many fears and doubts when first consulting a therapist or counselor. It is impossible to address them all in an initial session; establishing the rapport necessary to make clients comfortable working with you is an involved process (G. Weinberg, 1984). On the other hand, interviewers can begin rapport-building by acknowledging and sensitively addressing their clients' fears. Common client concerns and doubts follow (adapted from Othmer & Othmer, 1994; Pipes & Davenport, 1990; Wolberg, 1995):

Is this professional competent?
More important, can this person help *me?*
Will this person understand me and my problems?
Am I going crazy?
Can I trust this person to be honest with me?
Will this interviewer share or reject my values (or religious views)?
Will I be pressured to say things I don't want to say?
Will this interviewer think I am a bad person?

Interviewers can intimidate clients. It might be difficult for you to imagine yourself as an authority figure, but the truth is, power and authority reside in the mental health professional role. As you continue studying mental health, you will become an authority—a master of a certain knowledge base.

No matter what your theoretical orientation, you will be perceived by clients as an authority figure. Clients may believe they should act in a manner similar to the way they act around other authority figures, such as physicians and teachers. In addition, they may expect you to behave as previous authority figures in their lives have behaved. This can range from warm, caring, wise, and helpful, to harsh, cold, and rejecting. Because clients come into counseling with both conscious and unconscious assumptions about authority figures, you may need to help your client view you as a partner in the therapeutic process.

## Putting the Client at Ease

Putting clients at ease partly involves convincing them you are a "different kind" of authority figure. You must encourage new clients to be interactive, to ask questions, and to be open; these are behaviors they may have avoided with previous authority figures.

After explaining confidentiality to clients (see Chapters 2 and 5), you may wish to use a statement similar to the following:

"Counseling is a unique situation. We're strangers—I don't know you, and you don't know me. So this first meeting is a chance for us to get to know each other better. My goal is to understand whatever's concerning you. Sometimes I'll just listen, and other times I'll ask you some questions. This first session is also a chance for you to see how I work with people in counseling and whether that feels comfortable to you. If you have questions at any time, feel free to ask them."

This introduction may seem long, but it usually serves to put clients at ease. It acknowledges the fact that interviewers and clients are initially strangers and gives the client permission to evaluate the interviewer and ask questions about therapy.

### Conversation and Small Talk

Othmer and Othmer (1994) consider introduction, conversation, and initial informal chatting as methods to help put clients at ease. These efforts may involve the following:

- "You must be Steven Green." (initial greeting)
- "Do you like to be called Steven, Steve, or Mr. Green?" (clarifying how the client would like to be addressed, or how to correctly pronounce his name)
- "Were you able to find the office (or a place to park) easily?" (small talk and empathic concern)
- "Where are you originally from?" (Geographical origin is usually a safe place to start an interview; this question can be answered successfully and may allow for interviewer comment regarding what it was like to have been from a particular place.)
- (with children or adolescents) "I see you've got a Los Angeles Lakers hat on. You must be a Lakers fan." (small talk; an attempt to connect with the client's world)

Chatting is often held to a minimum with adult clients, unless they are uncooperative and resistant, in which case it may constitute your primary interviewing technique. On the other hand, as we discuss more thoroughly in Chapter 10, initial casual conversation can easily make or break an interview with a child or adolescent. Many interviews with young people succeed primarily because at the beginning of the first session, you take time to discuss with the child his or her views on television shows, race cars, favorite foods, music groups, sports teams, and so on. Similarly, in interviews with adolescents or preadolescents, we sometimes discuss what slang words are "in" and how to use them appropriately (e.g., "Now I want to make sure I'm using the right words here. When something is really good, what do you call it? Is it cool, bad, fresh, or sweet?").

Interviewers who are good at putting clients at ease are usually warm, sensitive, and flexible. They sense client discomfort by reading signals. For example, they may notice a client chooses a distant chair in the interviewing room or, conversely, that a client sits too close and seems to intrude on the interviewer's personal space. Flexible interviewers respect clients' interpersonal styles; they do not insist that a client sit in a particular chair or at a certain distance. They try to speak the client's nonverbal language.

A number of small talk topics are relatively safe and nonjudgmental and put clients at ease. These include the weather, recent news events, sporting event outcomes, whether the client was able to locate the office easily, and parking availability. However, even comments about the weather may not be without "baggage" in terms of meaning.

Some topics commonly discussed in social situations are not good interview small talk. For example, comments on adult clients' clothing can seem innocuous, but may be interpreted as judgmental, parental, or overly personal. After you're well acquainted with a client, a change in clothing style may be useful therapy material. Initially, especially with adults, it's wise to avoid comments on clothing, hair style, perfume, or jewelry. With younger clients, this guideline changes somewhat (see Chapter 11).

In addition, comments regarding similarities between you and your client usually are not warranted, as such comments may be based on your own social needs and not on the client's therapy needs. In social situations, it is common to share and compare ages of offspring, marital status, likes and dislikes of food, exercise, political figures, common places of origin, and so on. You may feel an urge, on seeing the husband of your client holding a toddler, to say something like, "We have a little one at home, too" or "Our little girl likes that same Sesame Street book." If your client is carrying a bike helmet, you may feel tempted to say, "I commute on my bike, too." Again, interviewing is not a simple social situation. Although you must try to put your client at ease and present a warm, reassuring image, you must do so through a rather narrow selection of comments and actions. We do not mean to say that interviewers should never mention similarities between themselves and their clients. We simply mean that interviewers should restrain themselves from acting on their initial social urges or impulses because following through on every social urge or impulse is often not the most therapeutically effective approach (see Putting It in Practice 6.1). For example, Weiner (1998) states:

> Just as a patient will have difficulty identifying the real person in a therapist who hides behind a professional facade and never deviates from an impersonal stance, so too he will see as unreal a therapist who ushers him into the office for a first visit saying, "Hi, my name is Fred, and I'm feeling a little anxious because you remind me of a fellow I knew in college who always made me feel I wasn't good enough to compete with him." (p. 28)

### Educating Clients and Evaluating Their Expectations

Final introductory phase tasks involve client education and evaluation of client expectations. Several rules apply. First, clients should be informed of confidentiality and its limits. This process should be simple, straightforward, and interactive. You should be clear about the concept of confidentiality before beginning an interview so you can explain it clearly (see Chapter 2). You should check with clients to determine if they understand confidentiality. A conversation similar to the following is recommended:

**Interviewer:** "Have you heard of the term *confidentiality* before?"
**Client:** "Uh, I think so."
**Interviewer:** "Well, let me briefly describe what counselors mean by confidentiality. Basically, it means what you say in here stays in here. It means what you talk about with me is private; I won't be casually discussing the information with other people. However, there are some limits to confidentiality. For example, if you talk about harming yourself or someone else or if you talk about child or elder abuse, then I have to break confidentiality and inform the proper authorities. Also, if you want me to provide information about you to another person, such as an attorney, insurance company, or physician, I can do that if you give me your written permission. So, although there are some limits, basi-

cally what you say in here is private. Do you have any questions about confidentiality?"

In some cases after a confidentiality explanation, clients make a joke (e.g., "Well, I'm not planning to kill my mother-in-law or anything.") to lighten up the situation. At other times, they respond with specific questions (e.g., "Will you be keeping records about what I say to you?" or "Who else has access to your files?"). When clients ask questions about confidentiality, it may mean they are especially conscious of trust issues. It may also mean they've had some suicidal or homicidal thoughts and want to further clarify the limits of what they should and shouldn't say to you. Whatever the case, as a professional interviewer, respond to their questions directly and clearly: "Yes, I will be keeping records about our meetings, but only my office manager and I have access to these files. And the office manager will also keep your records confidential."

Finally, if you are being supervised and your supervisor has access to your case notes and tape recordings, make that clear in your initial statement to your client. For example:

"Because I'm a graduate student, I have a supervisor who checks over my work, and sometimes there are group case discussions. However, in each of these situations, the purpose is to enable me to provide you with the best services possible. Other than the exceptions I mentioned, no information about you will leave this clinic without your permission."

The second rule with regard to client education and evaluation of client expectations is to inform clients of the interview's purpose. Perhaps the classic line to *avoid* in this respect was offered by Benjamin (1987): "We both know why you are here" (p. 14). As Benjamin suggests, this type of introductory line can destroy any hope of initial rapport. Instead of a cryptic statement about the purpose of the interview, be clear, straightforward, and honest.

Obviously, the explanation you provide regarding an interview's purpose varies depending on the type of interview you are conducting. A general statement regarding the interview's purpose helps put clients at ease by clarifying their expectations about what will happen during the session. For example, a therapist who routinely conducted assessment interviews of prospective adoptive parents made the following statement:

"The purpose of this interview is for me to help the adoption agency you're working with evaluate qualities that might affect your performance as adoptive parents. I like to start this type of interview in an open-ended manner by having you describe why you're interested in adoption and having each of you talk about yourselves, but eventually I'll get more specific and ask about your own childhoods. Finally, toward the end of the interview, I will ask you specific questions about your parenting attitudes and abilities. Do you have any questions before we begin?"

The third rule is to see if client expectations for the interview are consistent with your expectations or purpose. Usually a simple direct question, such as the one at the end of the previous example, serves this purpose. Essentially, you want to be sure clients understand the interview's purpose and that they feel free to ask any questions about what will happen.

Table 6.1 summarizes these introduction tasks in the form of a checklist.

**Table 6.1.    Checklist for Introduction Phase**

| Interviewer Task | Relationship Variables |
| --- | --- |
| _____ 1. Schedule a mutually agreed upon meeting time. | Working alliance, positive regard, mutuality |
| _____ 2. Introduce yourself. | Congruence, attractiveness, positive regard |
| _____ 3. Identify how the client likes to be addressed. | Positive regard, empowerment |
| _____ 4. Engage in conversation or small talk. | Empathy, rapport |
| _____ 5. Direct client to an appropriate seat (or let the client choose). | Expertness, empathy, rapport |
| _____ 6. Present your credential or status (as appropriate). | Expertness |
| _____ 7. Explain confidentiality. | Trustworthiness, working alliance |
| _____ 8. Explain the purpose of the interview. | Working alliance, expertness |
| _____ 9. Check client expectations of interview for similarity to and compatibility with your purpose. | Working alliance, mutuality, empowerment |

## THE OPENING

Shea (1998) writes that the opening begins with an interviewer's first questions about the client's current concerns and ends when the interviewer begins determining the interview's focus by asking specific questions about specific topics.

In Shea's (1998) model, the opening is a nondirective interview phase lasting about five to eight minutes. During this phase, the interviewer uses basic attending skills and nondirective listening responses to encourage client disclosure. The main interviewer task is to stay out of the way so that clients can tell their story. For example:

> You arrive in your office. You allow the client to choose a seat. (As discussed previously, even seating choices provide information. We have had clients choose our usual chair, even when the chair is sitting behind a desk!) Your client shifts uneasily, keeps her coat on, and grips a large purse tightly on her lap. She smiles nervously. You have the intake form she filled out. You ask her if she has any questions about it. She shakes her head. You review confidentiality. She nods, indicating it makes sense to her. You sense both her nervousness and sadness. She looks frightened and she is blinking rapidly, perhaps fighting back tears.

Given the observations listed in this example, the interviewer could form several hypotheses. It is through forming hypotheses regarding the meaning of your clients' behavior that you eventually come closer in your understanding of what clients are communicating to you about themselves.

### The Interviewer's Opening Statement

The opening statement signals the client that small talk, introductions, and explanations of confidentiality and the interview are over and it is time to begin. An opening statement consists of the interviewer's first direct inquiry into what brought the client to seek professional assistance. The statement can usually be delivered in a calm, easy manner, so it doesn't feel like an interruption in the flow. However, occasionally, you will need to be assertive as you start the interview.

Most counselors and psychotherapists develop a comfortable opening statement. A common prototype is: "Tell me what brings you to counseling (or therapy or help) at this time." The elements of import include:

1. *Tell Me:* The interviewer is expressing direct interest in hearing what the client has to say. In addition, the interviewer is making it clear that the client is responsible for doing the telling.
2. *What Brings You:* This is more specific than "Tell me about yourself," yet is open to the client's interpretation regarding which areas of life to begin sharing with the interviewer.
3. *To Counseling:* This phrase acknowledges that coming to the clinic or to see you is an action that is out of the ordinary. It suggests the client tell you about precipitating events that stimulated the client to seek help.
4. *At This Time:* This helps the client direct his or her comments to the pertinent factors leading up to the decision to come in. The interviewer is aware that the decision to seek help has been made based not only on causes but on timing. Sometimes, a problem has existed for years, but the time was never quite right to seek help until now.

You may not be comfortable with these particular words, but it is important to think about what you can say to convey the essential aspects of this message to your clients.

There are a variety of approaches to formulating the opening statement. Essentially, the opening statement should include either an open question (i.e., a question beginning with *what* or *how*) or a gentle prompt. The opening statement described is an example of a gentle prompt, which is a directive that usually begins with the words "Tell me." Other popular opening statements include the following:

What brings you here?

How can I be of help?

Maybe you could begin by telling me things about yourself, or your situation, that you believe are important.

So, how's it going?

What are some of the stresses you have been coping with recently? (Shea, 1998)

As you examine these potential openings, think about how you would respond to each one if you were the client. You may also want to try them out in practice interviews or role plays. Your opening statement influences how your clients begin talking about themselves or their problems; therefore, you should consciously choose the elements of the statement you use for your opening. For example, if you want to hear about stressors and coping responses, you could use the sample opening provided by Shea (1998). The opening recommended by Ivey (1988) is much more social in nature and communicates more of an informal, perhaps even chatty, style. "How can I be of help?" communicates an assumption that the client needs help and that you will be functioning as a helper. No opening is, of course, completely nondirective. In general, the opening statement's purpose is to help clients begin talking freely about personal concerns that have caused them to seek professional assistance.

## The Client's Opening Response

After you make your opening statement, the spotlight is on the client. How will the client respond? Will he or she take your opening statement and run with it, or hesitate, struggle for the right words, and perhaps ask for more direction or structure? As noted, some clients come to a professional interviewer expecting authoritative guidance; therefore, they may be surprised by a general and nondirective opening statement. Usually, their first response gives you clues about how they respond to unstructured situations. Some clinicians consider this initial behavior crucial in understanding the client's personality dynamics.

*Rehearsed Client Responses*

Clients may begin in a way suggesting they've rehearsed for their part in the interview. For example, we've heard clients begin with:

"Well, let me begin with my childhood."
"Currently, my symptoms include . . ."
"There are three things going on in my life right now that I'm having difficulty with."
"I'm depressed about . . ."

There are advantages and disadvantages to working with clients who begin in a straightforward and organized manner. The primary advantages are that these clients have thought about their personal problems and are trying to get to the point as quickly as possible. If they are relatively insightful and have a good grasp of why they want professional assistance, then you are at a distinct advantage and the interview should proceed smoothly.

On the other hand, sometimes client openings characterized by too much directness and organization may indicate the beginning of what Shea (1998) refers to as a "rehearsed interview" (p. 76). In such cases, clients may be providing stock interview responses out of defensiveness. They may give factual and informative, but emotionally distant, accounts of their problems. Emotional distance may, in fact, be a major part of the problem (e.g., the client could have trouble being emotionally connected in close relationships). A very organized and direct opening response sometimes reflects general discomfort with unstructured situations; clients may be reacting to an unstructured opening statement by providing excessive structure and organization.

*Helping Clients Who Struggle to Express Themselves*

Some clients struggle because an opening statement did not provide clear enough directions and they don't know how to proceed. For example, imagine your client falls silent, looks at you with a pained expression, and asks, "So what am I supposed to talk about?" or "I don't know what you want me to say." If you're faced with clients who appear uncomfortable with an unstructured opening, try the following sequence:

1. Assume a kind and attentive posture, but allow them to struggle for a few moments (while you evaluate their coping methods).
2. Provide emotional support regarding the difficulty of the task.
3. Provide additional structure.

Letting clients struggle with an unstructured opening provides an opportunity to assess general expressive abilities. If a client responds to your opening by asking, "What should I talk about?," respond warmly with "Whatever you'd like." This places the responsibility for identifying an appropriate place to start back on the client and provides an excellent test of the client's inner expressive resources. In essence, you're learning how much help the client needs to express himself or herself.

Another reason it is important to let clients struggle with an unstructured opening is that it allows them an opportunity to overcome their faltering start and recover by adequately identifying a place to begin their communications with you. If you assist too soon, you do not allow them to demonstrate their ability to recover and express themselves. Perhaps the client is simply a slow starter, which is important information in itself.

If your client falters a second time or begins to become visibly irritated with your unstructured opening, you should provide support:

**Client:** "Come on, really, I don't know where to start."
**Interviewer:** "Sometimes it's difficult to know what you want to say, but once you get started, it gets easier."

This interviewer statement is designed to acknowledge the difficulty of beginning an interview and to provide hope that the interview process will become smoother or easier.

Finally, if your client simply cannot seem to get started independently, then you should help by providing additional structure:

**Client:** "I still can't think of what to say."
**Interviewer:** "Sometimes it helps to begin with how things have been going at home (or work or school)."

By defining and narrowing the client's opening task, this interviewer statement provides structure and simplifies the demand placed on the client. In some cases, the interviewer may need to become even more structured to help clients succeed in expressing themselves (e.g., "Maybe you could begin by telling me about how your day has been going.").

### Other Client Responses to the Interviewer's Opening Statement

Some clients begin interviews in odd ways that give you reason to wonder about the "normality" of their current functioning. For example, imagine clients beginning sessions with the following statements:

"I have come because the others told me to come. You will be my witness."

"You're the doc, you tell me what's wrong with me."

"It's by the grace of Allah that I'm sitting before you right now. May I pray before we begin?"

"I have this deep ache inside of me. It comes over me sometimes like a wave. It's not like I have been a wellspring of virtue and propriety, but then really . . . I ask myself constantly, do I deserve this?"

Evaluating or judging client normality is a difficult and demanding task requiring good clinical judgment. We discuss evaluation procedures in more detail later in this chapter and in Chapter 8.

Ideal client responses to your opening statement usually reflect thoughtfulness and the initiation of a working alliance. For example:

"I'm not totally sure of all the reasons I'm here, or why I chose to come right now. Lately, I haven't been handling the stress at work very well and it's affecting my family life. I guess I'll start by telling you about work and family and as I go along maybe you can tell me if I'm talking about the things you need to know about me."

### Evaluating Client Verbal Behavior during the Opening

As clients proceed during the opening phase of the interview, you should evaluate their approach and begin to modify your responses accordingly. For instance, with clients who are very verbal and tend to ramble, you need to be ready to interject yourself into the interview whenever you get (or create) the chance. With such individuals, toward the end of the opening, you may be thinking about how to exercise additional control over the client's verbal behavior. Consider using more closed questions in an effort to direct an overly rambling client.

Similarly, it will become apparent that some clients are using an internal frame of reference to describe their problems. For example:

> "I don't know what's wrong with me. I feel anxious all the time . . . like someone's watching me and evaluating me, but I know that's not the case. And I feel so depressed. Nothing I do turns out quite right. I'm underemployed. I can't seem to get involved in a good relationship. I pick the wrong type of women, and I can't figure out why anyone who has anything going for them would want to go out with me anyway."

Clients who use an internal frame of reference tend to be self-critical and self-blaming. They may begin criticizing themselves and not stop until the end of the session. They are sometimes referred to as *internalizers* because they describe their problems as having an internal cause. Internalizing clients seem to be saying, "What's wrong with me?" or "There's something wrong with me that's making me feel this way."

On the other hand, some clients are more aptly described as *externalizers*. They communicate the message "What's wrong with *them*?" or "There's something wrong with all those other people in my life." For example, a client may begin by stating:

> "My problem is that I have a ridiculous boss. He's rude, stupid, and arrogant. In fact, men in general are insensitive, and my life would be fine if I never had to deal with another man again."

Externalizing clients tend to believe that their troubles stem from other people. Although certainly there may be truth to their complaints, it can be difficult to get them to accept responsibility and focus on their own feelings, thoughts, and behavior in a constructive manner.

Realistically, client problems usually stem from a combination of personal (internal) and situational (external) factors. It is useful, especially during the opening phase, to listen for whether your clients are taking too much or too little responsibility for their problems (see Individual and Cultural Highlight 6.2 later in this chapter for a different perspective on clients' taking responsibility for their problems).

It takes more than one piece of evidence to conclude even tentatively something about a client from a brief opening statement. Nonetheless, opening responses provide you with an initial glimpse of how clients perceive themselves and their problems and initial clinical hypotheses about the clients. Consider clients' openings with respect to the following questions:

Does the client express himself or herself in a direct and coherent manner?

Is the opening response overly structured, organized, and perhaps rehearsed?

Does the client struggle excessively with lack of structure?

**Table 6.2.    Checklist for Opening Phase**

| Interviewer Task | Technical Approaches |
|---|---|
| _____ 1. Continue working on rapport. | Nondirective listening |
| _____ 2. Focus on client's view of life and problems. | Open-ended questioning, gentle prompting |
| _____ 3. Provide structure and support if necessary. | Feeling reflections, clarify purpose of opening phase, narrow the focus of opening question |
| _____ 4. Help client adopt an internal, rather than external frame of reference, if necessary. | Nondirective listening, mild confrontation |
| _____ 5. Evaluate how the interview is proceeding and think about what approaches might be most effective during the body phase. | Paraphrasing, summarization, role induction |

If the client does struggle with lack of structure, what is the nature of the struggle (e.g., Does he or she ask you directly for more structure, become angry or scared in the face of low structure, digress into a disordered or confusing communication style)?

Is the client's speech characterized by oddities?

Does the client's response focus on external factors (other people or situations causing distress) or internal factors (ways the client may have contributed to his or her own distress)?

Table 6.2 lists interviewer tasks for the opening phase of the interview.

## THE BODY

The body of an interview is characterized primarily by information gathering. The quality and quantity of information gathered depends almost entirely on the interview's purpose. Shea (1998) states, "Like the Chinese artist, the goals of the clinician vary during the body of the interview depending upon the various therapeutic landscapes with which the clinician is presented" (p. 93). Sometimes, the interview's purpose dictates the therapeutic landscape; other times, as suggested by Shea, the therapeutic landscape shapes clinical goals.

If the purpose of a particular interview has to do with whether the client will make a good candidate for psychoanalytic psychotherapy, then the body of the interview will include asking questions designed to help you judge, among other things, whether the client is psychologically minded, motivated, and capable, both financially and psychologically, to seek such treatment (J. Gustafson, 1997). On the other hand, if the purpose of the interview is to determine a client's clinical diagnosis and formulate a treatment plan, the data gathered will focus much more on diagnostic clues and criteria (see Chapter 9). However, the purpose or focus of the interview body may change, depending on information shared by the client. For example, you may discover partway through an interview that your client is contemplating suicide; consequently, your general goal shifts to assessing suicide risk (see Chapter 8).

The body is the heart of the interview. As an interviewer, you must obtain certain information to formulate the case and make recommendations. Your ears are tuned to pick up information, and you use nondirective and directive responses discussed in earlier chapters to encourage your client to elaborate more fully in some areas than others.

## Sources of Clinical Judgment: Making Inferences

During the body phase, the interviewer gathers information to make professional inferences about the client. Depending on the interview's purpose, the inferences will relate to some of the following:

Statements about client personality style and functioning.

Recommendations on whether psychotherapy is needed.

Recommendations regarding the most appropriate psychotherapeutic approach.

Statements about the client's diagnosis, including diagnostic impressions.

Estimates of client intellectual or cognitive functioning.

Statements pertaining to parenting ability, attitudes, and adequacy.

Statements regarding possible addictions, past criminal behavior, past employment, and relationship and educational experiences.

Making statements, recommendations, estimates, or predictions based on a single clinical interview is risky. Describing, explaining, and especially predicting human behavior is a challenging task, often fraught with error (Caspi & Roberts, 2001; Paunonen, 2001). Nonetheless, after conducting an assessment-oriented interview, interviewers are often expected to make some statements or even decisions about the client. Consequently, the next section will help you become more capable of making accurate clinical inferences about client functioning. In Chapter 7, we discuss specific activities to engage in during an assessment interview's body.

## Defining Psychological and Emotional Disorders

All interviewers must distinguish normal and healthy emotional or psychological functioning from disturbed or disordered functioning (see Individual and Cultural Highlight 6.1 for additional information on this topic). The *Diagnostic and Statistical Manual of Mental Disorders,* fourth edition text revision (*DSM-IV-TR;* American Psychiatric Association, 2000), is the standard reference in the United States for diagnoses of mental disorders. The *International Classification of Diseases,* tenth edition, (*ICD-10;* World Health Organization, 1997a, 1997b) is the world standard for classification of mental disorders. Before you use these manuals to identify specific clinical diagnoses, however, you must be able to judge whether a client's behavior indicates a psychological disorder (disordered way of thinking, feeling, and behaving) at all. What follows are general standards for determining whether a client might be experiencing a disorder. These are not diagnostic criteria. Instead, they are general guidelines to aid your clinical judgment and thinking about normal and abnormal behavior (in Chapter 10, the *DSM's* approach to defining and identifying mental disorders is reviewed).

### Statistical Infrequency

Any behavior that your client experiences or engages in is subject to objective evaluation. Engaging in or experiencing a statistically infrequent or atypical behavior is one way of defining behavior disorders or psychopathology. For example, your client may

---

**INDIVIDUAL AND CULTURAL HIGHLIGHT 6.1**

### Sources of Clinical Judgment

Perhaps the most general question interviewers must be able to address is: How is normal and healthy emotional or psychological functioning distinguished from disturbed or disordered functioning? There are several sources of judgment on which interviewers base these clinical judgments, including:

- Graduate school classes and experiences.
- Personal experiences and opinions.
- Experiences and opinions of friends or family.
- Books, movies, television, radio, and other media.
- Supervisors.
- Research data.
- Cultural background and experiences.
- Colleagues.
- Previous clinical interviewing experiences.
- The *Diagnostic and Statistical Manual of Mental Disorders IV* (American Psychiatric Association, 1994).
- Intuition.

For interviewers to make reasonable judgments about clients, they need to have knowledge about norms. In other words, interviewers need to have a normative standard to which they can compare their client's interview behavior.

In many cases, interviewers rely on their own accumulated clinical experience to evaluate clients' behavior. Although relying on their own clinical judgment can be helpful, it may also be completely misleading because all interviewers have idiosyncratic personal biases that adversely affect their judgment (Binik, Cantor, Ochs, & Meana, 1997; K. Murphy & Davidshofer, 1988); interviewers also have imperfect memories that can further bias or distort what clients have said. Most beginning interviewers have no previous clinical experience or internalized standards to help in evaluating their clients. They must count on other information to support or bolster their judgment.

It is tempting for beginning interviewers to base their inferences on their own personal experiences. However, inferences are more accurate when interviewers use research reports, colleagues, and supervisors to enhance their clinical judgment. We recommend that you become aware of the norms you use for your clinical judgment. Awareness of normal functioning will help you come to more valid conclusions about whether dysfunctional or abnormal behavior is present.

---

report how many hours he sleeps each night, or how many beers he drinks each week. In each of these cases, as a clinical interviewer, you can compare his reports to statistical normality. If your client reports sleeping 12 hours nightly and drinking three cases of beer weekly, you can begin to establish that your client is behaving in an unusual or abnormal manner.

Obviously, all statistically infrequent behavior does not indicate a mental disorder. Such reasoning is too simplistic and can result in classifying exceptional, creative, or culturally divergent people as disordered (e.g., it would result in classifying most professional basketball players as having a height disorder and most published poets as having a thinking disorder). Behavior should never be considered indicative of a mental disorder simply because of statistical infrequency. Statistically infrequent behavior should be further examined for the following conditions:

### Disturbing to Self or Others

An individual might choose to sleep 12 hours nightly and drink large quantities of beer and feel just fine about that behavior. Other individuals may feel extreme personal distress because they slept more than 9 hours two nights in a row or because they drank excessively on a single occasion. It is difficult for evaluators to predict what behaviors might produce personal distress in particular individuals. Therefore, interviewers should ask clients directly whether they are bothered by their own behaviors.

Mental disorders may also be characterized by the fact that they disturb or bother others. Most family members would be at least a little concerned to observe a loved one sleeping and drinking alcohol excessively. In the case of personality disorders (one of the diagnostic categories identified in *DSM-IV-TR*), the people who live or work with a person who has a personality disorder often experience distress and eventually insist the person obtain counseling. Therefore, when evaluating clients for behavior disorders, be sure to ask whether anyone in their immediate environment is disturbed or bothered by their behavior.

### Maladaptive Behaviors

When individuals repeatedly engage in self-defeating behavior, hold self-defeating beliefs, or experience negative emotions, they are commonly considered to have a behavior or mental disorder. Usually, such thoughts, feelings, or actions serve some function in the person's life, but for the most part, the patterns are negative or dysfunctional. For instance, a parent may sincerely want a teenager to keep her room clean, but constant screaming and arguing about it may end up damaging the parent-child relationship and not achieve a clean room. In fact, our experience is that screaming, yelling, and striking children, especially teenagers, are maladaptive behaviors in that they are ineffective means of attaining desired goals. Similarly, a man may sincerely want to be in an intimate relationship, but his overly enthusiastic behavior could alarm potential partners and keep them from coming close to him. The man's intent is positive, but his approach is maladaptive; it results in his scaring potential partners away and, consequently, his increased loneliness. By definition, a behavior pattern is maladaptive when it interferes with effective occupational, social, physical, or recreational functioning.

### Rationally or Culturally Unjustifiable

If a client's behavior, thought, or feeling is unusual or maladaptive, you should ascertain whether there is any reasonable excuse or justification for it. Take the case of a client who claimed that because his wife was unable to determine when she was hungry or sleepy, he saw it as his responsibility to force her to eat or sleep when he judged it necessary to do so. Think about this scenario. Are there any rational justifications that a man might have for forcing his spouse to eat or sleep? In such a case, it is appropriate to focus on whether the spouse is capable of caring for herself. We asked several questions: How old is she? Is she able to work or perform other functions effectively? Does she have Alzheimer's or another brain disease or deficiency? The client could be asked to describe why he thought his wife was unable to determine appropriate times to eat and sleep. In this case, the answers were revealing. His wife was capable of working outside the home. She was in her mid-forties. She did not have any identifiable brain disease or damage. He attributed her inability to monitor her own needs for sleep and food to the fact that she had a brother who was "mentally retarded"; therefore, he concluded, she probably had similar genetic deficits (although she was a fully functioning person in virtually every sense of the word).

In this case, it was obvious after conducting a thorough interview that the client was behaving in an unusual and disturbing manner. His behavior was rationally unjustifiable (his wife was able to care for herself), statistically infrequent (not many people believe they need to regulate their spouse's eating and sleeping patterns), disturbing (to his wife), and maladaptive (it had precipitated a marital crisis).

Now we are left with a final question regarding the justifiability of the man's behavior. Namely, is his behavior culturally justified or sanctioned? Think about this standard. Can you think of any cultural situations that might adequately justify this man's rather controlling behaviors? We take up the issue of judging mental disorders in their cultural context to a greater extent in Individual and Cultural Highlight 6.2 and Chapter 13.

---

INDIVIDUAL AND CULTURAL HIGHLIGHT 6.2

## Exploring Society's Contributions to Client Problems

That client problems must be viewed in their social and cultural context is an unarguable fact. Articulating this point for families in particular, Goldenberg and Goldenberg (2000) describe the discoveries made by renowned family therapist Salvador Minuchin (Minuchin, Rossman, & Baker, 1978).

As Minuchin and his coworkers began to accumulate research and clinical data and to redefine the problem in family terms, successful interventions involving the entire family became possible. Later research expanded to include asthmatic children with severe, recurrent attacks as well as anorectic children; the additional data confirmed for Minuchin that the locus of pathology was in the context of the family and not simply in the afflicted individual (Goldenberg & Goldenberg, 2000, p. 197).

Minuchin argued the importance of seeing individual client symptoms from the family systems perspective. In contrast, the *DSM-IV-TR,* although including a section on cultural issues with each major diagnostic category, continues to define mental disorders as residing exclusively in the individual (American Psychiatric Association, 2000).

If you were aware of only the *DSM*'s perspective and Minuchin's perspective, you might conclude that they represent polar opposite ends of a conceptual continuum of clients' individual responsibility for their symptoms. In reality, both the *DSM* and Minuchin represent what might be considered "moderate" etiological perspectives. More extreme views have been articulated by biological psychiatry (where the cause of mental disorders is not only considered to reside in the individual, but also in his or her genes; Toates, 2001).

On the other extreme, British psychologist David Smail (1997, 2000) holds culture responsible for causing symptoms in an individual.

Emotional distress arises from painful struggles with a real world that causes real and often lasting damage. Life isn't easy and very few of us get through it without being

*(continued)*

---

INDIVIDUAL AND CULTURAL HIGHLIGHT 6.2 (continued)

marked by events which, however we look at them and whatever the colour of the light we try to cast on them, leave us worse off than we had hoped to be. The limitations of counseling to have any real impact on the kind of social, economic and health difficulties which may sap a person's confidence and ability to cope are obvious. What really helps in circumstances such as these is the availability of powers to tackle the problems themselves.

It's possible to identify at least four points on a continuum examining the causes of "mental disorders." Of course, the biological psychiatrists might even claim that the words *mental disorder* are inaccurate (and *mental illness* more accurate), while someone like David Smail (or Thomas Szasz; 1961) would claim that there is no such thing as mental illness. The following table briefly describes four viewpoints on causal factors in mental/behavioral problems.

| Biological Psychiatry | DSM-IV-TR | Minuchin | Smail |
|---|---|---|---|
| Client problems are a product of their individual genetic and biological make-up. | Client problems reside in the individual, but are sometimes provoked or maintained by social or cultural factors. | Client problems are primarily a function of family and environmental context. | Client problems are completely derived from social, cultural, and political context. |

As with so many issues in psychology and counseling, your beliefs about clients' responsibility for their problems will undoubtedly influence how you interact with them. Take time to examine (or discuss with friends or classmates) where you fall on this continuum of client responsibility.

---

The previous standards may be applied to almost any type of clinical observation that takes place in an interview. For example, if a client exhibits symptoms of depression or sadness during an interview, ask yourself the following questions:

Is this person's sadness unusual or extraordinary as compared to the emotional states of most people with similar life circumstances?

Is the sadness disturbing or upsetting to the client? Is it particularly disturbing to other people in the client's environment?

Is the sadness adversely affecting the client's ability to function at work, to carry on in interpersonal relationships, or to enjoy usually pleasurable recreational activities?

Is there a rational explanation for the client's sadness? That is, did an event occur that is logically associated with your client's sadness (e.g., a series of rejections or the death of a loved one)? Is there an adequate cultural explanation for the client's sadness?

You should not rely solely on any one of these criteria to determine that an individual has a psychological disorder. Each criterion has its shortcomings. Instead, examine

**Table 6.3.   Checklist for Body Phase**

| Interviewer Task | Interviewer Tools |
|---|---|
| ____ 1. Make the transition from nondirective to more directive listening. | Role induction; explain this shift of style to the client, if necessary. |
| ____ 2. Gather information. | Open and closed questions (see Chapter 8). |
| ____ 3. Obtain diagnostic information. | Use *DMS-IV, ICD-10,* or the four guiding principles discussed in this chapter to formulate useful questions. |
| ____ 4. Shift from information gathering to preparation for closing. | Acknowledge that time is passing; explain and discuss the need to summarize major issues. |

your client's thoughts, feelings, and behavior with respect to these standards to obtain a clearer sense of whether psychopathology is present in an individual case.

Tasks for the body phase of the interview are listed in Table 6.3.

## THE CLOSING

As time passes during the interview, both interviewer and client may feel pressure. Usually, the interviewer is tempted to fire a few more pertinent questions at the client; it becomes a race to see if you can fit everything into the 50- or 90-minute session. One key to a smooth closing is to consciously and skillfully stop gathering new information somewhere between 5 and 10 minutes before your interview time is over. Shea (1998) notes, "One of the most frequent problems I see in supervision remains the overextension of the main body of the interview, thus forcing the clinician to rush through the closing phase" (p. 130).

Clients may also feel increasing tension as time passes in the interview. They may wonder whether they have been able to express themselves adequately and whether the interviewer can provide help or adequate recommendations. Clients also may feel worse than they did at the outset of the interview because they have discussed their problems too graphically or simply because as they reflect on their problems, they begin feeling worse. Because clients are likely to feel such stresses and think such thoughts, interviewers should leave ample time for closure.

### Reassuring and Supporting Your Client

Clients need to be reassured and supported in at least two major areas. First, clients need to have their expressive capabilities praised. Nearly all clients who voluntarily seek professional assistance do the best they can during an intake interview. An intake interview is a challenging and sometimes anxiety-provoking experience. Therefore, during the closing, interviewers should make comments such as:

"You sure covered lots of ground today."
"I appreciate your efforts in telling me about yourself."

"First sessions are always difficult because there's so much to cover and so little time."

"I think you did a nice job describing yourself and your life in a very short time period."

"Thanks for being so open and sharing so much about yourself with me."

Comments such as these acknowledge that an interview situation is difficult and commend clients for their expressive efforts.

Second, most clients come to their first interview session with ambivalent feelings; they experience both hope and fear regarding the interview and the therapeutic experience. Therefore, the interviewer should support the client's decision to seek professional services, siding with the hope evidenced by that decision. For example:

"You made a good decision when you decided to come for an appointment here."

"I want to congratulate you for coming here today. Coming to someone for help can be hard. I know some people think otherwise, but I believe that getting help for yourself is a sign of strength."

These statements acknowledge the reality of how difficult it can be to seek professional help. Clients should be supported for making such a difficult decision. Providing support may help clients feel their decision to seek help was a good one.

In some cases, clients behave defensively and avoid disclosing information during the interview. Nonetheless, as a professional interviewer, you should recognize and acknowledge that clients are generally doing their best to interact with you on any given day. It is permissible to note the task's difficulty or to comment on how the client seemed to be reluctant to talk much, but take care to refrain from expressing anger or disappointment toward clients who are resistant or defensive. Instead, if your client is defensive, remain optimistic:

"I know it was hard for you to talk with me today. That's not surprising; after all, we're basically strangers. Usually, it gets easier over time and as we get to know each other."

## Summarizing Crucial Themes and Issues

As Shea (1998) points out, perhaps the most important task of the closing is "solidifying the patient's desire to return for a second appointment or to follow the clinician's referral" (p. 125). One of the best methods for enhancing a client's likelihood of returning for therapy is to clearly identify, during the closing phase, precisely why the client has come for professional assistance. This can be difficult because often clients themselves are not exactly sure why they've come for assistance. Variations on the following statement may be useful:

"Based on what you've said today, it seems you're here because you want to feel less self-conscious when you're in social situations. You'd like to feel more positive about yourself. I think you said, 'I want to believe in myself' and you also talked about how you want to figure out what you're feeling inside and how to share your emotions with others you care about."

Most clients come to professionals because they hope their lives can improve. If you can summarize how they would like to improve their lives, your clients are more likely to return to see you or follow your recommendations; they see you as a credible authority with useful information and skills.

## Instilling Hope

If appropriate, after you accurately summarize why your client has sought professional assistance, you should make a statement about how counseling or psychotherapy may help address the client's personal issues and concerns. It can be as simple as making the following very brief, but positive, statement: "I want you to know, I think therapy can help" (M. Spitzform, personal communication, October 1982).

In a sense, if we believe in our best clinical judgment that therapy can be helpful to a particular client, part of our task is to effectively communicate that belief. After all, most clients are somewhat naïve about the potential benefits (and detriments) of psychotherapy. It is our job to inform them of the potential effects:

"You've said you want to feel better, and I think therapy can help you move in that direction. Of course, not everyone who comes for therapy reaps great benefits. But most people who use therapy to improve their lives are successful, and I believe that you're the type of person who is very likely to get good results from this process."

## Guiding and Empowering Your Client

You have just spent 35 or 40 minutes with someone you had never met before, listening to his or her deepest fears, pain, confusion, and problems. You hope you have listened well, summarized along the way and, when necessary, guided him or her in talking about especially important material. In a sense, regardless of how accepting you may have been, you have sat in judgment of the client, her problems, and her life. No matter how well you've functioned as an interviewer, your client may still feel that the experience was overwhelmingly one-sided; after all, you know a fair amount about him or her, but he or she knows next to nothing about you. Therefore, it is often useful to consciously shift the focus and give your client the opportunity to have a bit more power and control as the interview closes. Some methods for such a shift follow:

"I've done all the questioning here. I wonder if you have any questions for me?"

"Has this interview been as you expected it to be?"

"Are there any areas that you feel we've missed or that you would like to discuss at greater length?"

These queries help give power and control back to the client. As Foley and Sharf (1981) point out, although it is important to maintain control toward the end of an interview, it is also important to share that control with the client. In most cases, clients don't ask many questions or make many comments; however, we have found clients respond positively to being offered such an opportunity. In addition, questions and comments from clients can augment our own professional growth.

**Table 6.4.   Checklist for Closing Phase**

| Interviewer Task | Interviewer Tools |
|---|---|
| _____ 1. Reassure and support the client. | Feeling reflection, validation; openly appreciate your client's efforts at expression. |
| _____ 2. Summarize crucial themes and issues. | Summarization; use interpretation to determine client's insight and ability to integrate themes and issues. |
| _____ 3. Instill hope. | Suggestion, explanation of counseling process, and how it is usually helpful. |
| _____ 4. Guide and empower your client. | Questions; ask client for comments or questions of you. |
| _____ 5. Tie up loose ends. | Clarify the nature of further contact, if any, and schedule next appointment. |

### Tying Up Loose Ends

The final formal task of the interviewer is to clarify whether there will be further professional contact. This involves specific and concrete steps such as scheduling additional appointments, dealing with fee payment, and handling any other administrative issues associated with working in your particular setting. Tasks associated with the closing phase are presented in Table 6.4.

## TERMINATION

Some professionals believe that each session termination we face is a mini-death (Maholick & Turner, 1979). Although comparing an interview's end with death is a bit dramatic, it does point out how important endings are in our lives. For many people, saying goodbye is difficult. Some bolt away, avoiding the issue altogether; others linger, hoping it will not have to happen; still others have strong emotional responses such as anger, sadness, or relief. Certainly, the way clients cope with a session's end may foreshadow the way therapy terminates. It may also represent our own or our clients' conflicts in the areas of separation and individuation. Termination is an essential and often overlooked component of clinical interviewing.

### Watching the Clock

Of course, interviewers should not literally watch the clock; however, they should promote timely session endings. It is crucial to begin the closing phase early enough so there is time to terminate the session well. If there is not adequate time and the client and interviewer are rushed through closing, the termination phase may be affected. The ideal is to finish with all clinical business on time so the client's termination behavior can be observed and evaluated. When it is time to end the session, clients often begin thinking, feeling, and behaving in ways that give the sensitive clinician clues regarding therapeutic issues, psychopathology, and diagnosis (see Putting It in Practice 6.2).

```
══════════ Putting It in Practice 6.2 ══════════

     Interpreting and Understanding Doorknob Statements

Statements made by clients at the very end of their sessions, as they are getting
up to leave or while they are walking out the door, are commonly referred to as
*doorknob statements*. Review the following doorknob statements and actions
and then discuss their potential clinical significance in a small group or with a
partner.

  • "Thank you." (accompanied by a handshake or even an attempt to give you
    a hug at the end of every session)
  • "By the way, my thoughts about killing myself have really intensified these
    past few days." (Clients sometimes wait until the final minute of a session to
    mention suicidal thoughts.)
  • "Maybe sometime we could get together for coffee or something."
  • "That was great! I feel lots better now."
  • "So when will I start feeling better?"
```

## Guiding or Controlling Termination

Interviewers need control over session termination. Session termination occurs as both parties acknowledge that the meeting is over. This may involve escorting the client out along with a comfortable farewell gesture or ritual. One of our colleagues always says "Take care" in a kind voice but with a tone of finality. Some interviewers like to set up the next appointment and finish by saying "See you then." We also recall, with some chagrin, a colleague who would peek her head out of her office as the client was leaving and say, "Hang in there!"

It is worth thinking about how you'd like to end your sessions. It's also worth taking time to practice various endings with colleagues. Find a comfortable method of bringing about closure firmly and gently.

In some cases, clients do not let interviewers have control over termination. A client may keep an eye on the clock and then, 2, 5, or even 15 minutes before the time is officially up, stand up abruptly, and state something like, "Well, I'm done talking for today." Obviously, at some point, it may be wise to explore what motivates such a client to terminate sessions early. As a rule, interview sessions have a designated ending time, and clients should not be excused early (although certain clients, such as adolescents, commonly claim that they have nothing else to talk about and request to be let out of their session early). When adult clients want to leave early, it may signal that important but anxiety-provoking material is near the surface; the desire to leave may be a defense—conscious or otherwise—designed to avoid experiencing and talking about their anxiety. As an interviewer, be prepared for the client who wants to leave early, as well as the client who wants to stay late. Following are several strategies that may be used alone or in combination when you encounter a client who wants to terminate an interview early.

  • Ask why the client wants to leave early.
  • Ask the client to talk about his or her thoughts or feelings in reaction to the interview process or in reaction to you.

- Find out whether your client usually ends relationships or says goodbye quickly.
- Gently ask the client to simply "say whatever comes to mind" right now.
- Consult a detailed outline you've prepared before the session to evaluate whether you've covered all the potential issues that you wanted to cover during the interview.
- Let the client know that there's no hurry by saying something like, "We still have plenty of time left," and then continue to go about the business of closure (see the previous discussion about closing).

In rare cases, your client may desperately want to leave the interview room early. Certainly, you should never engage in a power struggle aimed at keeping the client in the room. Instead, make a statement suggesting that, sometime in the future, he or she may decide to come back for another meeting or visit a different professional. For example:

"I can see you really want to leave right now, even though we still have time remaining. Your desire to leave could simply mean that you've talked about everything you wanted to talk about today or it could mean that you don't want to go deeper into personal issues. Obviously, I'm not going to force you to stay when you want to go. But I hope you can come back and meet with me, or perhaps someone else, in the future if there are some things you'd like to discuss more completely."

## Facing Termination

Often, our own issues affect the way we terminate with clients. If we are characteristically abrupt and hurried, it shows in the way we say goodbye. If we are unsure of ourselves or not convinced we did a good enough job, we may linger and "accidentally" go over time. If we are typically quite assertive, and the client attempts to share one last bit of information, we may reveal serious irritation and end up in a power struggle.

Time limits are important from both a practical and an interpretive perspective. For your own professional survival, stay in bounds with regard to beginning and ending on time. At a deeper level, model for your clients that therapy, too, is bound in time, place, and real-world demands. You are not omniscient; you are not the all-good parent, and you cannot give your clients extra time to make up for the difficult lives they've had. Your time with clients, no matter how good, must end. You must withstand your clients' efforts to push the time boundaries.

In our experience, students sometimes feel guilty for being firm and ending a session on time. They allow clients to go on, colluding with the client in breaking the rules just a little. This doesn't really serve clients well in the end, even though they may feel special or like they got a little extra for their money. In fact, their excessive need to feel special may be what they most need to face and work on. Reality is not always easy, and neither is closing an interview or therapy session, but by doing so in a kind, timely, professional manner, the message you give your client is: "I play by the rules, and I believe you can, too. I will be here next week. I hold you in positive regard and am interested in helping you, but I can't work magic or change reality for you."

The list of tasks for this final phase of the interview is presented in Table 6.5.

## THE SCIENCE OF CLINICAL INTERVIEWING

In this chapter, we reviewed a structural model for conducting clinical interviews. Theoretically, it should follow that if you practice the skills in the preceding five chapters

Table 6.5.    Checklist for Termination Phase

| Interviewer Task | Interviewer Methods |
|---|---|
| ____ 1. Watch the clock. | Place a clock where you can see it without straining. Explain that time is nearly up. |
| ____ 2. Observe for client's significant doorknob statements. | Paraphrase. Make feeling reflections. |
| ____ 3. Guide or control termination. | Use a standardized ending. Make a warm and comfortable termination statement. Discuss termination and time boundaries with your client. |
| ____ 4. Face termination. | Evaluate your own response to ending sessions. Stay within time boundaries. |

and then stick with the model presented in this chapter, you will conduct a successful interview. But is this really the case? And what do we mean by a "successful" interview?

The answers to these questions undoubtedly depend on the specific goal of your interview. For example, if your goal is to establish rapport and develop the beginning of a working relationship, then using the skills and structure contained thus far in this text will likely help you be successful. In contrast, if your goal is to assess your client for addiction potential, readiness for change, sexual deviance, or general health status, then simply following the outlined structure is inadequate for conducting a successful interview. As we have noted early and often, the purpose of your clinical interview drives your interviewing behavior and varies depending on your setting, client, theoretical orientation, and other factors.

Over the years, clinical interviewing has been subjected to extensive scientific research. Broadly speaking, research has focused on two primary areas, depending on the purpose of the interview. First, interviewing has been evaluated as a data gathering or assessment technique. Second, clinical interviewing has been evaluated as a method for helping or treating clients, as a specific counseling or psychotherapy technique. In this section and again in Chapter 10 (Diagnosis and Treatment Planning), we briefly examine the "state of the science" of clinical interviewing as an assessment procedure. The immense literature on interviewing as a therapy technique is available elsewhere (see Hubble et al., 1999).

## The Interview as a Data Collection Procedure

The interview has long been viewed as a natural, easy, and convenient method for gathering data. In a general sense, interviews are used throughout our society. For example, if a father wants to know what activities his teenage daughter engaged in during her school day, he's most likely to use one type of interview format. He will probably sit down with her and ask a few questions such as, "What did you do in school today?" and "Did you learn anything new?" In this instance, as a data-gathering technique, his interview approach will probably be an abysmal failure (his daughter will quickly answer "Nothing" and "Nope" and then either turn on the television or go out with her friends).

However, an interview is not the only method for obtaining information about someone. In some cases, professionals prefer administering self-report (or parent-report) questionnaires, physiological measures, role plays, or direct behavioral observations.

Examples include using the Suicidal Behaviors Questionnaire to evaluate suicide potential (Osman, Bagge, & Gutierrez, 2001) or using physiological measures, such as a plethismograph to measure sexual deviance. In the case of the father who wants to know about his daughter's school day, he could call her teacher or even, we suppose, ask his daughter to fill out a quick questionnaire.

Despite the presence of alternatives to clinical interviewing, for most mental health professionals, the interview is a natural and indispensable tool for information gathering. Many of us wouldn't want to be mental health professionals if it did not involve the kind of personal contact and intimacy that an interview can provide. However, the research question is still important: "Are clinical interviews a reliable and valid method for obtaining information?" As you might suspect, the answer to this question is complex and generally depends on the type of information you're trying to obtain.

In 1954, renowned psychologist Paul Meehl published what he referred to later as a "disturbing little book" titled *Clinical versus Statistical Prediction* (1954, 1986). This book took what was then the rather controversial position that tests and questionnaires are more accurate predictors of human problems and behaviors than clinical interviews and clinician intuition. Currently, contemporary scientific literature on assessment and prediction supports Meehl's groundbreaking conclusion (Garb, 1998; Karon, 2000). Statistics and computer models do a better job than clinicians or interviewers of objectively analyzing large amounts of data and accurately making predictive statements. The unpleasant scientific fact is that interviewers are more predisposed to subjectivity, bias, overconfidence, and other distinctly human failings than statistical or computer models.

However, as is well-known in many areas, there is no substitute for human contact or human reasoning. This is especially the case when it comes to establishing rapport, gathering deeply personal information, and generating hypotheses about an individual client. To date, strictly mechanized or computer models are lacking in these more human-oriented functions. As Karon (2000) states, "The rich qualitative data of a . . . clinical interview are what clinicians mean by *clinical data*—data that could be relevant to an infinite number of dimensions and that the human mind can sift through to decide what is relevant," (p. 231) and "Subjective clinical interpretations of qualitative clinical data are essential to the task of understanding the human personality in its diversity and richness" (p. 232).

As a data collection procedure in the twenty-first century, the clinical interview, despite its many strengths, may for a time fall out of favor. This would be unfortunate because, as a method for "casting a wide net" for potentially important information, the clinical interview remains a viable, even preferred, technique. Of course, interviewers must be careful about coming to inappropriate conclusions—because this is where research indicates we are most likely to go wrong. However, as a method for gathering an immense range of data and generating tentative hypotheses about human personality and behavior, the well-conducted clinical interview remains the centerpiece.

Finally, with all due respect to Meehl (1954, 1986) and his research in the area of clinical versus statistical approaches to assessment, to dichotomize these approaches—as if they were competing entities—may be the wrong way to look at the issue. Instead, as you may have already concluded, both clinical and statistical approaches to assessment can produce reliable, valid, and useful data. Consequently, in the real world of interviewing and therapy, mental health professionals will likely conduct interviews, administer questionnaires, and gather information from parents, teachers, or significant others, all to maximize the probability of obtaining all potentially relevant information. Additionally, as discussed in the next section of this text, modern approaches to assessment interviewing use many highly structured and standardization procedures; this is done, in part, to address problems with subjectivity inherent in the interview method. We return to the science of clinical interviewing in the context of diagnostic interviewing in Chapter 10.

## SUMMARY

Researchers and clinicians have developed many models to describe the temporal and substantive structure of what occurs during a clinical interview. A model described by Shea (1998) is used in this chapter as a means of highlighting the events and tasks in the typical interview.

The introduction phase begins with the client's first contact with the interviewer. It is important that interviewers plan how to handle first contacts with prospective clients. Some interviewers follow a standard procedure when first meeting clients, which may be perceived as artificial or sterile. Consequently, a balance between standardization and flexibility is recommended. During the introduction, interviewers should educate clients on key issues such as confidentiality and the interview's purpose.

All theoretical orientations emphasize the need for establishing rapport with clients. There are many different tactics or strategies interviewers use to establish rapport. Some of these strategies address client fears about therapy through education, reassurance, courteous introductions, conversation, and flexibility.

The opening phase of an interview begins when the interviewer first makes an open-ended inquiry into the client's condition. The opening phase typically consists of several activities, including the interviewer's opening statement, the client's opening response, and the interviewer's silent evaluation of the client's expressive abilities. The opening phase ends when the interviewer has listened adequately to the client's efforts to express, without much direction from the interviewer, the main reasons he or she has sought professional assistance.

The body of an interview focuses primarily on information gathering. Information to be gathered during an interview depends in part on the interview's purpose and in part on what clinical material is revealed during the interview. An important clinical interviewing component that occurs during the body of an interview is diagnosis and assessment of mental and emotional problems or disorders.

The closing phase of an interview consists of a shift from information gathering to activities that prepare clients for interview termination. Often, both clients and interviewers feel pressured during this part of the interview because time is running short, and there's usually much more information that could be obtained or additional feelings that could be discussed. Interviewers should summarize key issues discussed in the session, instill hope for positive change, and empower clients by asking them if they have questions or feedback for the interviewer.

Interview termination sometimes brings important separation or loss issues to the surface in both clients and interviewers. Clients may express anger, disappointment, relief, or a number of other strong emotions at the end of an interview. These emotions may reflect unresolved feelings that the client has concerning previous separations from important people in his or her life. It is important that interviewers plan how they can most effectively end their interviews.

## SUGGESTED READINGS AND RESOURCES

This chapter contains numerous topics woven together to form the structure and sequence of the clinical interview. The following readings may help further your understanding of these issues.

American Psychiatric Association. (2000). *Diagnostic and statistical manual of mental disorders* (4th ed., text rev.). Washington, DC: Author. All mental health professionals must be familiar with this standard for diagnostic classification of mental disorders.

Foley, R., & Sharf, B. F. (1981). The five interviewing techniques most frequently overlooked by primary care physicians. *Behavioral Medicine, 8,* 2631. This is a brief article outlining one temporal structure model for clinical interviews. The authors discuss the criteria they view as basic for effective client interviewing.

Meehl, P. E. (1954). *Clinical versus statistical prediction: A theoretical analysis and a review of the evidence.* Northvale, NJ: Jason Aronson, Inc. Although this is a dated publication, its arguments about the relative merits of clinical versus statistical prediction are still interesting and pertinent. In fact, in 1986, Meehl claimed that 90% of what he wrote in 1954 was still true.

Othmer, E., & Othmer, S. C. (1994). *The clinical interview using DSM-IV* (Vol 1: Fundamentals). Washington DC: American Psychiatric Press. Chapter 2 of this practical text discusses strategies for developing rapport.

Shea, S. C. (1998). *Psychiatric interviewing: The art of understanding.* Philadelphia: W. B. Saunders. Chapter 2 of Shea's book is titled "The Dynamic Structure of the Interview" and provides a thorough and practical discussion of the temporal structure typical of most diagnostic clinical interviews.

Smail, D. (1997). *Illusion & reality: the meaning of anxiety.* London: Constable and Company. Smail's work, although somewhat controversial, emphasizes the importance of examining the role of society and our current political systems in causing and contributing to human suffering and mental disorder.

# Chapter 7

# *INTAKE INTERVIEWING AND REPORT WRITING*

> *Interviewing is the foundation from which all of the outpatient's psychiatric care proceeds. It demands psychopathological knowledge, interpersonal skills, and intuitive abilities. Thus, it is a true blending of science, craft, and art.*
> —J. E. Mezzich and S. C. Shea, *Interviewing and Diagnosis*

---

### CHAPTER OBJECTIVES

In most clinical and counseling settings, treatment begins with an intake interview. During an intake interview, you are faced with the seemingly insurmountable task of gathering a large amount of information about the client and his or her situation, while maintaining client comfort and rapport at the same time. In this chapter, we review the nuts and bolts of conducting an intake interview. Information is also provided on preparing intake reports. After reading this chapter, you will know:

- The nature and objectives of a typical intake interview.
- Strategies for identifying, evaluating, and exploring client problems and goals.
- Strategies for obtaining historical information about clients, for evaluating their interpersonal styles, and for assessing their current level of functioning.
- Different agency or institutional guidelines and procedures that might affect your intake interviewing procedures.
- A brief or minimal intake interviewing procedure for working with clients in a managed care or time-limited model.
- How to write a professional, but client-friendly intake report.
- Special considerations when interviewing clients with substance abuse problems or recent trauma.

---

## WHAT IS AN INTAKE INTERVIEW?

The intake interview is primarily an assessment interview. Before initiating counseling, psychotherapy, or psychiatric treatment, it's usually necessary and always wise to conduct an intake interview. Intake interviews are designed to answer a number of critical questions, which typically include:

- Is the client suffering from a mental, emotional, or behavioral problem?
- If so, are his or her mental, emotional, or behavioral problems sufficient to require treatment?
- What form of treatment should be provided to the client?
- Who should provide the treatment and in what setting?

The advent of managed care has changed the types and duration of psychological help available to many people. Similar to psychotherapy, intake interview procedures have been affected by managed care mental health programs. Ages ago, back when we had to walk five miles through the snow to get to our graduate classes, our supervisors emphasized that several fifty-minute interviews were needed before enough assessment information could be obtained to diagnose the client, develop an adequate treatment plan, and initiate treatment. This was true even in the case of traditionally shorter therapies such as cognitive or behavioral therapy.

Today's managed care climate requires practitioners to be faster and more efficient in identifying client problems, establishing treatment goals, and outlining an expected treatment course. Speed and brevity are the order of the day. In addition, treatment goals are sometimes more modest in their depth and breadth.

Although it's reasonable for therapists to become more efficient in making treatment decisions, efficiency is not always enhanced by speed or brevity. For example, when individuals are pressured to work faster, it doesn't matter whether they're baking cakes, building cabinets, repairing automobiles, or doing intake interviews—the outcome is similar: Quality can be compromised.

As we discuss intake interview procedures in this chapter, be aware that we are describing an intake procedure that is more comprehensive and lengthy than is usually expected, or even tolerated, in managed care settings. We do so for several reasons. First, it's important to learn what *can* be accomplished in the context of an intake interview assessment, even though it may not accurately reflect what ordinarily *will* be accomplished. Second, it would be unethical to educate prospective mental health professionals using exclusively a "bare bones" intake assessment approach; trimming back and becoming more efficient is best done from a broad and thorough understanding of the entire process. However, we must be pragmatic; if you are in graduate school today, chances are you will, at some point in your clinical career, work in a managed care setting. Therefore, we provide an outline and checklist designed for performing abbreviated intake interviews toward the end of this chapter.

## Settings and Professional Groups

Whether the setting is a social service agency, hospital, mental health center, college counseling center, or a private office, some form of intake interview precedes treatment or disposition of each case. Similarly, it doesn't matter whether the interviewer is a social worker, psychiatrist, psychologist, or counselor—all practitioners must have the ability to conduct an adequate intake interview. Of course, the nature and focus of intake interviews vary depending on the type of practitioner, the setting, and purpose of the interview, but even so, there usually is, or should be, more consistency than variation.

In most settings, the intake interview is referred to simply as an *intake*. *Intake* is defined as "an act or instance of taking in" (Random House, 1993), which reflects how an intake is needed to get something into a system. The intake interview is the entry point for clients seeking professional mental health assistance. Intake data come from the client, the interviewer's observations of and reactions to the client, and referral or registration information. Although intake interviews sometimes help clients resolve their problems, or at least initiate the helping process, intakes usually are not designed to provide treatment or help. Intake interviews, in their purest sense, are designed for assessment. Consequently, interviewers rely heavily on questions when conducting intake interviews (J. Sommers-Flanagan & Means, 1987).

## OBJECTIVES OF INTAKE INTERVIEWING

Broadly speaking, the three basic objectives associated with an intake interview are:

1. Identifying, evaluating, and exploring the client's chief complaint and associated therapy goals.
2. Obtaining a sense of the client's interpersonal style, interpersonal skills, and personal history.
3. Evaluating the client's current life situation and functioning.

Achieving these objectives during an intake interview is difficult, requiring refined skills and attentiveness to interpersonal process and informational content.

An additional objective associated with intake interviewing involves communicating the results of your intake interview—most often to other professionals, but sometimes to other interested parties. In most mental health settings, you not only conduct the intake interview, but also write or dictate the *intake report* following your session.

### Identifying, Evaluating, and Exploring Client Problems and Goals

Your first, and perhaps primary, objective is to find out about your client's distress. As an interviewer, your exploration of a client's chief complaint begins with your opening statement (e.g., "What brings you here?" or "How can I be of help?"; see Chapter 6). After the opening statement, at least 5 to 15 minutes should be spent tracking the client and trying to understand exactly why he or she has come to see you (Shea, 1998). In some cases, clients clearly identify their reasons for seeking professional assistance; in other cases, perhaps more often, they are vague as to why they are in your office. As clients begin to articulate their problems, nondirective listening responses can be used to facilitate rapport. Then, after an initial impression of primary concerns is obtained, directive information-gathering responses, including questions, should be used more liberally.

Client problems are intimately linked with client goals (Jongsma & Peterson, 1995). Unfortunately, many clients who come to therapy are unable to see past their problems. Consequently, it is the interviewer's task to help clients orient toward goals or solutions early in the counseling process (Bertolino & O'Hanlon, 2002; Murphy, 1997). Remember that behind (or in front of) every client problem is a client goal.

Common problems presented by clients include anxiety, depression, and relationship conflicts. Other problems include eating disorders, alcoholism or drug addiction, social skill deficits, physical or sexual abuse, stress reactions, vocational confusion, and sexual dysfunction. Because of the wide range of symptoms or problems clients present, it is crucial that interviewers have at least a general knowledge of psychopathology and *DSM-IV-TR* (American Psychiatric Association, 2000). However, every problem has an inherent goal. Therefore, early in the intake, interviewers can help clients reframe their problem statements into goal statements. For example, when clients begin talking about anxiety, interviewers can translate such language into a positive framework:

> "I hear you talking about your feelings of nervousness and anxiety. If I understand you correctly, what you're saying is you really want to feel calm and relaxed more often. I guess maybe one of your general goals for therapy might be to feel calm and relaxed more often and to be able to bring on those calm and relaxed feelings yourself. Do I have that right?"

By reframing client problems into goal statements, interviewers help clients feel hopeful and also begin a positive, therapeutic goal-setting process (Selekman, 1993; J. Sommers-Flanagan & Sommers-Flanagan, 1997). Such goal-setting reframes can also provide useful assessment information regarding the client's openness, or resistance, to actually setting realistic goals for therapy.

### Prioritizing and Selecting Client Problems and Goals

Often, we wish clients would come to their intake interview with a single, easily articulated problem and associated goal. For example, it might be nice (though a bit intimidating) if a new client in the first session stated:

> "I have a social phobia. You see, when in public, I worry more than the average person about being scrutinized and negatively judged. My anxiety about this is manifest through sweating, constant worry about being inadequate, and avoidance of most, but not all, social situations. What I'd like to do in therapy is build my self-confidence, increase my positive self-talk, and learn to calm myself down when I'm starting to get upset."

Unfortunately, most clients come to their intake interview with either a number of interrelated complaints or with general vague symptoms. They usually use problem-talk (verbal descriptions of what's wrong) to express concerns about their lives. Consequently, after the initial 5 to 15 minutes of an intake interview, it's the interviewer's job to begin establishing a list of primary problems and goals identified by the client. Usually, when an interviewer begins helping a client make a problem/goal list, it signals a transition from general nondirective listening to specific identification and prioritization of emotional and behavioral problems and goals. Transitioning from client free expression to more structured interactions has a dual purpose. First, it allows the interviewer to check for any additional problems that the client has not yet talked about. Second, the transition begins the process of problem prioritization, selection, and goal setting:

> **Interviewer:** "So far, you've talked mostly about how you've been feeling so down lately, how it's so hard for you to get up in the morning, and how most things that are usually fun for you haven't been fun lately. I'm wondering if you have any other major concerns or distress in your life right now."
> **Client:** "As a matter of fact, yes, I do. I get awful butterflies. I feel so apprehensive sometimes. Mostly these feelings seem connected to my career . . . or maybe I should say lack of career."

During problem exploration, interviewers help clients identify their problems or concerns. This process is truly exploratory; interviewers listen closely to problems that clients discuss, paraphrase or summarize what problems have been identified, and inquire about the existence of any other significant concerns.

In the preceding exchange, the interviewer used an indirect question to continue exploring for problems. After several problems are identified, the interviewer then moves to problem prioritization or selection. Because all problems cannot be addressed simultaneously, interviewer and client must choose together which problem or problems receive most attention during an intake.

> **Interviewer:** "I guess so far we could summarize your major concerns as your depressed mood, anxiety over your career, and shyness. Which of these would you say is currently most troubling to you?"
>
> **Client:** "Well, they all bother me, but I guess my mood is worst. When I'm in a really bad mood and don't get out of bed all day, I end up never facing those other problems anyway."

This client has identified depression as his biggest concern. Of course, an alternative formulation of the problem is that social inhibition and anxiety produce the depressed mood and, therefore, should be dealt with first. Otherwise, the client will never get out of bed because of his strong fears and anxieties. However, it's usually (but not always) best to follow client leads and explore their biggest concerns first (psychiatrists refer to what the client considers the main problem as the *chief complaint*). In this example, all three symptoms may eventually be linked anyway. Exploring depression first still allows the clinician to integrate the anxiety and shyness symptoms into the picture.

Even if you believe an issue different from what the client identifies should be explored (e.g., alcoholism), it's best to wait and listen carefully to what the client thinks is the main problem (chief complaint). Acknowledging, respecting, and empathizing with the client's perspective and helps you be effective, gain trust, and keep the client in counseling. In time-limited circumstances (e.g., managed care), nondirective empathic responses arebrief and intermittent. Usually, there must be a quick transition from problems to goal setting (Jongsma & Peterson, 1995), which is reasonable given that goal setting has a positive effect on treatment outcome (Locke, Shaw, Saari, & Latham, 1981; J. Sommers-Flanagan & Sommers-Flanagan, 1996). Nonetheless, we proceed, for now, with a discussion of problem analysis, selection, and prioritization. In Chapter 10, goal setting is discussed more thoroughly—in the context of treatment planning.

## Analyzing Symptoms

Once you've identified a primary problem in collaboration with your client, attention should turn to a thorough analysis of that problem, including emotional, cognitive, and behavioral aspects. Seek answers to a list of questions similar to the following. As you read the questions, think about different client problems (e.g., panic attacks, low self-esteem, unsatisfactory personal relationships, binge eating or drinking, vocational indecision) that you might be exploring through the use of such questions:

1. When did the problem or symptoms first occur? (In some cases, the symptom is one that the client has experienced before. If so, you should explore its origin and more recent development and maintenance.)

2. Where were you and what exactly was happening when you first noticed the problem? (What was the setting, who was there, etc.?)
3. How have you tried to cope with or eliminate this problem?
4. Which efforts have been most effective?
5. Can you identify any situations, people, or events that usually precede your experience of this problem?
6. What exactly happens when the problem or symptoms begin?
7. What thoughts or images go through your mind when it is occurring?
8. Do you have any physical sensations before, during, or afterwards?
9. Where and what do you feel in your body? Describe it as precisely as possible.
10. How frequently do you experience this problem?
11. How long does it usually last?
12. Does the problem affect or interfere with your usual ability to function at work, at home, or at play?
13. In what ways does it interfere with your work, relationships, school, or recreational pursuits?
14. Describe the worst experience you have had with this particular symptom. When the symptom is at its worst, what are your thoughts, images, and feelings then?
15. Have you ever expected the symptom to occur and it did not occur, or it occurred only for a few moments and then disappeared?
16. If you were to rate the severity of your problem, with 1 indicating no distress and 100 indicating so much distress that it's going to cause you to kill yourself or die, how would you rate it today?
17. What rating would you have given your symptom on its worst day ever?
18. What's the lowest rating you would ever have given your symptom? In other words, has it ever been completely absent?
19. As we have discussed your symptom during this interview, have you noticed any changes? (Has it gotten any worse or better as we have focused on it?)
20. If you were to give this symptom and its effects on you a title, like the title of a book or play, what title would you give?

These questions are listed in an order that flows fairly well in many interviews. However, these particular questions and their order are not standard. Before conducting an intake interview, you might want to review a list of questions such as these and then reword them to fit your style. New questions can be added and others deleted until you believe you have a set of questions that meets your particular needs. We encourage you to continually revise your list so that you can become increasingly efficient and sensitive when questioning clients. A varying number of questions can be used during practice intake interviews so you can estimate how many specific questions you can fit reasonably into a single interviewing session.

Sometimes even best-laid plans fail. Clients can be skillful at drawing interviewers off-track. At times, it may be important for interviewers to allow themselves to be drawn off-track because diverging from your planned menu of questions can lead to a different and perhaps more significant area (e.g., reports of sexual or physical abuse or suicidal ideation). Therefore, you may not end up following your planned list of questions and content areas in a rigid manner. Although you should make efforts to stick with your planned task, at the same time, remain flexible so you do not inadvertently overlook important clues clients give about other significant problem areas.

## Using Problem Conceptualization Systems

Some authors recommend using organized problem conceptualization systems when analyzing client problems (Cormier & Cormier, 1998; Seay, 1978). Usually, these systems are theory-based, but several systems reflect a more eclectic orientation (Cormier & Cormier, 1998; Lazarus, 1976). Most conceptualization systems guide interviewers by analyzing and conceptualizing problems with strict attention to predetermined, specified domains of functioning.

Lazarus (1976, 1981) developed a "multimodal" behavioral-eclectic approach. He believes problems should be assessed and treated via seven specific modalities or domains. Lazarus (1976) developed the acronym *BASIC ID* to represent his seven-modality system:

B: *Behavior.* Specific, concrete behavioral responses are analyzed in Lazarus's system. He particularly attends to behaviors that clients engage in too often or too infrequently. These include positive or negative habits or reactions. A multimodal-oriented interviewer might ask: "Are there some things you'd like to stop doing?" and "Are there some things you'd like to do more often?" as a way of determining what concrete behaviors the client might like to increase or decrease through therapy.

A: *Affect.* Lazarus's definition of *affect* includes feelings, moods, and other self-reported and self-described emotions. He might ask, "What makes you happy or puts you in a good mood?" or "What emotions are most troubling to you?"

S: *Sensation.* This modality refers to the sensory processing of information. For example, clients often report physical symptoms associated with high levels of anxiety (e.g., choking, elevated temperature, heart palpitations). The multimodal interviewer might ask, "Do you have any unpleasant aches, pains, or other physical sensations?" and "What happens to cause you those unpleasant sensations?"

I: *Imagery.* Imagery consists of internal visual cognitive processes. Clients often experience pictures or images of themselves or of future events that influence their functioning. A multimodal interviewer could query, "When you're feeling anxious, what images or pictures pop into your mind?"

C: *Cognition.* Lazarus believes in closely evaluating client thinking patterns and beliefs. This process usually includes an evaluation of distorted or irrational thinking patterns that occur almost automatically and lead to emotional distress. For example, an interviewer could ask, "When you meet someone new, what thoughts go through your mind?" and "What are some positive things you say to yourself during the course of a day?"

I: *Interpersonal Relationships.* This modality concerns interpersonal variables such as communication skills, relationship patterns, and assertive capabilities as manifest during role play and as observed in the client-interviewer relationship. Possible relevant questions include, "What words would you use to describe the positive or healthy relationships that you have?" and "Who would you like to spend more time with, and who would you like to spend less time with?"

D: *Drugs.* This modality refers to biochemical and neurological factors that can affect behavior, emotions, and thinking patterns. It includes physical illnesses and nutritional patterns. Questions might include, "Are you participating in any regular physical exercise?" and "Do you take any prescription drugs?"

Lazarus's (1976) model is broad-based, popular, and useful to interviewers of different theoretical orientations. If you're interested in learning more about his model, his latest book is *Brief but Comprehensive Psychotherapy: The Multimodal Way* (1997; see Readings and Resources at the end of this chapter).

Lazarus's model slightly overemphasizes cognitive processes (two separate cognitive modalities exist in his seven-modality system: cognition and imaging) while neglecting or deemphasizing spiritual, cultural, and recreational domains. As suggested previously, similar to every system designed to aid in problem identification, exploration, and conceptualization, the multimodal system has its imperfections. It is important to be familiar with numerous systems so, as a competent professional interviewer, you can be flexible in your questioning and conceptualizing and adapt to your setting and individual client problems and needs.

Behavioral and cognitive theorists and practitioners emphasize the importance of antecedents and consequences in problem development and maintenance. This approach is founded on the belief that analyzing clients' environments and their interpretation of environmental stimuli allows counselors to explain, predict, and control specific symptoms. Behaviorists have called this model of conceptualizing problem behavior the *ABC model* (Thoresen & Mahoney, 1974): behavioral *A*ntecedents, the *B*ehavior or problem itself, and behavioral *C*onsequences. Although this model has been criticized (Goldfried, 1990), it is useful for all interviewers to explore—at the very least—the following ABCs with their clients:

- What events, thoughts, and experiences precede the identified problem?
- What is the precise operational definition of the problem (i.e., what behaviors constitute the problem)?
- What events, thoughts, and experiences follow the identified problem?

When following the ABC model, interviewers can be meticulous in their search for potential behavioral antecedents and consequences. For example, an interviewer could assess for behavioral antecedents and consequences using all modalities identified by Lazarus (1976):

| | |
|---|---|
| Behavior: | What behaviors precede and follow symptom occurrence? |
| Affect: | What affective experiences precede and follow symptom occurrence? |
| Sensation: | What physical sensations precede and follow symptom occurrence? |
| Imagery: | What images precede and follow symptom occurrence? |
| Cognitions: | What specific thoughts precede and follow symptom occurrence? |
| Interpersonal: | What relationship events or experiences precede or follow symptom occurrence? |
| Drugs: | What biochemical, physiological, or drug-use experiences precede or follow symptom occurrence? |

### The Diagnostic Look: Searching for a Syndrome

A *syndrome* is a set of symptoms that usually occur together. After you've identified a symptom, such as a sad or depressed mood, your next task is to explore it in greater depth. A client's reported depressed mood may represent nothing more than a single symptom (e.g., sadness) caused by the natural ups and downs of life. Alternatively, depressed mood may represent the tip of a diagnostic iceberg. Once a primary symptom has been identified and the client has acknowledged it as a significant concern, a search for accompanying symptoms is warranted (see Chapter 10 for more information on diagnostic interviewing).

The *DSM-IV-TR* (American Psychiatric Association, 2000) and the *ICD-10* (World Health Organization, 1997a, 1997b) provide contemporary standards for diagnostic classification of mental disorders. There are numerous structured diagnostic interview systems designed to reliably identify a client's *DSM* diagnosis (R. Rogers, 2001). Structured diagnostic interviewing is a particular type of interviewing designed to confirm or rule out psychiatric diagnoses (Vacc & Juhnke, 1997). To maximize the reliability of such procedures, many standardized approaches have been developed. These approaches are essentially menu-driven; for example, if a client responds to a particular question with a yes, there is a specific question the evaluator must subsequently ask. Obviously, rigid adherence to standardized diagnostic interviewing protocols has its costs and benefits. On the one hand, rigid, diagnosis-oriented approaches can adversely affect rapport. On the other hand, if clients are adequately informed of the nature and purpose of the structured diagnostic interview, such approaches can be effective, efficient, and reliable. Specific diagnostic interviewing and treatment planning procedures are the focus of Chapter 10.

## Obtaining Background and Historical Information

In an intake interview, three basic sources of information are used to assess the client's personality and mental condition:

1. The client's personal history.
2. The client's manner of interacting with others.
3. Formal evaluation of client mental status.

The remainder of this section discusses methods and issues related to obtaining a client's personal history and evaluating a client's interpersonal style (evaluating mental status is the focus of Chapter 8).

### *Shifting to the Personal or "Psychosocial" History*

After spending about 15 to 25 minutes exploring the presenting complaint, you should have a reasonable idea of the primary reasons the client is seeking counseling. It is time to consider shifting your focus. A useful bridge from problem exploration to personal or psychosocial history is *the question.* Say to the client something like:

> "I think I'm pretty clear on the main reasons you've come for counseling, but one thing I'd like to know more about is why you've chosen to come for counseling *now.*"

The purpose of this question is to determine what specific factors convinced the client to seek professional help at this *particular time* in his or her life. This question helps determine whether a specific precipitating event produced the referral. The client's response can also shed light on whether the client is a willing participant in the interview or perhaps was coerced by friends or family to come for assistance. If the client balks or scoffs at your question of *Why now?,* simply continue to pursue the question, perhaps through alternative approaches, such as:

"Why didn't you come in a few weeks ago when you were first jilted by your girl-friend?"

"You've had these symptoms so long, I'm still a little puzzled over exactly what prompted you to seek counseling now. Why not before? And why didn't you choose to wait and 'tough it out' as you have in the past?"

After your client has responded to the *Why now?* question (and after you've summarized or paraphrased that response), you can formally shift the interview's focus from the *problem* to the *person.* This shift can be made with a statement similar to the following:

"So far, we've spent most of our time discussing the concerns that caused you to come for counseling. Now I'd like to try to get a more complete sense of how you've become the person you are today. One of the best ways for me to do that is to ask you some questions about your past."

### Nondirective Historical Leads

Immediately following your shift to psychosocial history, in most cases, you should become very nondirective. This is because you are moving away from analyzing specific symptoms and entering a completely new domain

"How about if you begin by telling me some of your childhood memories?"

"Maybe it would be easiest if you started with where you were born and raised and then talk about whatever significant details come to mind."

"Tell me what you remember about growing up."

For assessment purposes, shifting to psychosocial history should be done as nondirectively as possible. Clients reveal significant information simply by what they choose to focus on and by what they choose to avoid. After a brief nondirective period (perhaps two to five minutes), you can provide clients with more structure and guidance and begin asking specific questions about their past.

As discussed in Chapter 6, many clients are hesitant to talk freely about their childhood experiences; they may ask for structure and guidance. For a few minutes during history taking, we believe it can be useful to avoid giving structure and guidance. If you provide structure and ask specific questions, you may never know what the client would spontaneously choose to talk about. If your client presses you on this issue, you can state directly:

"I'll ask you some specific questions about your childhood in a few minutes, but right now I'm interested in past experiences and memories that you would like to share. Just tell me a few memories that seem important to you."

After making such a statement, simply sit back and lend an interested ear. Clients may feel anxious and uncomfortable, but if you appear genuinely interested in hearing about their past, it helps ease their discomfort.

Still, many clients resist delving into their personal history. Personal histories are sometimes traumatic and disturbing. Significant historical experiences may be re-pressed or at least purposely not considered or remembered very often. In our experi-ence, clients frequently claim, "I really can't remember much of my past" or "My child-hood is mostly a blank." If this is the case, try to be supportive and reassuring:

> "You know, memory is a funny thing. Sometimes bits of it will come back to you as we discuss it. Of course, most of us have memories we would rather not recall because they are painful or traumatic. My job is not to force you into talking about difficult past experiences. But I hope you feel free to discuss whatever past events you want to discuss."

Obtaining a psychosocial history is a delicate and sensitive process. For the most part, intake interviews are not designed to dig deeply into specific trauma experiences. On the other hand, opening up and sharing about traumas can be a therapeutic and emotionally ventilating experience (M. Greenberg, Wortman, & Stone, 1996; Penne-baker, 1995). Effective intake interviewers give clients an opportunity to disclose past trau-matic events, but they do not require clients to do so.

Perhaps more than any other time during the intake, the interviewer must be ready during the personal history to shift back to nondirective listening. Many times, our stu-dents have asked, "What if my client has been sexually abused?" or "What if my client's parents died when she was a young child; what do I do then?" The fact is, when you delve into a client's personal history, you run the risk of stumbling onto emotionally charged or "hot" material. Be prepared; expect that you will come across at least a few emotionally warm, if not hot, memories. When you do run across such memories, simply listen well. You cannot fix the memories or change the past. When clients first disclose a traumatic experience to an interviewer, they need most of all a supportive and empathic ear. Comments that track your client's experience, such as "Sounds like that was an especially difficult time" or "That was a time when you were really down (or an-gry, or anxious)," might be all your client needs when disclosing traumatic experiences.

Some clients may have trouble pulling themselves out of their emotionally distress-ing memories. In such cases, clear distinctions can be made between what happened then and what's happening now. Explore with clients how they managed to handle the trying times in their lives. Exploring, identifying, and emphasizing how clients coped and survived during a difficult past situation is helpful and appropriate. In fact, you may be able to point out ways your clients were strong during their most difficult times. For example:

> "It sounds like you've been through some very hard times, there's no doubt about that. And yet, it's also clear to me, as I listen to you, that back then, when things were at their worst, you reached out and got help and got yourself back on your feet again."

It is also helpful to gradually lead clients back to the present as you gather historical in-formation. As you move into the present, your clients may be able to gain distance from painful past experiences. On rare occasions, a client will remain consumed with nega-tive emotions. Sometimes, this happens because of the powerful nature of traumatic memories. Other times, clients get stuck because they do not view the present as an im-provement over the bad times in the past. Whatever the case, when clients get stuck in their negative or traumatic memories, it can be disheartening or frightening to begin-ning interviewers. Consequently, strategies for assessing and managing clients who are overwhelmed by negative or suicidal thoughts are covered in Chapter 9.

## Directive Historical Leads

After briefly allowing your clients to freely discuss what they feel is significant in their past, initiate another transition in the interview and become a more directive explorer of your clients' past. You can potentially obtain literally a lifetime of historical material from a client. In a typical intake, you have a limited amount of time and, therefore, must decide which areas to focus on. A good place to begin your directive exploration of a client's past is with an early memory (A. Adler, 1931/1958):

> **Interviewer:** "What is your earliest memory—the first thing you can remember from your childhood?"
>
> **Client:** "I remember my brothers trying to get me to get into my dad's pickup. They wanted me to pretend I was driving it. They were laughing. I got into the cab and somehow got the truck's brake off, because it started to roll. My dad got pretty mad, but my brothers were always trying to get me to do these outrageous things."
>
> **Interviewer:** "How old were you?"
>
> **Client:** "I suppose about 4, maybe 5."

Often, memories reported by clients hold significance for their present lives; that is, the memories represent major themes or issues the client is currently struggling with (A. Adler, 1931/1958; Mosak, 1989; Parrott, 1992). For example, the client who revealed the preceding memory reported that his life was characterized by performances that he put on for others. He admitted having strong urges to do outrageous things to get the attention and approval of others.

When clients reveal memories that are either strikingly positive or strikingly negative, it is useful to follow up with questions that seek an opposite type of memory. Virtually everyone has both positive and negative childhood memories. A good practice is to assess whether your client can produce a balanced report of positive and negative childhood experiences. Clients who remember mostly negative childhood experiences may be suffering from a depressive disorder, whereas clients who never mention negative experiences may be using defense mechanisms of denial, repression, or dissociation (Mosak, 1989):

> **Client:** "I remember breaking a pipe down in the basement of my house. I had gotten into my dad's tools and was striking an exposed pipe with a hammer. It started leaking and flooded the basement. I was in big trouble."
>
> **Interviewer:** "It sounds like that memory was mostly of a negative time when you got in trouble. Can you think of an early memory of something with a more positive flavor?"
>
> **Client:** "Oh yeah, my memories of playing with my next-door neighbor are great. My mom used to have him over and we would play with every game and toy in the house."
>
> **Interviewer:** "Do you remember a specific time when he came over and you played?"
>
> **Client:** "Uh . . . yeah. He always wanted to play army, but I liked dinosaurs better. We got in a fight, and I ended up throwing all the army men out into the front yard. Then we stayed in and played dinosaurs."

Sometimes, even when you ask for a positive client memory, you will get a response with negativity and conflict. On the other hand, some clients deny they have ever had any negative memories. There is probably no use in pointing out to clients, unless they note it themselves, the fact that they reported another largely negative (or positive) event. Instead, merely take note of the quality of their memories and move on.

Another standard method for exploring childhood or, more specifically, parent-child relationships, is to ask clients to describe their parents with three words.

**Interviewer:** "Give me three words to describe your mother."
**Client:** "What do you mean?"
**Interviewer:** "When you think of your mother and what she's like, what three words best describe her?"
**Client:** "I suppose . . . clean, . . . and proper, and uh, intense. That's it, intense."

As noted, there is a high likelihood of stumbling into strong, affectively charged memories when exploring your clients' psychosocial histories. This is especially true when exploring parent-child relationships. The words used by clients to describe their parents may require follow up. You can do so by asking clients to provide examples of their descriptions:

"You said your mother was intense. Can you give me an example of something she did that fits that word?"

A natural flow while history taking is: (a) first memories, (b) memories of parents and siblings (if any), (c) school and peer relations, (d) work or employment, and (e) other areas (see Table 7.1). Psychosocial history information that might be covered in a very thorough intake interview is listed in Table 7.1. Note that this is a fairly comprehensive list of historical domains. In a typical clinical intake, you will need to be selective regarding history taking. It is a gross understatement to say that in most cases you cannot cover everything in the 15 to 20 minutes you have to devote to personal history taking. In fact, even in a 50-minute interview designed for specifically obtaining historical background information, judicious selection from the areas listed in Table 7.1 is necessary.

Table 7.1 should not be considered a rigid outline for the psychosocial history. Other interviewing guides are available for many of the content areas (or domains) listed in the table (see Suggested Readings and Resources at the end of the chapter).

Because it is often difficult to choose which domains to explore during the limited time available in an interview, agencies and individual clinicians often use registration forms or intake questionnaires for new clients. These forms are designed to provide interviewers with client information before they see the client for the first time. On the basis of such information, interviewers can select domains to emphasize with a new client. Additionally, a considerable amount of research has been carried out on computer administration of intake interviews and mental status examinations. Although this type of approach is impersonal, it has some advantages: Computers do not forget to ask particular questions, and some clients feel more comfortable disclosing their drug abuse history, sexual history, or other sensitive facts (e.g., HIV status) to a computer than to an interviewer (Binik, Cantor, Ochs, & Meana, 1997; Bloom, 1992; Dolezal-Wood, Belar, & Snibbe, 1998).

## Evaluating Interpersonal Style

The claim that individuals have personality traits resulting in consistent or predictable patterns of behavior is more or less controversial, depending on a person's theoretical

**Table 7.1    Personal History Interview Sample Questions**

| Content Areas | Questions |
|---|---|
| 1. First memories | What is your first memory?<br>How old were you then?<br>Do you have any very positive (or negative) early memories? |
| 2. Descriptions and memories of parents | Give me three words to describe your mother (or father).<br>Who did you spend more time with, Mom or Dad?<br>What methods of discipline did your parents use with you?<br>What recreational or home activities did you do with your parents? |
| 3. Descriptions and memories of siblings | Did you have any brothers or sisters? (If so, how many?)<br>What memories do you have of time spent with your siblings?<br>Who was your closest sibling and why?<br>Who were you most similar to in your family?<br>Who were you most dissimilar to in your family? |
| 4. Elementary school experiences | Do you remember your first day of school?<br>How was school for you? (Did you like school?)<br>What was your favorite (or best) subject in school?<br>What subject did you like least (or were you worst at)?<br>Do you have any vivid school memories?<br>Who was your favorite (or least favorite) teacher?<br>What made you like (or dislike) this teacher so much?<br>Were you ever suspended or expelled from school?<br>Describe the worst trouble you were ever in when in school.<br>Were you in any special or remedial classes in school? |
| 5. Peer relationships (in and out of school) | Do you remember having many friends in school?<br>What kinds of things did you do for fun with your friends?<br>Did you get along better with boys or girls?<br>What positive (or negative) memories do you have from relationships you had with your friends in elementary school? |
| 6. Middle school, high school, and college experiences | Do you remember having many friends in high school?<br>What kinds of things did you do for fun with your friends?<br>Did you get along better with boys or girls?<br>What positive (or negative) memories do you have from high school?<br>So you remember your first day of high school?<br>How was high school for you? (Did you like high school?)<br>What was your favorite (or best) subject in high school?<br>What subject did you like least (or were you worst at)?<br>Do you have any vivid high school memories?<br>Who was your favorite (or least favorite) high school teacher?<br>What made you like (or dislike) this teacher so much?<br>Were you ever suspended or expelled from high school?<br>Describe the worst trouble you were ever in when in high school.<br>What was your greatest high school achievement (or award)?<br>Did you go to college?<br>What were your reasons for going (or not going) to college?<br>What was your major field of study in college?<br>What is the highest degree you obtained? |

**Table 7.1    (Continued)**

| Content Areas | Questions |
|---|---|
| 7. First employment and work experience | What was your first job or the first way you ever earned money? <br> How did you get along with your coworkers? <br> What kinds of positive and negative job memories do you have? <br> Have you ever been fired from a job? <br> What is your ultimate career goal? <br> How much money would you like to make annually? |
| 8. Military history and experiences | Were you ever in the military? <br> Did you volunteer, or were you drafted? <br> Tell me about your most positive (or most negative) experiences in the military. <br> What was your final rank? <br> Were you ever disciplined? What was your offense? |
| 9. Romantic relationship history | Have you ever had romantic feelings for someone? <br> Do you remember your first date? <br> What do you think makes a good romantic or loving relationship? <br> What do you look for in a romantic (or marital) partner? <br> What first attracted you to your spouse (or significant other)? |
| 10. Sexual history (including first sexual experience) | What did you learn about sex from your parents (or school, siblings, peers, television, or movies)? <br> What do you think is most important in a sexual relationship? <br> Have you had any traumatic sexual experiences (e.g., rape or incest)? |
| 11. Aggressive history | What is the most angry you have ever been? <br> Have you ever been in a fight? <br> Have you ever been hit or punched by someone else? <br> What did you learn about anger and how to deal with it from your parents (or siblings, friends, or television)? <br> What do you usually do when you get angry? <br> Tell me about a time when you got too angry and regretted it later. <br> When was your last fight? <br> Have you ever used a weapon (or had one used against you) in a fight? <br> What is the worst you have ever hurt someone physically? |
| 12. Medical and health history | Did you have any childhood diseases? <br> Any medical hospitalizations? Any surgeries? <br> Do you have any current medical concerns or problems? <br> Are you taking any prescription medications? <br> When was your last physical examination? <br> Do you have any problems with eating or sleeping or weight loss or gain? <br> Have you ever been unconscious? <br> Are there any major diseases that seem to run in your family (e.g., heart disease or cancer)? <br> Tell me about your usual diet. <br> What kinds of foods do you eat most often? <br> Do you have any allergies to foods, medicines, or anything else? <br> What are your exercise patterns? <br> How often do you engage in aerobic exercise? |

*(continued)*

**Table 7.1    (Continued)**

| Content Areas | Questions |
| --- | --- |
| 13. Psychiatric or counseling history | Have you ever been in counseling before?<br>If so, with whom and for what problems, and how long did the counseling last?<br>Do you remember anything your previous counselor did that was particularly helpful (or particularly unhelpful)?<br>Did counseling help with the problem? If not, what did help?<br>Why did you end counseling?<br>Have you ever been hospitalized for psychological reasons? What was the problem then?<br>Have you ever taken medication for psychiatric problems?<br>Has anyone in your family been hospitalized for psychological reasons?<br>Has anyone in your family had significant mental disturbances? Can you remember that person's problem or diagnosis? |
| 14. Alcohol and drug history | When did you have your first drink of alcohol (or pot, etc.)?<br>About how much alcohol do you consume each day (or week or month)?<br>What is your "drink/drug of choice"?<br>Have you ever had any medical, legal, familial, or work problems related to alcohol?<br>Under what circumstances are you most likely to drink?<br>What benefits do you believe you get from drinking? |
| 15. Legal history | Have you ever been arrested or ticketed for an illegal activity?<br>Have you been issued any tickets for driving under the influence?<br>Have you been given any tickets for speeding?<br>How many or how often?<br>Have you ever declared bankruptcy? |
| 16. Recreational history | What is your favorite recreational activity?<br>What recreational activities do you hate or avoid?<br>What sport, hobby, or leisure time pursuit are you best at?<br>How often do you engage in your favorite (or best) activity?<br>What prevents you from engaging in this activity more often?<br>Whom do you do this activity with?<br>Are there any recreational activities that you'd like to do, but you've never had the time or opportunity to try? |
| 17. Developmental history | Do you know the circumstance surrounding your conception?<br>Was your mother's pregnancy normal?<br>What was your birth weight?<br>Do you know whether you were nursed or bottle-fed?<br>When did you sit, stand, and walk?<br>When did your menses begin? (for females) |
| 18. Spiritual or religious history | What is your religious background?<br>What are your current religious or spiritual beliefs?<br>Do you have a religious affiliation?<br>Do you attend church, pray, meditate, or otherwise participate in religious activities?<br>What other spiritual activities have you been involved in previously? |

orientation (Bem & Allen, 1974). Psychoanalytic and interpersonal psychotherapists base their therapy approaches on the assumption that individuals behave in highly consistent ways, depending on their personality or interpersonal style (Fairbairn, 1952; G. Kelly, 1955; Sullivan, 1970). In contrast, cognitive and behavioral psychotherapists are more likely to reject the concept of personality and claim that behavior is a function of the situation or a person's cognitions about the situation (Beck, 1976; Mischel, 1968; Ullmann & Krasner, 1965).

For the purposes of this section, we are assuming people do engage in consistent behavior patterns, but recognize that these patterns may vary greatly depending on particular persons and situations.

## Interpersonal Styles

People tend to assume specific roles in their interpersonal relationships. Some people behave in dominant ways; others are more submissive and self-effacing. Other individuals adopt a hostile or aggressive stance in interpersonal relationships; still others prefer to function in a warm and affiliative manner when relating to others. Some people seem to stay consistently in one role; others behave much differently depending on the situation and people involved. This interplay between consistency and variance can be informative and useful in assessing clients' interpersonal problem areas.

During an intake interview, three primary sources of data help interviewers evaluate client interpersonal style. First, obtain client descriptions of how he or she has related to others in the past (e.g., during childhood, adolescence, and young adulthood). Second, obtain information about how your client relates to others in his or her contemporary relationships. Third, observe client behavioral interactions that occur with you during the interview session.

Some contemporary forms of psychotherapy place great importance on evaluating a client's interpersonal style. Luborsky (1984) refers to a client's "core conflictual relationship theme" (p. 98). He believes the purpose of psychotherapy is to allow clients greater conscious choice regarding their interpersonal behavior (Kivlighan, 2002). Similarly, Schact, Binder, and Strupp (1984) consider the appropriate focus of psychotherapy to be "human actions, embedded in a context of interpersonal transactions, organized in a cyclical psychodynamic pattern, that have been a recurrent source of problems in living and are also currently a source of difficulty" (p. 70).

It is not necessary, and often not possible, to have a clear sense of a client's interpersonal style after only a single brief interview. The goal, instead, is to have a few working hypotheses about how your client generally relates to others. Further, as noted by Teyber (1997), interviewers should be "willing to work with their own emotional reactions to the feelings that clients present" (p. 150). In other words, clients affect others, including you, by behaving in ways that produce a distinct reaction. For example, some clients may cause you to feel bored, aroused, depressed, or annoyed. As noted previously, personal and emotional reactions you have toward clients are a sign of countertransference (Beitman, 1983).

## Exploring Underlying Dynamics

When interviewers begin to have a grasp of a client's interpersonal style, it is sometimes appropriate to explore dynamics that might underlie the pattern. One way of exploring underlying dynamics is to examine the nature of the client's early significant relationships. This process is straightforward, but unfortunately, clients tend to reconstruct or distort their early interpersonal relationships. Strupp and Binder (1984) comment on this issue:

A patient's memories of personally relevant events, particularly those referring to early childhood, are often subject to a variety of reconstructions. While such information may be useful for gaining a better understanding of a patient's emotional life, it is hazardous to rely on it as a primary source for formulating the patient's current problem. (p. 53)

A more effective way of exploring a client's underlying dynamics involves direct questioning about a client's thoughts, feelings, and memories that come up when he or she considers changing a deeply ingrained behavior pattern. This is an advanced form of interviewing involving questioning, trial interpretation of life patterns, and checking the client's ability to respond to this type of approach. Although this approach is not always advisable, it can provide important information when the situation is appropriate. For example:

**Interviewer:** "It seems that in many of your relationships you tend to wait for others to meet your emotional and sometimes physical needs."

**Client:** "Yeah, that's right . . . and I always end up waiting a long time too, don't I?"

**Interviewer:** "I wonder what would happen if you were to take a different, more active approach to having your needs met."

**Client:** "I don't know, I suppose it would be better, but I just can't seem able to pull it off when the time is right."

**Interviewer:** "Well, let's try something. Imagine your relationship with Sarah. What if, instead of waiting for her to call you, you took the initiative by calling her first and suggesting something you could do together? Imagine doing that and then describe to me what thoughts, feelings, and images come to mind."

**Client:** "Well . . . it's hard for me to even imagine doing that, but, well, she probably wouldn't want to do something I suggested. Or maybe she'd do it, but not enjoy it and then it would be my fault. I hate having all the responsibility for how things turn out."

In the preceding example, the interviewer traced the client's interpersonal pattern to thoughts and feelings related to fear of rejection and responsibility. This type of exploration can provide useful information to psychotherapists of virtually any theoretical orientation. Behaviorists could consider it an evaluation of a client's behavioral repertoire. Cognitive therapists could use this approach to examine a client's underlying irrational beliefs. Psychoanalytic therapists might focus on what underlies the client's irrational fears, perhaps traumatic events that occurred early in the context of significant interpersonal relationships (e.g., dependency issues related to repressed memories of being rejected when a person asks directly to have his or her needs met). Narrative therapists might see this approach as helping clients re-script or retell their story in a new and different way. Solution-oriented therapists would likely help clients view their behavior patterns differently by focusing on "exception sequences" or by using the "miracle question" (de Shazer, 1994; see Bertolino & O'Hanlon, 2002; D. Hillyer, 1996; Hoyt, 1996; O'Hanlon & Bertolino, 1998, for more detailed information on solution-oriented approaches to interviewing).

The previous client-interviewer exchange uses what psychoanalytic psychotherapists refer to as a *trial interpretation.* Some clinicians recommend using trial interpretations in initial sessions to determine whether a client is a good candidate for psychoanalytic psychotherapy (Helstone & van Zurren, 1996; Sifneos, 1987; Strupp & Binder, 1984). In the previous example, the client responds positively to the trial interpretation and, therefore, evidence to support his ability to engage in insight-oriented therapy is provided. However, it is also possible for clients to respond very negatively to trial interpretations. For example:

**Interviewer:** "It seems that in many of your relationships you tend to wait for others to meet your emotional and sometimes physical needs."

**Client:** "I don't know what you mean."

**Interviewer:** "In lots of the examples you've talked about in here, you've been waiting for someone to provide you with financial support, fix your car, or supply you with recreational entertainment. Seems like kind of a pattern in terms of how you relate to others."

**Client:** "That's ridiculous! Just because my parents are a couple of scrooges doesn't have the least bit to do with me."

This exchange not only provides important information about the client's capacity for insight, it also suggests that he is unable to take feedback or criticism well and that he may have a tendency to blame others for his personal situations. Traditionally, this client response would be viewed as an illustration of resistance or defensiveness.

Although it is possible that client resistance or defensiveness during an initial session illustrates how the client behaves outside therapy, it is also possible—because of anxiety or other factors—that the client is behaving unusually during the intake session. Consequently, therapists need to be cautious when speculating about what the new client's behavior might mean.

Once again, we are reminded that—in contrast to more psychoanalytic approaches—solution-oriented approaches deemphasize client pathology when dealing with what appear to be pervasive client behavior patterns. For example, a solution-oriented intake interviewer might query: "Suppose you were to go home tonight, and while you were asleep, a miracle happened and this problem was solved. How will you know the miracle happened? What will be different?" (de Shazer, 1985, p. 5). This "miracle question" reorients clients toward solutions, rather than problems and stuckness. It is important for therapists of all theoretical orientations to avoid perpetuating client maladaptive behavior patterns by assuming that such patterns are evidence for deeply ingrained personality defects.

Evaluating a client's personal history and interpersonal style are formidable tasks that can easily take several sessions, if you have such time to devote to assessment. However, contemporary limits on psychotherapy usually don't allow for lengthy assessment procedures. Traditionally, the main purpose of exploring interpersonal and historical issues during an intake has been to formulate hypotheses, not to provide definitive case formulations and not to advocate specific client actions or solutions. As time available to therapists has become more limited, approaches such as solution-oriented therapy are used to initiate therapeutic procedures in an intake session.

## Assessment of Current Functioning

After inquiring and exploring historical and interpersonal issues, interviewers should make one more major shift and focus on current functioning. Not only is it important to assess current functioning, but also it is equally important not to end an interview focused on the past. The shift to current functioning provides both a symbolic and a concrete return to the present. The end of the interview is also a time to encourage clients to focus on personal strengths and environmental resources, not on past problems.

Questions during this last portion of the intake focus on current client involvements or activities. Following are statements and questions to help clients talk about areas of current functioning:

> We've talked about your major concerns and a bit about your past. I'd like to shift to what's happening in your life right now.
> What kinds of activities fill up your usual day?
> Describe a typical day in your life.
> How much time do you spend at work?
> About how much time do you spend with your partner (spouse)?
> What kinds of things do you and your partner do together? How often do you do these activities?
> Do you spend much time alone?
> What do you most enjoy doing all by yourself?

Some clients have difficulty shifting from talking about their past to talking about their contemporary life. This can be especially true with clients who had difficult or traumatic childhoods. In such cases, you can use two primary strategies so clients can view their intake interviewing experience in an appropriate and realistic context. Specifically, when clients become upset during an intake interview, respond by (a) validating the client's feelings and (b) instilling hope for positive change. For example, in a case of a mother who comes to counseling shortly after losing her child to a tragic accident, you might state:

> "I can see that losing your son has been terribly painful. You probably already know that your feelings are totally normal. Most people consider losing a child to be the most emotionally painful experience possible. Also, I want you to know how smart it is for you to come and talk with me so openly about your son's death and your feelings. It won't make your sad and horrible feelings magically go away, but in almost every case, talking about your grief is the right thing to do. It will help you move through the grieving process."

Feeling validation, as discussed in Chapter 3, involves acknowledgment and approval of a client's feelings. This technique is generally reassuring to clients and is an appropriate tool toward the end of an intake when a client is experiencing painful or disturbing feelings. Another more general example of what an interviewer might say to a client who is in emotional pain or distress toward the end of an intake follows:

> "I can't help but notice that you're still feeling pretty sad about what we've talked about today. I want you to know that your sad or upset feelings are very natural. Most people who come in to talk to a counselor leave with mixed feelings. That's because it's hard to talk about your childhood or your personal problems without having uncomfortable feelings. You know, I think I'd be worried about you if you didn't feel some of what you're feeling. What you're feeling is natural."

It is normal to feel bad when talking about sad, disappointing, or traumatic events. Therapists should provide this factual information to clients in a reassuring, validating manner. Reassurance and support are essential parts of an effective closing.

## Reviewing Goals and Monitoring Change

Another key issue toward the end of the intake is the future. Clients come to counseling or therapy because they want change, and change involves the future.

Many interviewers pose some form of the following question toward the end of the intake: "Let's say that therapy is successful and you notice some major changes in your life. What will have changed?" Other future-oriented questions may also be appropriate, including "How do you see yourself changing in the next several years?" or "What kind of personal goals (or career goals) are you striving toward?" Discussion of therapy goals during an intake interview or in early therapy sessions provides a foundation for termination (Zaro, Barach, Nedelman, & Dreiblatt, 1977). Corey (1996) suggests that initial interview assessments include a question such as "What are the prospects for meaningful change, and how will we know when that change has occurred?" (p. 13). Through establishing clear definitions of desired change, clients and interviewers can jointly monitor the progress of therapy and together determine when the end of therapy is approaching. Client goals should be formulated from client problems at the beginning of an intake interview. It is also important to review client goals in a positive and upbeat manner toward the interview's end.

## FACTORS AFFECTING INTAKE INTERVIEW PROCEDURES

To conduct an intake interview that thoroughly covers each area described in this chapter within a traditional 50-minute period is impossible. As a professional interviewer, you must make choices regarding what to emphasize, what to deemphasize, and what to ignore. Several factors affect your choices.

## Client Registration Forms

Some agencies and practitioners rely on client registration forms or intake questionnaires for information about clients. This practice is especially helpful for obtaining detailed information that might unnecessarily extend the clinical hour. For example, registration forms that include space for listing names of previous therapists, names and telephone numbers of primary care physicians, and basic biographical information (e.g., date of birth, age, birthplace, educational attainment) are essential.

Although intake questionnaires are acceptable in moderation, when used excessively, they may offend or intimidate clients. For example, some agencies use 10- to 15-page intake questionnaires to screen potential clients. These questionnaires contain many extremely personal questions, such as "Have you experienced sexual abuse?" and "Describe how you were punished as a child." This type of questionnaire can be offensive and should not be used without first thoroughly explaining its purpose to clients. It also may be appropriate, depending on your setting, to include standardized symptom checklists or behavioral inventories as a part of a pretherapy questionnaire battery (although the purpose of these questionnaires should be explained to clients before completion).

## Institutional Setting

Often, information obtained in an initial interview is partly a function of agency or interviewer policy. Some institutions, such as psychiatric hospitals, demand diagnostic or historical information; other settings, such as health maintenance organizations, place greater emphasis on problem or symptom analysis, goal setting, and treatment planning. Consequently, your intake approach will vary depending on your employment setting.

## Theoretical Orientation

The interviewer's theoretical orientation can strongly influence both *what* information is obtained during an intake session and *how* it is obtained. Specifically, behavioral and cognitively oriented interviewers tend to focus on current problems, and psychoanalytically oriented interviewers downplay current problem analysis in favor of historical information. Person-centered therapists focus on the current situation and how clients feel about themselves (e.g., whether any discrepancies exist between clients' real and ideal selves). Solution-oriented therapists focus on the future and dwell on potential solutions rather than laboriously examining past or current problems. Psychoanalytic and person-centered interviewers are also less likely to make use of detailed client registration forms, computerized interviewing procedures, or standardized questionnaires.

## Professional Background and Professional Affiliation

Finally, your professional background and professional affiliation can have a strong influence on what information is obtained in an intake interview. Before writing this book, we asked professionals from different backgrounds for their opinions about what was most needed in an interviewing textbook. The correlation between response content and respondents' areas of professional training was strikingly high. Psychiatrists emphasized the importance of mental status exam and diagnostic interviewing, based on the *DSM-IV-TR*. Clinical psychologists were interested in assessment and diagnosis as well, but they also emphasized problem assessment and behavioral and cognitive analysis. Counselors and counseling psychologists focused less on formal assessment and more on listening skills and helping strategies; clinical social workers expressed interest in psychosocial history taking, treatment planning, and listening skills. Marriage and family therapists stressed the importance of understanding the family and social systems and milieu of the client. Actually, addressing all of these areas is important. Your training, theoretical orientation, and professional affiliations influence the major focus and proportion of attention paid in certain areas, but in reality, none of these areas should be neglected.

## INTERVIEWING SPECIAL POPULATIONS

The client, along with his or her particular presenting problem, is another crucial factor that influences your behavior during an intake. Obviously, reviewing every potential type of client you might face in an interview is beyond the scope of this text. However, as an example, we now focus on two specific client problems commonly seen during intake interviews: (1) clients who have substance use issues or problems and (2) clients who have experienced trauma. Chapters 10–13 are devoted entirely to interviewing youth, couples and families, and clients from divergent ethnocultural backgrounds.

## Interviewing Clients with Substance Issues or Problems

Interviewing clients with substance abuse or substance dependence problems requires specialized training and experience. The purpose of this brief section is to whet your appetite for interviewing this challenging population and to provide you with initial ideas and basic strategies for working with substance-abusing clients.

Many professionals who work with alcohol and substance-abusing clients have a personal history of substance abuse or dependence. Obviously, if you choose to work with this population, having your own substance abuse history can be a benefit or a liability. If you have experienced substance problems, you are more likely to know about the big issues from the inside out; and this can give you greater empathy for substance-abusing clients; and greater knowledge about how alcoholics or drug addicts typically avoid facing their problems. Alternatively, having had your own personal substance abuse problems makes it more likely for you to project your issues onto clients and view them less accurately (see Putting It in Practice 7.1).

---

**Putting It in Practice 7.1**

### Exploring Your Personal Attitudes Toward Substances

In one way or another, everyone has a personal substance use or abuse history and an attitude toward alcohol and drug use worth examining. Whether you grew up in a family with strong prohibitions against drinking alcohol or a family with members suffering from cocaine addiction, your family experiences undoubtedly shaped how you think about people who use (or do not use) alcohol, cocaine, and other drugs. To become more effective in working with substance-abusing clients, you should reflect on your personal alcohol and drug history, your current attitude toward substances, and your family's alcohol and drug history (almost every family has someone—perhaps an uncle, a father-in-law, or a sister-with substance use problems).

As you read further, examine your attitudes toward alcohol and drugs. Also, as you study approaches for assessing and working with substance-abusing clients, imagine yourself in both the interviewer's and the client's shoes. Ask yourself some of the following questions:

- Do I have any assumptions about how interviewers should act when interviewing substance-abusing clients?
- Is it necessary to be strongly confrontational—to get the client to "fess up" about his or her substance use? Or, will confrontational techniques increase client defensiveness and therefore reduce his or her honesty?
- If I stay nonconfrontational with clients who are addicted to substances, will they just avoid admitting they have any problems?
- What do I think about the CAGE assessment questions (see text)? How about the NIAAA criteria (see text) for alcohol consumption? How would I answer the questions? Do I, or have I ever had a problem with alcohol or other drugs?

Regardless of your specific answers to the preceding questions, be sure to talk with someone, privately or in class, about your attitudes toward and experiences with alcohol and other drugs. Becoming aware of and working through your issues is part of your continued development as a professional interviewer.

## The Traditional Substance Abuse Interviewing Approach

In the past, it was generally assumed that interviewing substance-abusing clients required strong, directive, confrontational interviewing techniques. It was thought that because individuals who abuse alcohol and other drugs are defensive—they deny or minimize their substance problems—direct confrontation was needed to break down or break through the client's defenses. For example, a traditional interview with an alcoholic from the "confrontation of denial" (Miller & Rollnick, 1991, p. 53) perspective might look like this:

> **Client:** Really, Doc, I'm just a social drinker; I don't have a big problem with it.
>
> **Interviewer:** Well, let me tell you what's true, because I'm the expert, and you're not. You can face your problem with booze or go on jeopardizing your health, your safety, and your family. If you do choose to face your problem, then you'll need to do as I say and follow our treatment program. If you don't, you'll probably end up in a gutter somewhere, lying in your own vomit. Or maybe you'll end up in jail—in the drunk tank. The fact is you've got a problem and you'll be better off admitting it right now.

As you can see, this approach to interviewing clients is very harsh. It rests primarily on presenting the client with evidence about his or her problem; this evidence is supposed to help the client accept the problem or diagnosis. Despite its popularity throughout the 1970s and early 1980s, research suggests that the confrontation of denial approach to evaluating and treating substance-using clients often results in negative outcomes (Annis & Chan, 1983; Lieberman, Yalom, & Miles, 1973). Interestingly, it appears, at least to some degree, that the strong denial and resistance displayed by alcohol and substance-using clients may occur *as a reaction* to harshly confrontive techniques (Miller & Rollnick, 1991, 2002).

## Motivational Interviewing: A Contemporary Approach to Substance Abuse Interviewing

Over the past 20 plus years, the most well-respected and empirically validated approach to interviewing clients about substance use is largely, and perhaps surprisingly, nonconfrontational. Drawing from his experiences treating "problem drinkers," William Miller (1983) began writing about his beliefs and practices, calling his methodology *motivational interviewing.* He and his colleague Stephen Rollnick published a book by that name in 1991 (a second edition in 2002), and published a number of articles in the years between. In 1995, concerned that the concept had broadened and become diluted and confusing in the literature, Rollnick and Miller offered the following definition: "Motivational interviewing is a directive, client-centered counseling style for eliciting behavior change by helping clients to explore and resolve ambivalence" (p. 326).

Miller and Rollnick (1998, 2002) stress that motivational interviewing is both a set of techniques and a philosophy, or style, with essential elements that are more important than any particular technique. These elements are central to the approach. First, they stress that motivation for change is not something the interviewer imposes on the client. It must be elicited, gently and with careful timing. Second, the ambivalence experienced and expressed by the client belongs to the client. It is not the counselor's job to resolve it, but rather to reflect it and join with the client as the client explores and resolves his or her ambivalence. Motivational interviewers do not use direct persuasion. The style is one of coming alongside, not of confronting head-on.

Central to motivational interviewing is the *readiness to change* concept articulated by Prochaska and DiClemente (1984). Essentially, this model suggests that clients often cycle through six stages of readiness to change: (a) precontemplation (when clients have not even considered change), (b) contemplation (when clients experience ambivalence about their behavior or habit), (c) determination (when clients feel, even briefly, determined to do something about their problem), (d) action (when clients engage in behaviors specifically designed to alleviate their problem), (e) maintenance (when clients use different skills for keeping the problem—or addiction—away), and (f) relapse (when clients slip back into the problem behavior).

Motivational interviewers recognize that readiness to change is not a static trait residing in the client, but rather ebbs and flows in the context of the therapeutic relationship, interview interactions, and client life experiences. Concepts often thought of as negative, such as resistance and denial, are reframed as signals that the interviewer can interpret and work with.

Motivational interviewers sidestep any attempt to make them the expert, seeing themselves instead as collaborators and helpers. They believe that working with the deep, confusing ambivalence people feel about changing habits or destructive ways of being is the central mission of the professional.

The approach draws largely and openly from the philosophies and techniques of person-centered therapy developed by Carl Rogers. As pointed out in a training video series, Carl Rogers was collaborative, safe, and caring, but in the fullest sense of the concept, he was not nondirective (Miller & Rollnick, 1998). Instead, Rogers gently guided people to the places they were most confused, or in most pain, and helped them stay there and work it through.

The last decade has seen a remarkable growth in the motivational interviewing approach for clients from various backgrounds. Addictions, changing HIV risk behaviors, smoking, diet/exercise, domestic violence, criminal justice, and juvenile justice are all problem areas in which motivational interviewing is being used as an approach with significant research to support it (Dunn, Deroo, & Rivara, 2001). A video training series is available, as are intensive training workshops, for adding this approach to your skill and knowledge base (see Suggested Readings and Resources). Professionally, we find it quite appealing and in keeping with our own beliefs about how and why people change, as well as our beliefs about the professional's role in the change process.

## Motivational Interviewing Procedures and Techniques

Although motivational interviewing procedures are largely nondirective and nonconfrontational, conducting a substance-related interview requires that the interviewer structure the interview around a number of substance use and abuse questions and issues. Rollnick and Bell (1991) recommend covering 10 different content areas.

1. Bring up the subject of substance use. Do this gently and openly. For example, following about 5 to 10 minutes of building rapport and establishing a minimal amount of trust, transition to the substance issue by using a summary statement and swing question:

   "We've been talking a while in general about how your life is going. It sounds like you've had a bit of stress lately. Would you mind if I asked you now about your use of alcohol?"

In most cases, clients—even alcohol-abusing clients—cooperate with a gentle effort to explore their drinking patterns. As you can see, this approach is tentative and gives clients a sense of control over the interview. From the motivational interviewing perspective, this approach allows the client to become engaged in a conversation. In contrast, the confrontation of denial approach tends to elicit denial and resistance by using more accusatory questions or only closed questions.

2. Ask about substance abuse in detail. Rollnick and Bell (1991) suggest questions such as, "What kind of a drinker are you?" or "Tell me about your use of marijuana; what effect does it tend to have on you?" (p. 206). The purpose of these questions is to let clients talk about their view of their drinking. These questions can be followed up with more specific queries: "You said you like to have a few beers with your friends after work. What's a 'few beers' for you?"

3. Ask about a typical day/session. When clients are habitual users, they often use in ways that are characterized by clear patterns. For example, if you prompt your client with, "Tell me about your drinking patterns on a typical day," you are likely to hear about usual or regular use, which is useful assessment information. Additionally, you can follow these more general queries with specifics, "About how much does it take for you to get high?" or "When you're at your favorite bar, what's your favorite drink, who's your best buddy, and how many do you have?"

4. Ask about lifestyle and stress. From both conceptual and practical perspectives, during a clinical interview, it is important not to become preoccupied with asking about substances. Consequently, by moving away from talking about substances—to talking about life stress—and then back again, you help the client know you are interested in more than just gathering information about substance use. This often has the effect of opening the client up to talking more about the substances, rather than less. For example, if your client talks about using substances to help himself or herself cope with stress (e.g., "It's nice just to have a drink/smoke and relax," Rollnick & Bell, 1991, p. 207), you can expand the discussion into covering life stressors by saying something like:

> "It sounds like kicking back and relaxing is important to you. What kinds of things are happening in your life that are so nice to get away from when you kick back and smoke?"

5. Ask about health, then substance use. If your client has health issues related to substance use, it is helpful to focus first on the health issues and then to gently explore the relationship between health and substance use. For example, you might ask, "How does your marijuana use work with the asthma problems we've been talking about?"

6. Ask about the good things and the less good things. Miller and Rollnick (1991) discuss this strategy in detail in their book. Briefly, the point of this strategy is to get clients to willingly discuss what they like about their substance use (what is good) as well as some of the less good things about their substance use. Eventually, the goal is to get clients to expand on what is less good to the point that they can be conceptualized as "concerns." For example, a client may love the feeling of getting high and identify it as a good thing, but also identify the "munchies," the expense, and negative feedback from his girlfriend as less good. Also, Rollnick and Bell (1991) suggest that it is better to explore what is good/less good about "having a drink," rather than "your drinking" (p. 207).

7. Ask about substance use in the past and now. In many cases, client substance use patterns shift over the years. By asking, "How have your drinking patterns

changed over the years?" interviewers can open up the discussion to a variety of issues such as blackouts, tolerance, reverse tolerance, eye openers, and so on.

8. Provide information and ask, "What do you think?" When interviewers assume an expert role and begin explaining about addiction concepts and problems to clients, they risk increasing client defensiveness. Therefore, if you provide addiction information or addiction education, do so in an open and collaborative manner. For example, you might say:

> "I recently came across some interesting information on marijuana potency and this thing experts refer to as amotivational syndrome. Would you mind if I shared some of this information with you?" (Then, after sharing the information, you should follow up with a question like, "What do you think about all this?")

9. Ask about concerns directly. At some point in a substance use interview, directly inquire about your client's concerns about his or her use patterns. Rollnick and Bell (1991) suggest using an open question such as "What concerns do you have about your alcohol use?" rather than a closed question such as "Are you concerned about your use of alcohol?" (p. 208).

10. Ask about the next step. After a client has identified concerns about using a particular substance, you can broach the issue of what actions might be taken to address the stated concerns. Once again, Rollnick and Bell (1991) provide an example. They use an elegantly worded paraphrase, followed by an indirect question for inquiring about the next step: "It sounds like you are concerned about your use of marijuana. I wonder, what's the next step?"

The motivational interviewing approach is a gentle, yet powerful, method for working effectively with clients who are using substances. Several resources for studying this method in detail are listed in the Suggested Readings and Resources at the end of this chapter.

### Other Interview-Based Procedures

Gathering valid information from substance-abusing clients can be challenging. Consequently, numerous brief interview approaches to gathering diagnostic information about substance use have been developed over the years (Cherpitel, 1997; Seppae, Lepistoe, & Sillanaukee, 1998). These approaches are especially important for professionals working in psychiatric and managed care settings, where obtaining diagnostic information quickly and efficiently is a higher priority than pursuing the sort of positive therapeutic relationship associated with motivational interviewing strategies.

Determining whether an individual is suffering from a substance use disorder is a specific diagnostic procedure. We know some therapists who, when faced with this task, simply pull out their *DSM-IV-TR* and ask clients questions based on the manual's diagnostic criteria. In contrast, alcohol and drug researchers are likely to use a specific, and sometimes lengthy, diagnostic interview as their "gold standard" for determining whether a substance abuse disorder exists (Friedmann, Saitz, Gogineni, Zhang, & Stein, 2001).

The question of "How much is too much?" substance use is often not answerable. However, several useful methods, aside from the *DSM* criteria and extensive structured interviews, have been developed. The most commonly used brief interview technique for determining whether a given client has an alcohol problem is the CAGE questionnaire. The letters C-A-G-E form an acronym to help you remember four important questions to ask clients about their alcohol use. The questions are:

C: Have you ever felt that you should CUT DOWN on your drinking?

A: Have people ANNOYED you by criticizing your drinking?

G: Have you ever felt GUILTY about your drinking?

E: Have you ever had an EARLY morning (eye opener) drink first thing in the morning to steady your nerves or to get rid of a hangover?

Although diagnosis of an alcohol disorder should never be based on a single, brief interview procedure such as the CAGE questionnaire, many interviewers, as well as the National Institute on Alcoholism and Alcohol Abuse (NIAAA), consider a "yes" to any one of the CAGE questions to be evidence of an alcohol problem. Additionally, the NIAAA has established use criteria; for men, in excess of 14 drinks a week or 4 drinks per occasion is considered a sign of alcohol abuse or alcoholism. For women, more than 7 drinks per week or 3 drinks per occasion is considered problematic (Friedmann et al., 2001).

Before moving on to the next section on interviewing trauma survivors, make sure you have read and responded to the activity in Putting It in Practice 7.1.

### Interviewing Trauma Survivors

Many clients come to therapy because they are struggling with an experience of trauma. When individuals are exposed to traumatic events, such as natural disasters, school or workplace shootings, sexual assault, or war-related violence, they often experience immediate and longer term emotional and psychological symptoms. In this section, we briefly review issues associated with interviewing trauma survivors.

*What Is Trauma?*

In 1980, when posttraumatic stress disorder was first included in the *DSM, trauma* was defined as an event "outside the range of usual human experience" (p. 236). As Judith Herman (1992) wrote in her powerful book, *Trauma and Recovery,* "Sadly this definition has proved to be inaccurate" (p. 33). The sad part of this inaccuracy is the fact that many individuals, particularly women, experience sexual abuse, rape, and/or physical battering as a part of their usual human experience (Herman, 1992). Additionally, soldiers, police officers, and emergency personnel experience trauma as a part of their occupational roles (Pearn, 2000).

The newer definition for trauma, first included in *DSM-IV* (1994) has been more widely accepted by mental health professionals. This definition includes two main components:

1. The traumatized person "experienced, witnessed, or was confronted with an event or events that involved actual or threatened death or serious injury, or a threat to the physical integrity of self or other" (p. 427).

2. The person experienced "intense fear, helplessness, or horror" (p. 428).

As you reflect on these diagnostic criteria, you can probably see why individuals who experience trauma bring unique issues with them to a clinical interview.

*Trauma Interviewing: Issues and Challenges*

The benefits of talking about trauma are virtually indisputable (Everly & Boyle, 1999; Pennebaker, 2000). Everyone who experiences trauma should talk about it—sometime, somehow, some way. Despite the benefits of talking, traumatized people are often reluctant to talk about their horrific thoughts and feelings for at least three reasons: (a) thinking about and talking about trauma brings up extremely uncomfortable feelings;

(b) trauma often involves a violation of trust or betrayal (e.g., sexual assault), making it difficult for trauma victims to trust anyone, and especially difficult to trust and confide in a virtual stranger (a mental health provider); and (c) trauma survivors frequently feel guilty about surviving and sometimes ashamed that the traumatic event happened to them (Foa & Riggs, 1994). Therefore, when working with traumatized clients, emphasize rapport and trust building; otherwise, clients may be unwilling to share their stories or, if they do, they may feel retraumatized by your questioning.

Another factor that makes working with trauma survivors problematic is the fact that traumatized clients often benefit from talking about their experiences very soon, usually within 48 hours after the traumatic event (Campfield & Hills, 2001). Consequently, for interviewers, there is a major conflict between trying to establish trust (which often takes time) and yet encouraging the client to begin talking about traumatic experiences right away.

Keep in mind that when a client discloses a trauma, you have heightened professional responsibility to make sure the sharing of the trauma does not adversely affect the client. A calm, caring demeanor is essential. A good sense of time boundaries is important as well. It is irresponsible to allow someone to go too far into the deep emotions surrounding a trauma and conclude the session without adequate time for the client to regroup emotionally. Moving gently away from the trauma itself to problem-solving about the most therapeutic way to work on the effects of the trauma can be a good strategy if a client discloses a painful trauma in a first session. In addition, getting a clear picture of trauma symptoms is important.

If you want to work with traumatized clients, we recommend advanced training in critical incidence stress debriefing procedures (Mitchell & Everly, 1993), eye movement desensitization reprocessing (Shapiro, 1995), and more general advanced training in the developmental effects of trauma. To work effectively with traumatized clients, it is essential to have advanced understanding about the effects of trauma and a clear model for providing support and treatment.

*Critical Incident Stress Debriefing (CISD).*    The critical incident stress debriefing movement began in the early 1980s and has continued to the present (Mitchell & Everly, 1993). Mitchell and Everly's approach, usually implemented with emergency and disaster personnel in group settings, involves having all group members talk about experiences associated with a traumatic event. For example, following a school shooting, natural disaster, or terrorist attack, trained debriefers meet with the affected individuals in small to medium-sized groups to review each individual's personal experiences. For additional information, see Mitchell and Everly's work listed in the Suggested Readings and Resources Section.

*Eye Movement Desensitization Reprocessing (EMDR).*    Trauma symptoms typically center around emotionally powerful memories. In particular, traumatized individuals frequently either avoid thinking about trauma experiences, or trauma memories intrude on their consciousness, either via flashbacks or nightmares. Trauma memories take up significant emotional and psychological energy and resources.

In the mid-1990s, Francine Shapiro developed EMDR, a procedure designed to take the emotional power out of traumatic memories (Shapiro, 1995, 2001). The procedure includes eight basic phases, including both cognitive and behavioral components, as well as a phase that involves brief visualization of the traumatic memory followed by rhythmic horizontal eye movements.

Research on EMDR has been largely positive. Some studies indicate that EMDR treatments, properly delivered, alleviate posttraumatic stress disorder symptoms in 70% to 100% of treated clients (Barker & Hawes, 1999; Marcus, Marquis, & Sakai,

1997; Rothbaum, 1997). These studies included rape victims, single trauma victims, and multiple trauma victims. EMDR use with traumatized clients is justified, and in many cases, is the treatment of choice, for both youth and adults (Lovett, 1999). Consequently, if you have a strong interest in evaluating and treating trauma victims, you should explore further training in this area.

## BRIEF INTAKE INTERVIEWING: A MANAGED CARE MODEL

Given the current managed care and cost containment climate in all aspects of health care, it is essential for interviewers to be trained to conduct more abbreviated intake interviews. Intake interview objectives remain the same when operating under a managed care philosophy. Obtaining information about clients' problems and goals, the clients themselves, and clients' current situation is essential. However, three primary modifications are necessary for obtaining this information within managed care guidelines. First, interviewers must rely more extensively on registration forms and questionnaire data obtained from clients before an initial meeting. Second, interviewers must use more questions and permit less time for client-directed self-expression. Third, interviewers must reduce time spent obtaining personal history and interpersonal-style information. Because using registration forms and questionnaires and asking more questions are both relatively straightforward modifications, the following discussion focuses on how to briefly obtain personal history and interpersonal style information. Subsequently, an outline for conducting brief intake interviews is provided.

### Obtaining Historical and Interpersonal Style Information

Part of the managed care mental health philosophy involves placing responsibility for client well-being back on the client (Hoyt, 1996). In some ways, this model empowers clients to make greater contributions to their own mental health. To stay within this model, when reviewing a client's history, you might state:

> "We have only a few minutes to discuss your childhood and things that have happened to you in the past. So, very briefly, tell me the most crucial things about your past. What are the most essential things I need to know about your past?"

Often, when given this assignment, clients can successfully identify a few critical incidents in their developmental history. Alternatively, if an interviewer is the client for a second or follow-up session, he or she can ask for a one- to two-page biographical summary. We have used this technique successfully with clients when time is at a premium. It offers clients an opportunity to communicate essential historical information in a time-sensitive manner.

Information pertaining to client interpersonal style is minimally relevant in a managed care environment. Therefore, although gathering information associated with client interpersonal dynamics may be a part of a managed care intake, little or none of the interviewer's time is devoted to this task. Several approaches to dealing with this issue may be employed. First, interpersonal information may be ignored unless clients exhibit *DSM-IV-TR* personality disorder characteristics. In such cases, a checklist format can be employed wherein an intake interviewer simply indicates whether a client exhibits interpersonal behaviors consistent with one or more of the personality disorder clusters. If the presence of a personality disorder is suspected, further and more definitive assessment may or may not be pursued, depending on the particular managed care policy.

Second, interviewers may employ an abbreviated mental status examination format.

In such cases, notes or reports about the client would briefly state the nature and quality of a client's "attitude toward the interviewer" (see Chapter 8 for detailed information regarding mental status examinations).

Third, interviewers may reflect, after the session, on how they were affected by their client. After this reflection, some hypotheses can be generated and written down to assure that, if necessary, attention can be paid to further understanding of interpersonal dynamics during the next session.

## A Managed Care Intake Checklist

A managed care intake outline is included in Table 7.2. We recommend that you practice full-scale intake interviews as well as scaled-down managed care intake interviews (see Putting It in Practice 7.2).

**Table 7.2.    A Managed Care Intake Checklist**

When necessary, the following topics may be covered quickly and efficiently within a managed care setting.

_____ 1. Obtain presession or registration information from the client in a sensitive manner. Specifically, explain: "This background information will help us provide you with services more efficiently."

_____ 2. Inform clients of session time limits at the beginning of their session. This information can also be provided on the registration materials. All policy information, as well as informed consent forms, should be provided to clients prior to meeting with their therapist.

_____ 3. Allow clients a brief time period (not more than 10 minutes) to introduce themselves and their problems to you. Begin asking specific diagnostic questions toward the 10-minute mark, if not before.

_____ 4. Summarize clients' major problem (and sometimes a secondary problem) back to them. Obtain agreement from them that they would like to work on their primary problem area.

_____ 5. Help clients reframe their primary problem into a realistic long-term goal.

_____ 6. Briefly identify how long clients have had their particular problem. Also, ask for a review of how they have tried to remediate their problem (e.g., what approaches have been used previously).

_____ 7. Identify problem antecedents and consequences, but also ask clients about problem exceptions. For example: "Tell me about times when your problem is not occurring. What happens that helps you eliminate the problem at those times?"

_____ 8. Tell clients that their personal history is important to you, but that there is obviously not time available to explore their past. Instead, ask them to tell you two or three critical events that they believe you should know about them. Also, ask them about (a) sexual abuse, (b) physical abuse, (c) traumatic experiences, (d) suicide attempts, (e) episodes of violent behavior or loss of personal control, (f) brain injuries or pertinent medical problems, and (g) current suicidal or homicidal impulses.

_____ 9. If you will be conducting ongoing counseling, you may ask clients to write a brief (2–3 pages) autobiography.

_____ 10. Emphasize goals and solutions rather than problems and causes.

_____ 11. Give clients a homework assignment to be completed before they return for another session. This may include behavioral or cognitive self-monitoring or a solution-oriented exception assignment.

_____ 12. After the initial session, write up a treatment plan that clients can sign at the outset of the second session.

---

**Putting It in Practice 7.2**

### Prompting Clients to Stick With Essential Information About Themselves

Using the managed care intake interviewing checklist provided in Table 7.2, work with a partner from class to streamline your intake interviewing skills. Interviewers working in a managed care environment must stay focused and goal-directed throughout the intake interview. To maintain this crucial focus, it may be helpful to:

1. Inform your client in advance that you have only a limited amount of time and therefore must stick to essential issues or key factors.
2. If your client drifts into some less essential area, gently redirect him or her by saying something such as:
   "You know, I'd like to hear more about what your mother thinks about environmentalism (or whatever issue is being discussed), but because our time is limited, I'm going to ask you a different set of questions. Between this meeting and our next meeting, I want you to write me an autobiography—maybe a couple of pages about your personal history and experiences that have shaped your life. If you want, you can include some information about your mom in your autobiography and get it to me before our next session."

Often, clients are willing to talk about particular issues at great length, but when asked to write about those issues, they are much more succinct.

Overall, the key point is to politely prompt clients to only discuss essential and highly relevant information about themselves. Either before or after practicing this activity with your partner, see how many gentle prompts you can develop to facilitate managed care intake interviewing procedures.

---

## THE INTAKE REPORT

Report writing constitutes a unique challenge to clinicians. You must consider at least five dimensions:

1. Determining your audience.
2. Choosing the structure and content of your report.
3. Writing clearly and concisely.
4. Keeping your report confidential.
5. Sharing the report with your client.

Before discussing these dimensions, it should be emphasized that interviewers have a responsibility to keep and maintain client records. Although this responsibility varies depending on your professional affiliation and theoretical orientation, failure to maintain appropriate records is unethical and, in some cases, illegal. The American Psychological Association's (1992) ethical code states:

Psychologists appropriately document their professional and scientific work in order to facilitate provision of services later by them or by other professionals, to ensure accountability, and to meet other requirements of institutions or the law. (p. 1602)

The American Counseling Association (ACA; 1995) includes an almost identical statement in its ethical code:

Counselors maintain records necessary for rendering professional services to their clients and as required by laws, regulations, or agency or institution procedures. (p. 4)

The guidelines as written by the American Counseling Association and American Psychological Association imply a balancing act; they suggest, but do not directly state, that written documents must meet standards set by more than one entity. This leads us to a discussion of the first challenge of report writing: Determining your audience.

## Determining Your Audience

Consider this question: When you write an intake report, are you writing it for yourself, for another professional, for your client, for your supervisor, or for your client's insurance company? In other words, as you write, who might be looking over your shoulder?

Having a diverse audience may be the hardest part of report writing. For example, imagine giving your report to a supervisor. Depending on your supervisor, you might emphasize your diagnostic skills through a sophisticated discussion of your client's psychopathology or you might try using behavioral jargon such as "consequential thinking, response cost, and behavioral rehearsal." On the other hand, if you imagine your client reading your report, you may choose to avoid the behavioral jargon—and certainly you will deemphasize complex discussions of psychopathology.

After contemplating these issues, some beginning interviewers throw up their hands in frustration and consider writing two versions of the same report. This solution might be fine, except it requires far too much extra work and, in the end, your client has a right to read whatever you write about him or her anyway (even the version of the report solely aimed at impressing your supervisor).

The stark fact is that your intake report must be written for a diverse audience—and this greatly complicates your task. The answer to the question posed earlier, "Who's looking over your shoulder?" is this: Just about everybody. As you write, include the following list of people and agencies in your imagined audience:

- Your client
- Your supervisor
- Your agency administrator
- Your client's attorney
- Your client's insurance company
- Your professional colleagues
- Your professional association's ethics board
- Your state or local ethics board

After the preceding discussion, you should feel either motivated to write a carefully crafted intake report or flagrantly paranoid. We hope it is the former. For additional guidance regarding intake report writing, closely review Putting It in Practice 7.3: The Intake Report Outline, as well as the case example at the end of this chapter.

# The Intake Report Outline

Use the following intake report outline as a guide for writing a thorough intake report. Keep in mind that this outline is lengthy and therefore, in practical clinical situations, you will need to select what to include and what to omit in your client reports.

** C O N F I D E N T I A L **
Intake Report

NAME:                    James A. Johnson
DATE OF BIRTH:           17 August 1977
AGE:                     25
DATE OF INTAKE:          13 October 2002
INTAKE INTERVIEWER:      Andrew Potter, M.A.
DATE OF REPORT:          14 October 2002

I.   Identifying Information and Reason for Referral
     A. Client name
     B. Age
     C. Sex
     D. Racial/Ethnic information
     E. Marital status
     F. Referral source (and telephone number, when possible)
     G. Reason for referral (why has the client been sent to you for a consultation/intake session?)
     H. Presenting complaint (use a quote from the client to describe the complaint)
II.  Behavioral Observations (and Mental Status Examination)
     A. Appearance upon presentation (including comments about hygiene, eye contact, body posture, and facial expression)
     B. Quality and quantity of speech and responsivity to questioning
     C. Client description of mood (use a quote in the report when appropriate)
     D. Primary thought content (including presence or absence of suicide ideation)
     E. Level of cooperation with the interview
     F. Estimate of adequacy of the data obtained
III. History of the Present Problem (or Illness)
     A. Include one paragraph describing the client's presenting problems and associated current stressors
     B. Include one or two paragraphs outlining when the problem initially began and the course or development of symptoms
     C. Repeat, as needed, paragraph-long descriptions of additional current problems identified during the intake interview (client problems are usually organized using diagnostic—DSM—groupings, however, suicide ideation, homicide ideation, relationship problems, etc., may be listed)
     D. Follow, as appropriate, with relevant negative or rule-out statements (e.g., with a clinically depressed client, it is important to rule out mania: "The client denied any history of manic episodes.")

## Putting It in Practice 7.3 (continued)

IV. Past Treatment (Psychiatric) History And Family Treatment (Psychiatric) History
   A. Include a description of previous clinical problems or episodes not included in the previous section (e.g., if the client is presenting with a problem of clinical anxiety, but also has a history of treatment for an eating disorder, the eating disorder should be noted here)
   B. Description of previous treatment received, including hospitalization, medications, psychotherapy or counseling, case management, etc.
   C. Include a description of all psychiatric and substance abuse disorders found in all blood relatives (i.e., at least parents, siblings, grandparents, and children, but also possibly aunts, uncles, and cousins)
   D. Also include a list of any significant major medical disorders in blood relatives (e.g., cancer, diabetes, seizure disorders, thyroid disease)
V. Relevant Medical History
   A. List and briefly describe past hospitalizations and major medical illnesses (e.g., asthma, HIV positive, hypertension)
   B. Include a description of the client's current health status (it's good to use a client quote or physician quote here)
   C. Current medications and dosages
   D. Primary Care Physician (and/or specialty physician) and telephone numbers
VI. Developmental History (This section is optional and is most appropriate for inclusion in child/adolescent cases: See Chapter 10.)
VII. Social and Family History
   A. Early memories/experiences (including, when appropriate, descriptions of parents and possible abuse or childhood traumatization)
   B. Educational history
   C. Employment history
   D. Military history
   E. Romantic relationship history
   F. Sexual history
   G. Aggression/violence history
   H. Alcohol/Drug history (if not previously covered as a primary problem area)
   I. Legal history
   J. Recreational history
   K. Spiritual/Religious history
VIII. Current Situation and Functioning
   A. A description of typical daily activities
   B. Self-perceived strengths and weaknesses
   C. Ability to complete normal activities of daily living
IX. Diagnostic Impressions (This section should include a discussion of diagnostic issues or a listing of assigned diagnoses.)
   A. Brief discussion of diagnostic issues
   B. Multiaxial diagnosis

*(continued)*

---

**Putting It in Practice 7.3 (continued)**

X.   Case Formulation and Treatment Plan
  A. Include a paragraph description of how you conceptualize the case.
     This description will provide a foundation for how you will work with
     this person. For example, a behaviorist will emphasize reinforcement
     contingencies that have influenced the client's development of symp-
     toms and that will likely aid in alleviation of client symptoms. Alter-
     natively, a psychoanalytically-oriented interviewer will emphasize
     personality dynamics and historically significant and repeating rela-
     tionship conflicts.
  B. Include a paragraph description (or simple list) of recommended
     treatment approaches

Andrew Potter, M.A., Rita Sommers-Flanagan, Ph.D., Supervisor

---

## Choosing the Structure and Content of Your Report

The structure of your intake report varies based on your professional affiliation, professional setting, and personal preferences. For example, psychiatrists are more likely
to emphasize medical history, mental status, and diagnosis, while social workers are
more inclined to include lengthier sections on social and developmental history. The
following suggested structure (and accompanying outline in Putting It in Practice 7.3)
will not please everyone, but it can be easily modified to suit your particular needs and
interests. Also, keep in mind that the following structure errs on the side of being thorough; more abbreviated intake reports may be required by particular settings.

### Identifying Information and Reason for Referral

After listing your client name, date of birth, age, date of the intake session, date of the
report, and interviewer's name and professional credentials, most intake reports begin
with a narrative section designed to orient the reader to the report. This section is typically one or two short paragraphs and includes identifying information and a summary of the reasons for referral. Psychiatrists usually label this initial section *Identifying Information and Chief Complaint,* but the substance of the section is essentially the
same as described here. It might read something like:

> John Smith, a 53 year-old married Caucasian male, was referred for psychotherapy by his
> primary care physician, Nancy Jones, MD (509-555-5555). Dr. Jones described Mr. Smith
> as "moderately depressed" and as suffering from "intermittent anxiety, insomnia, and gen-
> eral distress associated with his recent job loss." During his initial session, Mr. Smith con-
> firmed these problems and added that "troubles at home with the wife" and "finances"
> were furthering his overall discomfort and "shame."

### Behavioral Observations (and Mental Status Examination)

The intake report begins with concrete, objective data and eventually moves toward
more subjective interviewer judgments. After the initial section, the intake report turns
to specific behavioral observations made by the interviewer. Depending on your institutional setting, these specific observations may or may not include a complete mental
status report (i.e., if you are in a medical setting, inclusion of a mental status examination is more likely, and possibly required). However, because we discuss mental status

examinations in the next chapter, the following example includes a basic description of the interviewer's behavioral observations, with only minor references to mental status.

> Mr. Smith presented as a somewhat short and slightly overweight man who looked approximately his stated age. His hygiene was somewhat poor, as his hair looked greasy and unkempt and he had slight body odor. Mr. Smith's eyes were sometimes downcast and sometimes focused intensely on the interviewer. He also engaged in frequent hand wringing, and his crossed legs bounced continuously. He spoke deliberately and consistently answered interview questions briefly and to the point; he responded directly and immediately to all interviewer questions. He described himself as feeling "pathethic" and "antsy." He acknowledged suicidal ideation, but denied suicidal intent, stating, "I've thought about ending my life, but I'm the kind of person who would never do it." Mr. Smith was cooperative with the interview process; the following information is likely an adequate representation of his past and present condition.

## History of the Present Problem (or Illness)

Traditionally, psychiatrists include a section in the intake report entitled, "History of the present illness." This terminology reflects a medical model orientation and may or may not be comfortable for nonphysicians or appropriate for nonmedical settings. This section is for stating the client's particular problem in some detail, along with its unique evolution. The history and description of several problems may be included.

> Mr. Smith reported that he's been feeling "incredibly down" for the past six weeks, ever since being laid off from his job as a millworker at a local wood products company. Initially, after losing his job, Mr. Smith indicated he was "angry and resentful" at the company. For about two weeks, he aggressively campaigned against his termination, and along with several coworkers, consulted an attorney. After it became apparent that he would not be rehired and that he had no legitimate claim against the company, he went for two job interviews, but reported "leaving in a panic" during the second interview. Subsequently, he began having difficulty sleeping, started snacking at all hours of the day and night, and quickly gained 10 pounds. He also reported difficulty concentrating, feelings of worthlessness, suicide ideation, and minimal constructive activity during the course of a typical day. He stated: "I've lost my confidence. I got nothing to offer anybody. I don't even know myself anymore."
>
> When asked if he had ever previously experienced such deep sadness or anxiety, Mr. Smith responded by saying, "Never." He claimed that this is the "first time" he's ever had any "head problems." Mr. Smith denied experiencing recurrent panic attacks and minimized the significance of his "panic" during the job interview by claiming "I was just getting in touch with reality. I don't have much to offer an employer."

## Past Treatment (Psychiatric) History and
## Family Treatment (Psychiatric) History

For many clients, this section is brief or nonexistent. For others, it is extensive, and you may need to reference other records you've reviewed regarding the client. For example, you might simply make a summary statement such as: "This client has been seen previously by a number of mental health providers for the treatment of posttraumatic stress disorder, substance abuse, and depression" unless there is something in particular about the treatment that warrants specification (e.g., a particular form of treatment, such as "dialectical behavior therapy" was employed and associated with a positive or negative outcome). In this section, we also include information on any family history of psychiatric problems (although some report writers devote a separate section to this topic).

Mr. Smith has never received mental health treatment previously. In the referral note from his primary physician, it was acknowledged that he was offered antidepressant medications at his outpatient appointment, but refused to take them in favor of a trial of psychotherapy.

Initially, Mr. Smith reported that no one in his family had ever seen a mental health professional, but later admitted his paternal uncle suffered from depression and received "shock therapy" back in the 1960s. He denied the existence of any other mental problems with regard to both himself and his family.

## Relevant Medical History

Depending on how much information you have obtained from your client's physician and on how closely you have covered this area during the intake, you may or may not have much medical history to include. At minimum, ask your client about (a) his or her general health, (b) any recent or chronic physical illnesses or hospitalizations, (c) prescription medications, and (d) when he or she last had a physical. Additionally, if you have the name (and telephone number) of your client's primary physician, include that information as well.

> Very little information was provided by Mr. Smith's primary care physician regarding his medical history. During the interview, Mr. Smith described himself as in generally good health. He denied having major illnesses or hospitalizations during his childhood or teen years. He noted that he rarely "gets sick" and that his employment attendance was exceptionally good. To the best of his recollection, his only major medical problems and associated treatments were for kidney stones (1996) and removal of a benign polyp from his colon (1998). He reported taking vitamins and glucosamine sulfate (for general health and joint pain), but currently does not take any prescription medications. Mr. Smith's primary care physician is Dr. Nancy Jones.

## Developmental History

The developmental history begins before birth and focuses primarily on the achievement of specific developmental milestones. A developmental history is most appropriate when working with child or adolescent clients. Consequently, we discuss the developmental history in Chapter 11.

## Social and Family History

Writing a social and family history about your client can be like writing a full-length novel. Everyone's life takes many twists and turns; your goal, as a historian, is to condense the client's life into a tight narrative. Be brief, relevant, organized, and whenever possible, summarize or present highlights (or low spots) of the client's history. Once again, the depth, breadth, and length of your social/developmental history depends on the purpose of your intake and your institutional setting. Specific topics to be covered are listed in Putting It in Practice 7.3).

> Mr. Smith was born and raised in Kirkland, Washington, a suburb of Seattle. He was the third of five children born of Edith and Michael Smith. His parents, now in their late 70s, have remained married and continue to live in the Seattle area, although they're beginning to experience significant health problems. Mr. Smith remains close to them, visiting several times a year and expressing concern about their well-being. He reported no significant conflicts or problems in his relationships with his parents or siblings.
>
> Early childhood memories were characterized by Mr. Smith as "normal." He described his parents as "loving and strict." He denied any experiences or knowledge of sexual or physical abuse in his family of origin.

Mr. Smith attended school in his hometown and graduated from high school in 1966. He described himself as "an average student." He had some minor disciplinary problems, including numerous detentions (usually for failing to turn in his homework) and one suspension (for fighting on school grounds).

Following high school graduation, Mr. Smith moved to Spokane, Washington, and briefly attended Spokane Falls Community College. During this time, he met his eventual wife and decided to seek employment, rather than pursue college. He worked briefly at a number of jobs, including as a service station attendant and roofer, eventually obtaining employment at the local wood products plant. He reported working at the plant for 31 years. He emphasized that he has always been a hard worker and has never been fired from a job. Mr. Smith was not drafted and never served in the military.

In terms of overall demeanor, Mr. Smith indicated that he has always been (until recently) "friendly and confident." He dated a number of young women in high school and continued to do so after moving to Spokane. He met Irene, the woman he married, in 1967, shortly before turning 20 years old. He described her as "the perfect fit" and described himself as a happily married man. He denied any sexual difficulties, but acknowledged diminished sexual interest and desire over the past month or so. He stated that his "pathetic condition" following his job loss had put a strain on his marriage, but he believed his marriage is still strong.

Mr. Smith and his wife have been married for 35 years. They have three children (two sons and one daughter; ages 28 to 34), all of whom live within 100 miles of Mr. and Mrs. Smith. According to Mr. Smith, all of his children are doing fairly well. He reported regular contact with his children and seven grandchildren.

Mr. Smith occasionally got in "fights" or "scuffles" during his school years, but emphasized that such behavior was "normal." He denied ever using a weapon in a fight and reported that his most recent physical altercation was just after quitting college, "back when I was about 20."

Alcohol and drugs have never been a significant problem for Mr. Smith. He reported drinking excessively a number of times in high school and a number of times in college. He also noted that he went out with his buddies for "some beers" every Friday after work and that he also would have a few beers on Tuesdays, associated with his and his wife's participation in a bowling league. He briefly experimented with marijuana while enrolled in college, but claimed "I didn't like it." He's never experimented with any "harder" drugs and denied any problems with prescription drugs, stating: "I avoid 'em when I can."

Other than a few speeding tickets (usually on the drive from Spokane to Seattle), Mr. Smith denied legal problems. His only nonvehicular-related citation was in his "college days" when he was cited for "disorderly conduct" while "causing a ruckus" outside a bar with a group of his "drinking buddies." He was required to pay a small fine and write a letter of apology to the business owner.

Mr. Smith reported that his favorite recreational activities include bowling, fishing, and duck hunting. He also acknowledged that he and his wife enjoy traveling together and gambling small amounts of money at casinos. He denied ever losing more money than he could "afford to lose" and said he does not consider his small-scale gambling to be a problem. He admitted that recently he has not been interested in "having any fun." Consequently, his involvement in recreational activities has been curtailed.

Mr. Smith was raised Catholic and reported attending church "off and on" for most of his life. He said he is currently in an "off" period, as he has not attended for about nine months. His wife attends regularly, but he indicates that his irregular attendance has not really been a problem in their relationship. He considers himself a "Christian" and a "Catholic."

## Current Situation and Functioning

This section of the intake report focuses on three main topics: (a) usual daily activities, (b) client self-perception of personal strengths, and (c) apparent ability to adequately perform usual age-appropriate activities of daily living. Depending on your setting and preference, it is also possible to expand on this section by including a description of the client's psychological functioning, cognitive functioning, emotional functioning, or personality functioning. This provides the interviewer with an opportunity to use more of a subjective appraisal of current client functioning in a variety of areas.

> Currently, during a typical day, Mr. Smith rises at about 7 A.M., has coffee and breakfast with his wife, reads the newspaper, and then moves to the living room to watch the morning news. He indicated that he usually reads the "classified" section closely for job opportunities, circling the positions he may be interested in. However, after moving into the living room, he reports doing everything he can to avoid having to go out and seek employment. Sometimes he watches television, but he reports being too "pent up" to sit around too long, so he goes out to the garage or into his backyard and "putters around." He usually makes himself a sandwich or a bowl of soup for lunch and then continues his puttering. At about 5:30 P.M., his wife returns home from her job as an administrator at a local nonprofit corporation. Occasionally, she reminds him of his plans to get a new job, but Mr. Smith indicated that he usually responds with irritation ("It's like I try to bite her head off") and then she retreats to the kitchen and makes dinner. After dinner with his wife, he "continues to waste time" by watching television, until it's time to retire. His usual routine is interrupted on the weekends, often by visits from his children and grandchildren and sometimes when he and his wife venture out to a local casino to "spend a few nickels" (however, he indicated their weekend activities are diminishing because of tightening finances).
>
> Mr. Smith sees himself as ordinarily having numerous personal strengths, although he needed prompting to elaborate on his positive qualities. For example, he considers himself an honest man, a hard worker, and a devoted husband and father. He further believes he is a good buddy to several friends and fun to be around ("back when I was working and had a life"). In terms of intelligence, Mr. Smith claimed he is "no dummy" but that he is having some trouble concentrating and "remembering anything" lately. When asked about personal weaknesses, Mr. Smith stated, "I hope you got lotsa ink left in that pen of yours, Doc," but primarily focused on his current state of mind, which he described as "being a problem of not having the guts to get back on that horse that bucked me off."
>
> Despite his poor hygiene and general lack of productiveness, Mr. Smith seems capable of adequately performing most activities of daily living. He reported occasionally cooking dinner, fixing the lawnmower, and taking care of other household and maintenance tasks. His perception, and it may be accurate, is that he is less efficient with most tasks because of distractibility and intermittent forgetfulness. His interpersonal functioning appears somewhat limited, as he described relatively few current outside involvements.

## Diagnostic Impressions

For good reason, students are often reluctant to assign a diagnosis to clients. Nonetheless, most intake reports should include some discussion of diagnostic issues, even if you discuss only broad diagnostic categories, such as depression, anxiety, substance use, eating disorders, and so on. Although simply listing your diagnostic considerations is acceptable in some circumstances and including only a multiaxial diagnosis is preferred by managed care companies, our preference is for a brief discussion of diagnostic issues followed by a *DSM* multiaxial diagnosis. The brief discussion orients the reader to how you conceptualized your diagnosis, and it can even include an explanation of why you chose one particular diagnostic label over another. In the following description, we use Morrison's (1993) guidelines of assigning the least severe label that adequately explains the symptom pattern.

> This 53-year-old man is clearly suffering from an adjustment disorder. Although he also meets the diagnostic criteria for major depression, I am reluctant to assign this diagnosis

because his depressive symptoms are so strongly associated with his recent life change, and he has no personal and minimal family history of a mood disorder. Mr. Smith is also experiencing numerous significant anxiety symptoms, which may actually be more central than his depressive symptoms in interfering with his ability to seek new employment. Similarly, a case could also be made for assigning him an anxiety disorder diagnosis, but again, the abrupt onset of these symptoms in direct association with his job loss suggests that his current mental state is better accounted for with a less severe diagnostic label.

His provisional *DSM-IV-TR* multiaxial diagnosis follows:

Axis I:    309.28   Adjustment Disorder with Features of Anxiety and Depression (Provisional)
           Rule Out (R/O)    296.21     Major Depressive Disorder, Single Episode, Mild
Axis II:   No Diagnosis on Axis II (V71.09)
Axis III:  None
Axis IV:   Severe: Recent job loss after 31 years of employment
Axis V:    GAF = 51–60

Note that in the preceding multiaxial diagnosis, we used a number of procedures provided by the *DSM* for indicating diagnostic uncertainty. Specifically, we used the "provisional" tag and included a "rule out" diagnostic possibility (major depression). Additionally, for the Global Assessment of Functioning (GAF) rating, we used a range (which we often recommend because of the inherent subjectivity of GAF ratings; Piersma & Boes, 1997).

## Case Formulation and Treatment Plan

For this section, include a paragraph description of how you conceptualize the case. This description provides you an opportunity to describe how you view the case and how you are likely to proceed in working therapeutically with this client. Not surprisingly, behaviorists describe their cases in behavioral terminology, while psychoanalytically oriented therapists describe their cases using psychoanalytic terminology. Generally, keep your theoretical jargon to a minimum, in case your client requests a copy of your intake report.

Mr. Smith is a stable and reliable individual who is currently suffering from severe adjustment to sudden unemployment. It appears that, for many years, much of his identity has been associated with his work life. Consequently, he feels depressed and anxious without the structure of his usual workday. Furthermore, his depression, anxiety, and lack of perceived constructive activities have considerably shaken his confidence. For a variety of reasons, he feels unable to go out and pursue employment, which, especially because of his strong value of normality and employment, further reduces his confidence in and respect for himself.

Psychotherapy with Mr. Smith should focus on two simultaneous goals. First, although it is impossible to provide him with new employment, it is crucial that Mr. Smith begin making a consistent effort to seek and obtain employment. It seems unrealistic to simply suggest to him (after 31 years of employment) that he reconstruct his identity and begin valuing himself as an unemployed person. The treatment objectives associated with this general goal include:

1. Analyze factors preventing Mr. Smith from following through on his daily job searches.
2. Develop physical anxiety coping strategies (including relaxation and daily exercise).
3. Develop and implement cognitive coping strategies (including cognitive restructuring and self-instructional techniques).

4. Develop and implement social coping strategies (including peer or spousal support for job-seeking behaviors).
5. Develop and implement social-emotional coping strategies. (Mr. Smith needs to learn to express his feelings about his personal situation to close friends and family without pushing them away through irritable or socially aversive behaviors).

The second general goal for Mr. Smith is to help him expand his identity beyond that of a man who is a long-term employee at a wood products company. Objectives associated with this second goal include:

1. Helping Mr. Smith recognize valuable aspects of relationships and activities outside an employment situation.
2. Helping Mr. Smith identify how he would talk with a person in a similar situation, and then have him translate that attitude and "talk" into a self-talk strategy with himself.
3. Exploring with Mr. Smith his eventual plans for retirement.

Although Mr. Smith's therapy will be primarily individually oriented treatment, it is recommended that his spouse accompany him to some sessions for assessment and support purposes. As he noted, there have been increasing conflicts in their relationship and it should prove beneficial for them to work together to help him cope more effectively with this difficult and sudden life change.

Overall, it is important to encourage Mr. Smith to use his already-existing positive personal skills and resources to address this new challenge in his life. If, after 6 to 10 sessions using this approach, no progress has been attained, I will discuss the possibility of medication treatment and/or an alternative change in approach to his treatment.

## Writing Clearly and Concisely

Writing a clear and concise intake report is very difficult. Do not expect to sit down and write the report perfectly the first time. It may take several drafts before you get it to the point where you want anyone else to see it. We have several recommendations for making the writing process more tolerable.

- Write the report as soon as possible (immediately following the session is ideal; the longer you wait, the harder it is to reconstruct the session in your mind and from your notes).
- Write an immediate draft without worrying about perfect wording or style; then store it in a confidential location and return to it soon for editing.
- Closely follow an outline; although we recommend the outline in Putting It in Practice 7.3, using any outline is better than simply rambling on about the client.
- Try to get clear information from your supervisor or employer about what is expected. If a standard format is available, follow it.
- If your agency has sample reports available, look them over and use them as a model for your report.
- Remember, like any skill, report writing becomes easier with practice; many seasoned professionals dictate a full intake report in 20 to 30 minutes—and someday you may do so as well.

Another issue associated with writing concisely involves choosing what information to put into your intake report. How brief and how detailed should you be? How much deeply personal information should be included in the report? These are difficult questions, and we suggest you explore them in Individual and Cultural Highlight 7.1.

=========== INDIVIDUAL AND CULTURAL HIGHLIGHT 7.1 ===========

## Choosing What to Include in Your Intake Report

The ethical guidelines of the National Association of Social Workers (NASW; 1996) provide a good foundation for a discussion of what to include in the content of your report. They state:

> Social workers' documentation should protect clients' privacy to the extent that it is possible and appropriate, and should include only that information that is directly relevant to the delivery of services. (p. 13)

Notice the emphasis by NASW of two particular points. First, they state that we need to "protect clients' privacy." Second, they note that we need to stay with "information that is directly relevant." As you contemplate these two points, read the following intake report excerpt.

> Jane Doe, a 21-year-old, single, Hispanic female, reported being raped by her stepfather when she was age 16. Following the rape, Ms. Doe was examined at the Baylor Medical Center emergency room. This examination revealed vaginal tearing and semen residue. Eventually, Ms. Doe's stepfather was arrested and convicted of sexual assault. His conviction followed a lengthy trial, during which he denied the assault, even in the face of positive DNA evidence. Currently, Ms. Doe's symptoms, including anxiety, hypervigilence, nightmares, flashbacks of the rape incident, and ruminative guilt, seem to have resurfaced in direct association with her stepfather's scheduled release from the Texas state penitentiary.
>
> During the past five years, there has been extensive conflict between Ms. Doe and her biological mother. She reports that her mother has "never believed" her account of the rape and remains committed to her stepfather. Ms. Doe's mother is a Hispanic immigrant who works at the local K-Mart store and has struggled financially ever since her husband's incarceration. These conflicts and financial difficulties eventually led to Ms. Doe's being permanently placed in foster care for about one to two years (until she turned 18 years old).
>
> Ms. Doe reports she is currently in a committed romantic relationship with a man by the name of William Mills. She notes that Mr. Mills is "White," which her mother finds undesirable. However, Ms. Doe describes Mr. Mills as sensitive and supportive of her "sexual hang-ups," but adds that "William has a number of sexual problems himself." As Mr. Mills's problems interact with Ms. Doe's sexual anxiety, it appears that her sense of guilt is significantly increased. For example, she believes she is an inadequate sexual partner for Mr. Mills and this further ignites the mix of guilt and resentment she feels toward her mother and stepfather.

In every case, as you write and proofread your intake report, ask yourself, "Am I respecting and protecting my client's privacy" and "Am I including in the report only information that is essential and relevant to her treatment?"

Do you think there is anything in the preceding report excerpt that could jeopardize the client's confidentiality? Is there any irrelevant information in the report? How would you feel if the client requested to review the report? To whom would you feel comfortable releasing this report?

## Keeping Your Report Confidential

It is hard to overemphasize confidentiality. We all need to be reminded that our clients are disclosing personal information about their lives, and we need to treat that information like precious jewels. To help assure intake report confidentiality, we always type or stamp the word *CONFIDENTIAL* on our reports. Obviously, this is no guarantee of confidentiality, but it is a step in the right direction.

In addition, be sure to have an adequately secure place for storing client records. Do not leave your report on your desk or open on your computer where clients and unauthorized colleagues might accidentally discover it. Keeping your records stored securely is simpler if you keep paper records (a locked file drawer in a locked office should suffice), but can get more complex if you maintain electronic records (Bartlett, 1996; Welfel & Heinlen, 2001).

Organizations and individuals who rely on computer systems for maintaining confidential records face unique problems. If reports are stored exclusively on floppy disks or hard drives, there is always the possibility of permanently losing that information (floppy disks become damaged and hard drives go down). Consequently, it is always necessary to maintain at least two electronic copies of client records.

Limiting access to electronic records is another problem linked to the computer age. At the very least, computer files should be managed with access codes and/or passwords, although some computer specialists recommend using a removable storage drive that can be locked up after hours. Welfel and Heinlen (2001) also recommend keeping a paper copy and floppy disk record with code numbers or pseudonyms for identification purposes.

## Sharing the Report with Your Client

Although clients have a legal right to access their medical/psychological/counseling records, it may not be in their best interests to have copies of your report for themselves. The ACA (1995) ethical guidelines articulate this concern:

> Counselors recognize that counseling records are kept for the benefit of clients, and therefore provide access to records and copies of records when requested by competent clients, unless records contain information that may be misleading and detrimental to the client. (p. 5)

This guideline means that, if you release client records to clients, you must take utmost care and caution. Once again, it is a balancing act. Because of consumer rights, clients have a right to their records. On the other hand, some clients may misunderstand or misinterpret what you have written—meaning you can get yourself in trouble by releasing the information.

In most cases, we follow these guidelines:

- Inform clients at the outset of counseling that you will keep records and that they have access to them.
- When appropriate, inform clients that some portions of the records are written in language designed to communicate with other professionals; consequently, the records may not be especially easy to read or understand.
- If clients request their records, tell them you would like to review the records with them before releasing them, so as to minimize the possibility that the records are misinterpreted—you can even say that such a practice is suggested in your professional ethical guidelines.

- When clients request records, schedule an appointment (free of charge) with them to review the records together.
- If your client is no longer seeing you, is angry with you, or refuses to meet with you, you can (a) release the records to them without a meeting (and hope the records are not misinterpreted), (b) agree to release the records *only* to another competent professional (who will review them with the client), or (c) refuse to release the records (based on justifiable professional grounds).
- Whatever the situation, always discuss the issue of releasing records with your supervisor, rather than acting impulsively on your client's request.

When clients request to see their records, it is important to remain calm and acknowledge your clients' rights. It is also important to have a procedure for sharing the records and to follow that procedure closely. Most clients will be satisfied if you treat them with compassion and respect *and* you have written compassionate and respectful documents about your contact with them.

## SUMMARY

The intake interview is probably the most basic type of interview conducted by mental health professionals. It usually involves obtaining information about a new client to identify what type of treatment, if any, is most appropriate. The intake is primarily an assessment interview. Consequently, it usually involves the liberal use of questions.

The three major objectives of intake interviewing are evaluating: (a) the client's problems and goals, (b) the client's personality, personal history, and mental condition, and (c) the client's current situation.

Evaluating a client's problems and goals requires that interviewers identify the client's main source of personal distress as well as the range of other problems contributing to the discomfort. Problems and goals need to be prioritized and selected for potential therapeutic intervention. Many systems are available to help interviewers analyze and conceptualize client symptoms. Usually, these systems involve identifying the factors or events that precede and follow occurrence of client symptoms.

Obtaining personal history information about clients is a sensitive and challenging process, so interviewers should begin nondirectively. Personal history flows from earliest memories to descriptions of parents and family experiences to school and peer relationships to employment. Interviewers must be selective and flexible regarding the historical information they choose to obtain from their clients; there is too much information to cover in a single interview.

The last major area of focus in an intake is the client's current functioning. Interviewers should focus on current functioning toward the interview's end because it helps bring clients back in touch with their current situation, both liabilities and assets. The end of the interview should slightly emphasize client personal strengths and environmental resources and should focus on the future and on goal setting.

Client registration forms and intake questionnaires can help interviewers determine in advance some of the areas to cover in a given intake. The interviewer's theoretical orientation, therapeutic setting, and professional background and affiliation also guide the focus of intake interviews. An approach to providing an initial interview within managed care guidelines is outlined.

Clients come for intake interviews for many reasons. Substance abuse and trauma are two common presenting problems you will see when interviewing new clients.

Methods for interviewing clients who have substance abuse and trauma problems are discussed.

Writing the intake report is a major challenge for most interviewers. When preparing an intake report, consider your audience, the structure and content of your report, how to write clearly and concisely, and how you will keep the report confidential.

## SUGGESTED READINGS AND RESOURCES

Gustafson, J. P. (1997). *The complex secret of brief psychotherapy: A panorama of approaches.* New York: Aronson. Gustafson eloquently describes brief psychoanalytically oriented approaches to psychotherapy. He includes discussions of preliminary interviews and trial therapy from a brief psychoanalytic perspective.

Hack, T. F., & Cook, A. J. (1995). Getting started: Intake and initial sessions. In D. G. Martin & A. D. Moore (Eds.), *First steps in the art of intervention* (pp. 46–74). Pacific Grove, CA: Brooks/Cole. In this chapter, the authors briefly outline issues they consider important in an intake interview. It also provides a sample intake report as a model for students' report writing.

Lazarus, A. A. (1976). *Multimodal behavior therapy.* New York: Springer. This is Lazarus's classic text on multimodal behavior therapy, in which he details his BASIC ID model.

Lazarus, A. A. (1997). *Brief but comprehensive psychotherapy: The multimodal way.* New York: Springer. This text is the most recent description of Lazarus's multimodal assessment and treatment model.

Miller, W. R., & Rollnick, S. (2002). *Motivational interviewing: Preparing people for change* (2nd ed.). New York: Guilford. This is the latest edition of Miller and Rollnick's groundbreaking approach to interviewing clients with substance abuse problems.

Mitchell, J., & Everly, G. S. (1993). *Critical incidence stress debriefing.* New York: Chevron Publishing. This book outlines the critical incidence stress debriefing process as it applies to emergency service personnel.

Ponterotto, J. G., Rivera, L., & Sueyoshi, L. A. (2000). The career-in-culture interview: A semi-structured protocol for the cross cultural intake interview. *Career Development Quarterly, 49,* 85–96. The article presents a novel idea, a structured career-oriented interview for administration to clients of divergent cultures. It illustrates one particular approach—standardizing interview approaches for addressing cultural sensitivity issues.

Teyber, E. (1997). *Interpersonal process in psychotherapy: A relational approach.* Pacific Grove, CA: Brooks/Cole. This book focuses on assessment from the interpersonal perspective in Chapters 6 through 8. It's a good source for beginning graduate students who want to employ interpersonal psychotherapeutic approaches.

Takushi, R. Uomoto, J. M. (2001). The clinical interview from a multicultural perspective. In L. A. Suzuki & J. G. Ponterotto (Eds.), *Handbook of multicultural assessment.* San Francisco: Jossey-Bass. This book chapter provides a glimpse of the variations required to conduct a multicultural intake interview.

# Chapter 8

# *THE MENTAL STATUS EXAMINATION*

*There are some who make a point of trying to investigate the world we live in with full
scientific rigour without becoming estranged from it. This is never easy: is it possible?*
—R. D. Laing, *The Voice of Experience*

---

### CHAPTER OBJECTIVES

Your professional identity as a mental health professional requires that you have
the skills to evaluate and communicate about your client's mental status. In this
chapter, we discuss the basic components of a typical mental status examination.
In particular, you will learn practical approaches for evaluating client mental status. After reading this chapter, you will know:

- The definition of a mental status examination.
- Individual and cultural issues to consider when conducting a mental status examination.
- Basic components of a generic mental status examination, including client appearance; behavior; attitude; affect and mood; speech and thought; perceptual
disturbances; orientation and consciousness; memory and intelligence; and
client reliability, judgment, and insight.
- When you do and do not need to administer a complete mental status examination.
- What to include in and how to write a brief mental status examination report.

It is important to be careful when assuming an objective stance. Good *interviewers*
make emotional connections with their clients. Good *evaluators* may or may not establish emotional connections with their clients. Some evaluators believe that such connection might interfere with objectivity, so they minimize rapport and emotional involvement.

We believe that you need not sacrifice human connection for objectivity. Maintaining objectivity takes up evaluator energy and can cause clients to actually reveal less information, rather than more. Consciously allowing a little emotional connection and
subjectivity into an evaluation is more humane and, if done professionally, can often
result in more accurate, extensive information. Too much emotional connection with
clients can disrupt objectivity.

If it were possible, total objectivity would require emotional neutrality. It may be that neither total objectivity nor complete emotional neutrality exists in any human endeavor. Fritjof Capra in *The Tao of Physics* (1975) eloquently addresses this issue:

> A careful analysis of the process of observation in atomic physics has shown that the subatomic particles have no meaning as isolated entities, but can only be understood as interconnections between the preparation of an experiment and the subsequent measurement . . . . In atomic physics, we can never speak about nature without at the same time speaking about ourselves. (p. 19)

Even in precise scientific enterprises such as subatomic physics, human elements such as emotion and belief influence and give meaning to what is being observed. When studying humans, excessive emotional distance or neutrality is neither desirable nor useful. Instead, interviewers must *use* emotional connection and emotional reactions to help understand the human in question. The critical challenge of mental status evaluations is to combine emotional sensitivity with an appropriate degree of objective detachment.

## WHAT IS A MENTAL STATUS EXAMINATION?

The mental status examination is a method of organizing and evaluating clinical observations pertaining to mental status or mental condition. The primary purpose of the mental status exam is to evaluate current cognitive processes (Strub & Black, 1977). However, in recent years, mental status exams have become increasingly comprehensive; and some now include sections on historical information, treatment planning, and diagnostic impressions (D. Robinson, 2001; Siassi, 1984). The mental status exam described in this chapter is a generic model in the tradition of Strub and Black, emphasizing assessment of *current* cognitive functions. Other chapters of this text are devoted to historical and psychodiagnostic interviewing and to treatment planning.

The mental status exam is common in medical settings: "In the psychiatric evaluation the mental status examination is considered to be analogous to the physical examination in general medicine" (Siassi, 1984, p. 267). In hospital settings, it is not unusual for admitting psychiatrists to request or administer daily mental status examinations for acutely disturbed patients. The results are reported in concise descriptions of approximately one medium-length paragraph per patient (see Putting It in Practice 8.1). Communication of mental status is a basic procedure in medical settings. Anyone seeking employment in the medical mental health domain should be competent in communicating with other professionals via mental status examination reports.

## THE GENERIC MENTAL STATUS EXAMINATION

The main categories covered in a basic mental status examination vary slightly among practitioners and settings. In our work, we find the following list of categories most useful:

1. Appearance
2. Behavior/psychomotor activity
3. Attitude toward examiner (interviewer)
4. Affect and mood

5. Speech and thought
6. Perceptual disturbances
7. Orientation and consciousness
8. Memory and intelligence
9. Reliability, judgment, and insight

---

**Putting It in Practice 8.1**

## Mental Status Examination Reports

Following are sample mental status reports. A good report is brief, clear, concise, and addresses all the areas noted in this chapter.

### Mental Status Report 1

Gary Sparrow, a 42-year-old Caucasian male, was disheveled and unkempt on presentation to the hospital emergency room. During the interview, he was agitated and restless, frequently changing seats. He was impatient and sometimes rude in his interactions with this examiner. Mr. Sparrow reported that today was the best day of his life, because he had decided to join the professional golf circuit. His affect was labile, but appropriate to the content of his speech (i.e., he became tearful when reporting he had "bogeyed number 15"). His speech was loud, pressured, and overelaborative. He exhibited loosening of associations and flight of ideas. Mr. Sparrow described grandiose delusions regarding his sexual and athletic performance. He reported auditory hallucinations (God had told him to quit his job and become a professional golfer) and was preoccupied with his athletic and sexual accomplishments. He was oriented to time and place, but claimed he was the illegitimate son of Arnold Palmer. He denied suicidal and homicidal ideation. He refused to participate in intellectual- or memory-related portions of the examination. Mr. Sparrow was unreliable and exhibited poor judgment. Insight was absent.

### Mental Status Report 2

Ms. Helen Jackson, a 67-year-old African American female, was evaluated during routine rounds at the Cedar Springs Nursing Home. Her grooming was adequate and she was cooperative with the examination. She reported her mood as "desperate" because she had "recently misplaced her glasses." Her affect was characterized by intermittent anxiety, generally associated with having misplaced items or with difficulty answering the examiner's questions. Her speech was slow, halting, and soft. She repeatedly became concerned with her personal items, clothing, and general appearance, wondering where her scarf "ran off to" and occasionally inquiring as to whether her appearance was acceptable (e.g., "Do I look okay? You know, I have lots of visitors coming by later."). Ms. Jackson was oriented to person and place, but indicated the date as January 9, 1981 (today is July 8, 2002). She was unable to calculate serial sevens and after recalling zero of three items, became briefly anxious and concerned, stating "Oh my, I guess you pulled another one over me, didn't you, sonny?" She quickly recovered her pleasant style, stating "And you're such a gem for coming to visit me again." Her proverb interpretations were concrete. Judgment, reliability, and insight were significantly impaired.

During a mental status examination, observations are organized to establish hypotheses about the client's *current mental functioning.* Although mental status examinations provide important diagnostic information, administration of the exam is not primarily or exclusively a diagnostic procedure, nor is it a formal psychometric procedure (Polanski & Hinkle, 2000). After a brief discussion of individual and cultural considerations, each assessment domain covered during a traditional mental status examination is described in the following section.

## Individual and Cultural Considerations

Like most assessment procedures, mental status examinations are vulnerable to error because of interviewer cultural insensitivity. To claim that client mental states are partly a function of culture is an understatement; an individual's culture can determine his or her mental state.

Despite potential misuse or abuse, mental status examinations can be highly useful, provided the examiner is knowledgeable and sensitive about multicultural issues. After all, as captured by the following excerpt from Nigerian novelist Chinua Achebe (1959/1994), the perception of madness depends on a person's perspective:

> After the singing the interpreter spoke about the Son of God whose name was Jesu Kristi. Okonkwo, who only stayed in the hope that it might come to chasing the men out of the village or whipping them, now said:
>
> "You told us with your own mouth that there was only one god. Now you talk about his son. He must also have a wife, then." The crowd agreed.
>
> "I did not say He had a wife," said the interpreter, somewhat lamely . . .
>
> The missionary ignored him and went on to talk about the Holy Trinity. At the end of it Okonkwo was fully convinced that the man was mad. He shrugged his shoulders and went away to tap his afternoon palm-wine. (pp. 146–147)

Sometimes specific cultural beliefs, especially spiritual beliefs, sound like madness (or delusions) to outsiders. The same can be said about beliefs and behaviors associated with physical illness, recreational activities, and marriage and family rituals. For example, in some cases, fasting might be considered justification for involuntary hospitalization, while in other cases, fasting—even for considerable time periods—is associated with spiritual or physical practices (B. Falloon & Horwath, 1993; Polanski & Hinkle, 2000). Overall, as with most assessment procedures, the mental status examiner must sensitively consider individual and cultural issues before coming to strong conclusions about his or her client's mental state (see Individual and Cultural Highlight 8.1 on page 239).

## Appearance

In mental status examinations, interviewers take note of their client's general appearance. Observations are limited primarily to physical characteristics, but some demographic information is also included in this domain.

Physical characteristics commonly noted on a mental status exam include grooming, dress, pupil dilation/contraction, facial expression, perspiration, make-up, presence of body piercing or tattoos, height, weight, and nutritional status. Interviewers should closely observe not only how clients look, but also how they physically react or interact with the interviewer. Morrison (1993) recommends: "When you shake hands during your introductions, notice whether the patient's palms are dry or damp" (p. 106). Similarly, Shea (1998) states: "The experienced clinician may note whether he or she encounters the iron fingers of a Hercules bent upon establishing control or the dampened palm of a Charlie Brown expecting imminent rejection" (p. 9).

A client's physical appearance may be a manifestation of mental state. Further, physical appearance may be indicative of particular psychiatric diagnoses. For example, dilated pupils are sometimes associated with drug intoxication and pinpoint pupils, with drug withdrawal. Of course, dilated pupils should not be considered conclusive evidence of drug intoxication; this is only one piece of the puzzle and would require further evidence before you could legitimately reach such a conclusion.

Client sex, age, race, and ethnic background are also concrete variables noted during a mental status exam. Each of these factors can be related to psychiatric diagnosis and treatment planning. For example, base rates of various *DSM* diagnoses vary with regard to sex. Also, as Othmer and Othmer (1994) note, the relationship between appearance and biological age may have significance: "A patient who appears older than his stated age may have a history of drug or alcohol abuse, organic mental disorder, depression, or physical illness" (p. 114).

In a mental status report, a client's appearance might be described with the following narrative:

> Maxine Kane, a 41-year-old Australian American female, appeared much younger than her stated age. She arrived for the evaluation wearing a miniskirt, spike heels, excessive makeup, and a contemporary bleached-blonde hairstyle.

A client's physical appearance may also be a manifestation of his or her environment or situation (Paniagua, 2001). In the preceding example, it would be important to know that Ms. Kane came to her evaluation appointment directly from her place of employment—the set of a television soap opera.

## Behavior or Psychomotor Activity

This category is concerned with physical movement. Client activity throughout the evaluation should be noted and recorded. Examiners watch for excessive or limited body movements as well as particular physical movements, such as absence of eye contact (keeping cultural differences in mind), grimacing, excessive eye movement (scanning), odd or repeated gestures, and posture. Clients may deny experiencing particular thoughts or emotions (e.g., paranoia or depression), although their body movements suggest otherwise (e.g., vigilant posturing and scanning or slowed psychomotor activity and lack of facial expression).

Excessive body movements may be associated with anxiety, drug reactions, or the manic phase of bipolar disorder. Reduced movements may represent organic brain dysfunction, catatonic schizophrenia, or drug-induced stupor. Depression can manifest either via agitation or psychomotor retardation. Sometimes, paranoid clients constantly scan their visual field in an effort to be on guard against external threat. Repeated motor movements (such as dusting off shoes) may signal the presence of obsessive-compulsive disorder. Similarly, repeated picking of imagined lint or dirt off clothing or skin is sometimes associated with delirium or toxic reactions to drugs/medications.

## Attitude toward Examiner (Interviewer)

Parents, teachers, and mental health professionals often overuse the word *attitude*. When someone claims a student or client has an "attitude problem" or a "bad attitude," it can be difficult to determine precisely what is being communicated.

In the mental health field, "attitude toward the interviewer" refers to how clients *behave* in relation to the interviewer; that is, *attitude* is defined as behavior that occurs in an interpersonal context. Observation of concrete physical characteristics and physical movement provides a foundation for evaluating client attitude toward the interviewer. Additionally, observations regarding client responsiveness to interviewer questions, including nonverbal factors such as voice tone, eye contact, and body posture, as well as verbal factors such as response latency and directiveness or evasiveness of response, all help interviewers determine their client's attitude.

This portion of the mental status exam benefits from the emotional subjectivity discussed earlier. Interviewers must allow themselves to respond honestly to clients and then scrutinize their own reactions for clues to clients' attitudes. Such judgments are based on the interviewer's internal cognitive and emotional processes and, consequently, are subject to personal bias. For example, a male interviewer may infer seductiveness from the behavior of an attractive female because of his wish that she behave seductively, rather than any actual seductive behavior. Furthermore, what is considered seductive by the examiner may not be considered seductive by the client. Differences may be based on individual or cultural background. It is the interviewer's professional responsibility to avoid overinterpreting client behavior by attributing it to a general client attitude or, in some cases, a personality trait. When making judgments or attributions about client behavior, you should recall the criteria for disordered behavior presented in Chapter 6 and ask yourself:

Is the behavior unusual or statistically infrequent?

Is the behavior disturbing to the client or to others in the client's environment at home or work?

Is the behavior maladaptive; that is, does it contribute to the client's difficulty?

Is the client's behavior justifiable based on present environmental or cultural factors?

There are many ways a client can relate to an interviewer. Words commonly used to describe client attitude toward the interview or interviewer are listed in Table 8.1.

## Affect and Mood

*Affect* is defined as the prevailing emotional tone observed *by the interviewer* during a mental status examination. In contrast, *mood* is the client's *self-reported* mood state.

### Affect

Affect is usually described in terms of its (a) content or type, (b) range and duration (also known as variability and duration), (c) appropriateness, and (d) depth or intensity. Each of these descriptive terms is discussed further.

*Affect Content*    To begin, you should identify what affective state you observe in the client. Is it sadness, euphoria, anxiety, fear, anger, or something else? Affective content indicators include facial expression, body posture, movement, and your client's voice tone. For example, when you see tears in your client's eyes, accompanied by a downcast gaze and minimal movement (psychomotor retardation), you will likely conclude your client has a "sad" affect. In contrast, clenching fists, gritted teeth, and strong language will bring you to the conclusion that your client is displaying an "angry" affect.

**Table 8.1.    Descriptors of Client Attitude Toward the Examiner**

*Aggressive:* The client attacks the examiner physically or verbally or through grimaces and gestures. The client may "flip off" the examiner or simply say in reply to an examiner response, "That's a stupid question" or "Of course I'm feeling angry, can't you do anything but mimic back to me what I've already said?"

*Cooperative:* The client responds directly to interviewer comments or questions. He or she may openly try to work with the interviewer in an effort to gather data or solve problems. Frequent head nods and receptive body posture are common.

*Hostile:* The client is indirectly nasty or biting. Sarcasm, rolling back one's eyes in apparent disgust over an interviewer comment or question, or staring off with a sour grimace may represent subtle, or not so subtle, hostility. This behavior pattern is especially common among delinquent teenagers (J. Sommers-Flanagan & Sommers-Flanagan, 1998).

*Impatient:* The client is on the edge of his or her seat. The client is not very tolerant of pauses or of times when interviewer speech becomes deliberate. He or she may make statements about wanting an answer to concerns immediately. There may be associated hostility and competitiveness in the case of Type A personality styles.

*Indifferent:* The client's appearance and movements suggest lack of concern or interest in the interview. The client may yawn, drum fingers, or become distracted by irrelevant issues or details. The client could also be described as apathetic.

*Ingratiating:* The client is obsequious and overly solicitous of approval and interviewer reinforcement. He or she may try to present self in an overly positive manner, or may agree with everything and anything the interviewer says. There may be excessive head nodding, eye contact, and smiles.

*Intense:* The client's eye contact is constant, or almost so; the client's body leans forward and listens intensely to the interviewer's every word. Client voice volume may be loud and voice tone forceful. The client is the opposite of indifferent.

*Manipulative:* The client tries to use the examiner for the client's own purpose or edification. He or she may interpret examiner statements to represent own best interests. Statements such as "His behavior isn't fair, is it Doctor?" are efforts to solicit agreement and may represent manipulation.

*Negativistic:* The client opposes virtually everything the examiner says. The client may disagree with reflections, paraphrases, or summaries that are clearly accurate. The client may refuse to answer questions or be completely silent throughout an interview. This behavior is also called oppositional.

*Open:* The client openly and straightforwardly discusses problems and concerns. The client may also be open to examiner suggestions or interpretations.

*Passive:* The client offers little or no active opposition or participation in the interview. The client may say things like, "Whatever you think." He or she may simply sit passively until told what to do or say.

*Seductive:* The client may touch self in seductive or suggestive ways (e.g., rubbing body parts). He or she may expose skin or make efforts to be "too close" to or to touch the examiner. The client may make flirtatious and suggestive verbal comments.

*Suspicious:* The client may look around the room suspiciously (some even actively check for hidden microphones). Squinting or looking out of the corner of one's eyes also may be interpreted as suspiciousness. Questions about what the examiner is writing down or about why such information is needed may also signal suspiciousness.

Although people use a wide range of feeling words in conversation, affective content usually can be accurately described using one of the following:

| | |
|---|---|
| Angry | Guilty or remorseful |
| Anxious | Happy or joyful |
| Ashamed | Irritated |
| Euphoric | Sad |
| Fearful | Surprised |

*Range and Duration*    A client's range and duration of affect, under normal conditions, varies depending on the client's current situation and the subject under discussion. Generally, the ability to experience and express a wide range of emotional states—even during the course of a clinical interview—is associated with positive mental health (Pennebaker, 1995). However, in some cases, a client's affective range may be too variable; and in others, it may be very constricted. Typically, clients with compulsive traits exhibit a constricted affect, while manic clients or clients with histrionic traits act out an excessively wide range of emotional states, from happiness to sadness and back again, rather quickly. Clients with this pattern are referred to as having a *labile affect.*

Sometimes clients exhibit little or no affect during the course of a clinical interview—as if their emotional life has been turned off. This absence of emotional display is commonly described as having a *flat affect.* The term is used to describe clients who seem unable to relate emotionally to other people. Examples include individuals diagnosed with schizophrenia, severe depression, or a neurological condition such as Parkinson's disease.

At times, when clients take antipsychotic medications, they experience and express minimal affect. This condition, which is very similar to flat affect, is often described as a *blunted affect* because an emotional response appears present, but in a restricted, minimal manner.

*Appropriateness*    The appropriateness of client affect is judged in the context of his or her speech content and life situation. Most often, inappropriate affect is observed in very disturbed clients who are suffering from severe mental disorders such as schizophrenia or bipolar disorder.

Determining the appropriateness of client affect is a subjective process that is sometimes more straightforward than at other times. For example, if a client is speaking about a clearly tragic incident (e.g., the death of his child) and inexplicably giggling and laughing without rational justification, the examiner would have substantial evidence for concluding the client's affect was "inappropriate with respect to the content of his speech." Alternatively, sometimes clients have idiosyncratic reasons for smiling or laughing or crying in situations where it does not seem appropriate to do so. For example, when a loved one dies after a long and protracted illness, it may be appropriate for a client to smile or laugh, either for reasons associated with relief, religious beliefs, or some other factor. Similarly, clients from various cultures may react in ways that most mainstream North American mental health professionals find unusual. What is important is that we remain sensitive and cautious in our judgments about the appropriateness or inappropriateness of client affective expressions.

One particular form of inappropriate affect deserves further description. Specifically, some clients exhibit a striking emotional indifference to their personal situation. Although profound indifference may occur in a diverse range of client types, it is most common, as Morrison (1993) describes, in the somatizing client: "Patients with somatization disorder will sometimes talk about their physical incapacities (paralysis, blindness) with the nonchalance that usually accompanies a discussion of the weather. This special type of inappropriate mood [*sic*] is called *la belle indifference* (French for "lofty indifference")" (p. 112).

*Depth or Intensity*   It is also typical for examiners to describe client affect in terms of depth or intensity. Some clients appear profoundly sad, while others seem to experience a more superficial sad affect. Determining the depth of client affect can be difficult, because many clients make strong efforts to "play their affective cards close to the vest." However, through close observation of client voice tone, body posture, facial expressions, and ability to quickly move (or not move) to a new topic, examiners can obtain at least some evidence regarding client affective depth or intensity. Nonetheless, we recommend limiting affective intensity ratings to situations when clients are deeply emotional or incredibly superficial.

When describing client affect in a mental status report, it is not necessary to use all of the dimensions described previously. It is most common to describe client affect content. The next most common dimension included is affective range and duration, with affective appropriateness and affective intensity included somewhat less often. A typical mental status report of affect in a depressed client who exhibited sad affective content, a narrow band of expression, and speech content consistent with sad life circumstances, might state:

> Throughout the examination, Ms. Brown's affect was occasionally sad, but often constricted. Her affect was appropriate with respect to the content of her speech.

In contrast, a client who presents with symptoms of mania might have much different affective descriptors:

> *Euphoric* (content or type): referring to behavior suggestive of mania (e.g., the client claims omnipotence, exhibits agitation or increased psychomotor activity, and has exaggerated gestures).
>
> *Labile* (range and duration): referring to a wide band of affective expression over a short time period (e.g., the client shifts quickly from tears to laughter).
>
> *Inappropriate with respect to speech content and life situation* (appropriateness): (e.g., the client expresses euphoria over job loss and marital separation; in other words, client's affective state is not rationally justifiable).
>
> *Shallow* (depth or intensity): referring to little depth or maintenance of emotion (e.g., the client claims to be happy because "I smile" and "smiling always takes care of everything").

The preceding client might be described as having a

> . . . labile, primarily euphoric affect that showed signs of being inappropriate and shallow.

## Mood

In a mental status exam, mood is different from affect. *Mood* is defined simply as the client's self-report regarding his or her prevailing emotional state. Mood should be evaluated directly through a simple, nonleading, open-ended question such as, "How have you been feeling lately?" or "Would you describe your mood for me?" rather than a closed and leading question that suggests an answer to the client: "Are you depressed?" When asked about their emotional state, some patients respond with a description of their physical condition or a description of their current life situation. If so, simply listen and then follow up with, "And how about emotionally? How are you feeling about (the physical condition or life situation)?"

It is desirable to record a client's response to your mood question verbatim. This makes it easier to compare a client's self-reported mood on one occasion with his or her self-reported mood on another occasion. In addition, it is important to compare self-reported mood with your evaluation of client affect. Self-reported mood should also be compared with self-reported thought content, because the thought content may account for the predominance of a particular mood.

Mood can be distinguished from affect on the basis of several features. Mood tends to last longer than affect. Mood changes less spontaneously than affect. Mood constitutes the emotional background. Mood is reported by the client, whereas affect is observed by the interviewer (Othmer & Othmer, 1994). Put another way (for you analogy buffs), mood is to affect as climate is to weather.

## Speech and Thought

In mental status exam formulations, speech and thought are intimately linked. It is primarily through speech that mental status examiners observe and evaluate thought process and content. There are, however, other ways for interviewers to observe and evaluate thought processes. Nonverbal behavior, sign language (in deaf clients), and writing also provide valuable information about client thinking processes. In a mental status exam, speech and thought are evaluated both separately and together.

### Speech

*Speech* is ordinarily described in terms of rate, volume, and amount. *Rate* refers to the observed speed of a client's speech. *Volume* refers to how loud a client talks. Both rate and volume can be categorized as:

High (fast or loud)
Medium (normal or average)
Low (slow or soft)

Client speech is usually described as pressured (high speed), loud (high volume), slow or halting (low speed), or soft or inaudible (low volume).

When clients speak freely, interviewers are more able to evaluate speech and thought. Usually, mental status reports describe speech that occurs without direct prompting or questioning as spontaneous. Clients whose speech is described as *spontaneous* are easy to interview and provide interviewers with excellent access to their internal thought processes. However, some clients resist speaking openly and may respond only briefly to direct questioning. Such clients are described as exhibiting "poverty of speech." Some clients who respond very slowly to questions may be described as having an increased *latency* or long response latency.

Distinct speech qualities or speech disturbances also should be noted. These may include an accent, high and screeching or low and gravelly pitch, and poor or distorted enunciation. In many cases, the examiner may comment, "The patient's speech was of normal rate and volume." Speech disturbances include dysarthria (problems with articulation or slurring of speech), dysprosody (problems with rhythm, such as mumbling or long pauses or latencies between syllables of words), cluttering (rapid, disorganized, and tongue-tied speech), and stuttering. Dysarthria, dysprosody, and cluttering are often associated with specific brain disturbances or drug toxicity; for example, mumbling may occur in patients with Huntington's chorea and slurring of speech in intoxicated patients.

## Thought Process

Observation and evaluation of thought is usually broken into two broad categories: thought process and thought content. *Thought process* refers to *how* clients express themselves. In other words, does thinking proceed in a systematic, organized, and logical manner? Can clients "get to the point" when expressing themselves? In many cases, it is useful to obtain a verbatim sample of client speech to capture psychopathological processes. The following sample was taken from a client's letter to his therapist, who was relocating to seek further professional education.

Dear Bill:

My success finally came around and I finally made plenty of good common sense with my attitude and I hope your sister will come along just fine really now and learn maybe at her elementary school whatever she may ask will not really develop to bad a complication of any kind I don't know for sure whether you're married or not yet but I hope you come along just fine with yourself and your plans on being a doctor somewhere or whatever or however too maybe well now so. I suppose I'll be at one of those inside sanitariums where it'll work out . . . and it'll come around okay really, Bye for now.

The client who wrote this letter clearly had a thinking process dysfunction. His thinking is disorganized and minimally coherent. Initially, his communication is characterized by a loosening of association; then, after writing the word *doctor,* the client decompensates into complete incoherence (i.e., "word salad"; see Table 8.2).

There are many ways to describe speech or thought processes. Some of the most common thought process descriptors are listed and defined in Table 8.2. When describing client speech and thought process, a mental status examiner might state:

The client's speech was loud and pressured. Her communication was sometimes incoherent; she exhibited flight of ideas and neologisms.

Sometimes clients from nondominant cultural backgrounds have difficulty responding quickly and smoothly to mental status examination questions. For example, as noted by Paniagua (2001), "Clients who are not fluent in English would show thought blocking" (p. 34). This particular phenomenon, characterized by a sudden cessation of thought or speech, may signal symptoms of anxiety, schizophrenia, or depression. However, "African American clients who use Black English in most conversational contexts would . . . spend a great deal of time looking for the construction of phrases or sentences in Standard American English when they feel that Standard American English is expected" (p. 34).

## Thought Content

*Thought content* refers to specific meaning expressed in client communication. Whereas thought process constitutes the *how* of client thinking, thought content constitutes the

**Table 8.2.   Thought Process Descriptors**

*Blocking:* Sudden cessation of speech in the midst of a stream of talk. There is no clear external reason for the client to stop talking and the client cannot explain why he or she stopped talking. Blocking may indicate that the client was about to associate to an extremely anxiety-laden topic. It also can indicate intrusion of delusional thoughts or disturbed perceptual experiences.

*Circumstantiality:* Excessive and unnecessary detail provided by the client. Sometimes, very intellectual people (e.g., scientists or even college professors) can become circumstantial; they eventually make their point, but they do not do so directly and efficiently. Circumstantiality or overelaboration also may be a sign of defensiveness and can be associated with paranoid thinking styles. (It can also simply be a sign the professor was not well-prepared for the lecture.)

*Clang Associations:* Combining unrelated words or phrases simply because they have similar sounds. Usually, this is manifest through rhyming or alliteration; for example: "I'm slime, dime, do some mime" or "When I think of my dad, rad, mad, pad, lad, sad." Some clients who clang are also perseverating (see below). Clanging usually occurs among very disturbed clients (e.g., schizophrenics). Of course, with all psychiatric symptoms, sometimes a specific situation or subculture encourages the behavior, in which cases it should not be considered abnormal (e.g., clanging behavior of rap group members is not abnormal).

*Flight of Ideas:* Continuous and overproductive speech in which the client's ideas are fragmented. Usually, an idea is stimulated by either a previous idea or an external event, but the relationship among ideas or ideas and events may be weak. In contrast to loose associations (see below), there are some perceivable connections in the client's thinking. However, unlike circumstantiality, the client never gets to the original point or never really answers the original question. Clients who exhibit flight of ideas often appear overenergized or overstimulated (e.g., manic or hypomanic clients). Many normal people, including one of the authors, exhibit flight of ideas after excessive caffeine intake.

*Loose Associations:* A lack of logical relationship between thoughts and ideas. Sometimes, interviewers can perceive the connections but must strain to do so; for example: "I love you. Bread is the staff of life. Haven't I seen you in church? I think incest is horrible." In this example, the client thinks of attraction and love, then of God's love as expressed through communion, then of church, and then of a presentation he heard in church about incest. The associations are loose but not completely nonexistent. Such communication may be an indicator of schizotypal personality disorder, schizophrenia, or other psychotic or pre- or postpsychotic disorder. Of course, some extremely creative people regularly exhibit loosening of associations, but most are able to find a socially acceptable vehicle through which to express their ideas.

*Mutism:* Virtually total unexpressiveness. There may be some signs that the client is in contact with others, but these are usually limited. Mutism can indicate autism or schizophrenia, catatonic subtype.

*Neologisms:* client-invented words. They are more than mispronunciations and are also rather spontaneously created; in other words, they are products of the moment rather than of a thoughtful creative process. We have heard words such as "slibber" and "temperaturific." It is important to check with the client with regard to word meaning and origin. Unusual words may be real words, or they may be taken from popular songs, television shows, or other sources. Neologisms are usually unintentionally created. They are associated with psychotic disorders.

*Perseveration:* Involuntary repetition of a single response or idea. The concept of perseveration may apply to speech or movement. Perseveration is often associated with brain damage or disease and with psychotic disorders. After being told no, teenagers often engage in this behavior, although normal teenagers are being persistent rather than perseverative; that is, if properly motivated, they are able to stop themselves voluntarily.

*Tangentiality:* Similar to circumstantiality, but the client never returns to his or her central point and never answers the original question. Tangential speech represents greater thought disturbance and disorganization than circumstantial speech, but less thought disturbance than loose association. Tangential speech is discriminated from flight of ideas because flight of ideas involves greater overproductivity of speech.

*Word Salad:* a series of words that seem completely unrelated. Word salad represents probably the highest level of thinking disorganization. Clients who exhibit word salad are incoherent. (For an example of word salad, see the second half of client letter above.)

*what* of client thinking. What clients talk about can give interviewers valuable information about mental status.

Clients can talk about an unlimited array of subjects during an interview. However, several specific content areas should be noted and explored in a mental status exam. These include delusions, obsessions, suicidal or homicidal thoughts or plans, specific phobias, and preoccupation with any emotion, particularly guilt (see Chapter 9 for ideas regarding inquiries about suicidal ideation). Although it is important in most mental status exams to ask a routine question regarding suicidal thoughts or impulses, we delay our discussion of suicide assessment until Chapter 9. The remainder of this section focuses on evaluating for delusions and obsessions.

*Delusions* are defined as false beliefs. They are deeply held and represent a break from reality; they are not based on facts or real events. For a particular belief to be a delusion, it must be unexplained by the client's cultural, religious, and educational background. Examiners may find it useful to record client reports of delusions verbatim. Examiners should not directly dispute clients' delusional beliefs. Instead, a question that explores a client's belief, such as the following, may be useful: "How do you know this [the delusion] is the case?" (Morrison, 1993, p. 119).

Clients may refer to many different types of delusions. *Delusions of grandeur* are false beliefs pertaining to a person's own ability or status. Most frequently, clients with delusions of grandeur believe they have extraordinary mental powers, physical strength, wealth, or sexual potency. They are usually unaffected by discrepancies between their beliefs and objective reality. In some cases, grandiose clients begin to believe they are a specific historical or contemporary figure (Napoleon, Jesus Christ, and Joan of Arc are particularly common).

Clients with *delusions of persecution* or *paranoid delusions* hold false beliefs that others are "out to get them" or are spying on them. Clients with such delusions may falsely believe that their home or telephone is bugged or that they are under surveillance by a neighbor whom they believe to be an FBI agent. Clients with paranoid delusions often have ideas of reference, which means that clients erroneously believe that ordinary events or occurrences are actually making reference to them. For example, many paranoid clients believe the television, newspaper, or radio is talking to or about them. A hospitalized man who was seeing his counselor twice a week complained bitterly that the television news was broadcasting his life story every night and thereby humiliating him in front of the rest of the patients and community.

Feelings and beliefs of being under the control or influence of some outside force or power characterize *delusions of alien control*. Symptoms usually involve a disowning of the client's own volition and personal responsibility. Clients report feeling as if they are puppets, passive and unable to assert personal control. In years past, it was popular to report being controlled by the Russians or Communists; in recent years, delusions of being possessed, abducted by aliens, or controlled by supernatural or alien forces appear to have increased in frequency.

*Somatic delusions* usually involve false beliefs about having a medical condition or disease, such as cancer, a heart condition, or obstructed bowels. Not surprisingly, AIDS has become a frequent preoccupation for clients with somatic delusions. It is not uncommon for very disturbed clients to believe they have AIDS despite the fact that they have never used intravenous drugs or engaged in sexual relations (Nash, 1996). Similarly, clients may believe they are pregnant when they have not had intercourse. Anorexic clients may falsely believe they are grossly overweight when, in fact, they are dying of malnutrition. Somatic delusions, like other delusions, sometimes may have a bizarre quality, as in a case we worked with wherein a woman believed a fetus was growing in her brain.

Depressed clients often manifest *delusions of self-deprecation.* They may believe they are the "worst case ever" or that their skills and abilities are grossly impaired (when they are not impaired). Common self-deprecating comments include statements about sinfulness, ugliness, and stupidity. In some cases, clients have engaged in behaviors or thoughts that cause them to feel negative about themselves.

It is always important to seek factual evidence to determine whether a client is truly delusional, especially in cases of suspected somatic delusions. Clients with somatic delusions should be examined by a physician to rule in or rule out the presence of a medical condition. Exploring delusional beliefs can also provide examiners with insights into client thought processes and personal experiences. The client who claims the "body snatchers" are making him shout profanities at his parents may feel overly controlled by his parents. He may also feel extremely angry toward them and find it less threatening to disown his impulses by ascribing the shouted profanities to some peculiar evil force; similarly, the grandiose client may feel unimportant or neglected. The paranoid client cannot trust anyone and, therefore, projects her feelings of distrust onto others and comes to believe others are constantly watching her.

On the other hand, we must also entertain the possibility that client delusions have a basis in reality rather than in the client's psychological dynamics. For example, the young man shouting obscenities at his parents may have Tourette's syndrome, and the woman who is paranoid and distrustful may have good reasons (i.e., she is actually being followed).

## Obsessions

*Obsessions* are recurrent and persistent ideas, thoughts, and images. True obsessions are involuntary and usually viewed as senseless or irrational *even by those who are experiencing them.* Clients may intentionally ruminate about a wide variety of issues. If they lose voluntary control over whether they think a particular thought, then they are considered obsessional. One obsessive-compulsive client we worked with had obsessions about being contaminated by "worms" and "germs" (Sommers, 1986). He reported that once, as he rode his bicycle down the street, he noticed an open garbage dumpster on the opposite side of the street and immediately became overwhelmed with the thought that somehow, he had "gotten some of the garbage on [his] lips." Intense obsessions are often followed by compulsive behaviors. In the same case, the client felt compelled to ride back and forth down the street past the garbage dumpster to determine whether he possibly could have reached his head across the street and into the garbage. Such a case illustrates the irrational and sometimes almost delusional nature of obsessions.

A child client we worked with had become obsessed with thoughts of keeping her ailing grandmother alive. She believed that if she thought continuously about her grandmother and engaged in various magical rituals every day, her grandmother's cancer would not progress. Her rituals, of course, would be categorized as *compulsions.* She also had begun scratching a certain spot on her cheek so the pain would make her remember to think of her grandmother. The scratching, too, would be considered a compulsion; her frantic, nonstop thinking of her grandmother and her beliefs about her power to keep her grandmother alive would be considered obsessions.

Most individuals who present with compulsions exhibit either washing or checking behavior. They continually feel the need to wash or clean something, or they constantly need to check whether a particular event has occurred or is going to occur. The most common examples are compulsions to wash hands, clean house, check the locks, and check to see if an intruder has gained entry into a bedroom or house. Clinically significant compulsions are virtually always preceded by clinically significant obsessions.

Obsessions are characterized primarily by a sense of doubt. Commonly, obsessive-compulsive clients wonder:

Are my hands clean?
Have I been contaminated?
Did I remember to lock the front door?
Did I remember to turn off the oven (lights, stereo, etc.)?
Is anyone under my bed?

Although everyone experiences obsessive thoughts on occasion, such thoughts may or may not be clinically or diagnostically significant. Information is of *clinical* significance if it contributes to the treatment process; information is of *diagnostic* significance if it contributes to the diagnostic process. During a mental status exam, it is always important to evaluate obsessions because they reveal to an examiner what the client spends time thinking about. Such information may be clinically significant; that is, it may enhance empathy and treatment planning. However, the same obsessions may or may not be diagnostically significant. For example, if a client describes occasional obsessions that do not interfere with his or her ability to function at work, school, home, or play, they may not be diagnostically significant.

## Perceptual Disturbances

There are two major types of perceptual disturbances: hallucinations and illusions. *Hallucinations* are defined as false sensory impressions or experiences. *Illusions* are defined as perceptual distortions, causing existing stimuli to appear quite different from what they are in reality.

Hallucinations may occur in any of the five major sensory modalities: visual, auditory, olfactory, gustatory, and tactile. Auditory hallucinations are most commonly reported. Clients who report hearing things (usually voices) that others do not hear usually suffer from either an affective disorder or schizophrenia. However, on occasion, such experiences may be produced by states of chemical intoxication or because of acute traumatic stress. In other instances, clients may report having especially good hearing or they may report listening to their own "inner voice." Although such reports are worth exploring, they are not in and of themselves signs of perceptual disturbance. In addition, people often report odd perceptual experiences, similar to hallucinations, that occur as they fall off to sleep or when they are just waking up. Such perceptual disturbances are normal—and occur during the hypnogogic or hypnopompic sleep states—and are a consistent part of many people's sleep patterns (Rosenthal, Zorick, & Merlotti, 1990). Therefore, when evaluating for hallucinations, interviewers should always determine *when* such experiences usually occur. If they occur exclusively when a client is in a stage of sleep, they are less diagnostically relevant.

Because of the psychotic nature of delusions and hallucinations and the bizarre nature of some obsessive-compulsive symptoms, interviewers should approach questioning in these areas with an especially gentle and explorative manner. The following sample interview dialogue illustrates how interviewers can help clients admit their unusual or bizarre experiences:

**Interviewer:** "I'm going to ask you some questions about experiences you may or may not have in your life. Some of the questions may seem odd or unusual, and others may fit some personal experiences you've had but haven't yet spoken about."

**Client:** "Okay."

**Interviewer:** "Sometimes radio broadcasts or television newscasts or programming can feel very personal, as if the people in them were speaking directly to you. Have you ever thought a particular program was talking about you or to you on a personal basis?"

**Client:** "That program the other night was about my life. It was about me and Cindy Crawford.

**Interviewer:** "You know Cindy Crawford?"

**Client:** "I sure do; she's my woman."

**Interviewer:** "And how did you meet her?"

**Client:** "We met when I was her director in about five or six movies she filmed."

The next dialogue models an evaluation for auditory perceptual disturbances:

**Interviewer:** "I've noticed you seem to be a pretty sensitive person. Is your hearing especially good?"

**Client:** "Yes, as a matter of fact, I have better hearing than most people."

**Interviewer:** "Really? What kinds of things do you hear that most people can't hear?"

**Client:** "I can hear people talking through walls, in the next room."

**Interviewer:** "Right now?"

**Client:** "Yeah."

**Interviewer:** "What are the voices saying?"

**Client:** "They're talking about me and Cindy . . . about our sex life."

**Interviewer:** "How about your vision? Is it especially keen too? Can you see things that other people can't see?"

The next dialogue models an evaluation for obsessions:

**Interviewer:** "You know how sometimes people get a song or tune stuck in their head and they can't stop thinking about it? Have you ever had that kind of experience?"

**Client:** "Sure, doesn't everybody?"

**Interviewer:** "Yeah, that's true. I'm wondering if you ever have some particular thoughts, kind of like a musical tune, that you wish you could get rid of, but can't?"

**Client:** "Maybe sometimes, but it's no big deal."

**Interviewer:** "How about images? Do you have any images that seem to intrude into your mind and that you can't get rid of?"

Notice how the interviewer in these preceding examples normalizes each type of pathology by saying things like, "you seem sensitive" and "you know how sometimes people get a song or tune stuck in their head. . ." and then inquiring about the symptoms present.

Visual or tactile hallucinations are often linked to organic conditions. These conditions may include drug intoxication or withdrawal, brain trauma, or brain disease. Clients in acute delirious states may pick at their clothes or skin in an effort to remove objects or organisms (e.g., insects) they believe are producing their sensory experiences. Similarly, clients may reach out or call out for people or objects that do not exist. Obviously, when clients report such experiences or you observe clients as they experience such perceptual disturbances, the disorder is usually of a very serious nature. Immediate medical evaluation and intervention is warranted.

## Orientation and Consciousness

Mental status examiners routinely evaluate whether clients are oriented to (i.e., aware of) their current situation. The question of whether a client is oriented involves evaluating basic cognitive functions. The examiner asks a client three simple questions:

What is your name?
Where are you (i.e., what city or where in a particular building)?
What is today's date?

When a client answers these queries correctly, the examiner might write in the progress notes that the client was "OX3" (oriented times three), referring to the fact that the client is aware of who and where he or she is, and what day it is. Evaluating a client's orientation is a direct way to assess level of confusion or *disorientation*. Extremely disturbed clients may not be able to respond accurately to one or more of these simple questions. Resisting (or refusing to answer) questions about orientation may indicate disorientation. In the following example, a hospital patient with a recent head trauma was interviewed regarding orientation:

**Interviewer:** "I'm going to ask you a few questions that may seem a bit strange. Just do the best you can in answering them. Tell me, what day is it today?"
**Client:** "They told me I was riding my bike and that I didn't have my helmet on."
**Interviewer:** "That's right. I'm still curious, though. What day is it today?"
**Client:** "Could I get a glass of water?"

After several minutes of this client's interview, it became apparent that he was evading the question about orientation to time. Note also that the examiner began with a simple orientation to time question (i.e., a question about the day of the week instead of a question about today's date). When clients are resistant to answering orientation questions, you may tentatively conclude they are disoriented, especially if additional evidence suggests disorientation.

Orientation levels can be pursued in greater or lesser depth. For example, clients can be asked what county they are in, who the governor of the state is, and the name of the mayor or local newspaper. They also can be asked if they recognize hospital personnel, visitors, and family. However, these additional questions may be confounded by factors such as the client's level of intelligence, social awareness, or cultural background, and, therefore, they are not always accurate indicators of orientation.

Clients can become disoriented for a number of reasons. Common causes include drug intoxication, recent brain trauma, and dementia (e.g., Alzheimer's). It is not the mental status examiner's task to determine the cause of a client's disorientation, but to accurately and briefly document presence or absence of disorientation.

In cases of delirium, acutely disoriented clients may experience a gradual clearing of consciousness. When clients become disoriented, they usually lose their sense of time first, then of place, and finally of person. Orientation is recovered in reverse order (person, then place, then time).

Questioning for orientation can be viewed as offensive by fully oriented clients. They may feel belittled by the simple questions. On the other hand, cognitively impaired clients sometimes act indignant about having to answer simple questions, partly as a defensive ploy, because they cannot recall the correct answer. Therefore, questioning for orientation should always be approached gently with clients. It helps to inform clients that questions about orientation are simply a routine evaluation procedure. The client's orientation to self should be checked at the beginning of an interview. Questions on the following list can be used in combination with more chatty or social questions or statements.

**Self/Person**

What is your name? Where are you from?

Where do you currently live?

What kinds of activities do you engage in during your free time?

Are you employed? (If so) What do you do for a living?

Are you married? (If so) What is your spouse's name?

Do you have any children?

**Place**

There's been a lot happening these past few days (or hours); I wonder if you can describe for me where you are?

Do you recall what city we're in?

What's the name of the building we're in right now?

Do you know what part of the hospital we're in?

**Time**

Have you been keeping track of the time lately?

What's today's date? (If client claims not to recall, ask for an estimate; estimates can help assess level of disorientation.)

Do you know what day of the week it is?

What month (or year) is it?

How long have you been here?

Consciousness is usually evaluated along a continuum from alert to comatose. Examiners evaluate level of consciousness as well as degree of orientation, because although the two concepts are related, they are not identical. As examiners observe clients' responses and behaviors during an interview, they select a descriptor of consciousness. Descriptors include:

Alert

Confused

Clouded

Stuporous

Unconscious

Comatose

After evaluating a client who is relatively cognitively intact, a mental examiner might state, "The client was alert and oriented to person, place, and time." In contrast, an acutely delirious client might be described as: "The client's consciousness was clouded; she was oriented to person (OX1), but incorrectly identified the year as '1993' instead of 2003 and was unable to identify the city where her examination was taking place."

## Memory and Intelligence

Mental status examinations include a cursory assessment of more advanced client cognitive abilities, usually including assessments of memory and general intelligence.

### Memory

A mental status exam can provide a quick memory screening, but it does not provide a definitive answer as to whether a specific memory impairment exists. Formal neuropsychological assessment is required to specify the nature and extent of memory impairment.

*Memory* is broadly defined as the ability to recall past experiences. Three types of memory are typically assessed in a mental status examination: remote, recent, and immediate. *Remote memory* refers to recall of events, information, and people from the distant past. *Recent memory* refers to recall of events, information, and people from the prior week or so. *Immediate memory* refers to retention of information or data to which one was exposed only minutes previously.

Recall of remote events involves reviewing chronological information from the client's history. Some clinicians simply weave an evaluation of remote memory into the history-taking portion of the intake interview. This type of assessment involves questions about time and place of birth, names of schools attended, date of marriage, age differences between client and siblings, and so forth. The problem with basing an assessment of remote memory on self-report of historical information is that the examiner is unable to tell if the client is recalling historical experiences and information accurately. This problem reflects the main dilemma in assessment of remote memory impairment: the possibility of confabulation.

The term *confabulation* refers to spontaneous fabrication or distortion of memories. Confabulation often occurs during recall. To some extent, a certain amount of confabulation is normal (Loftus, 2001). In fact, we have found that intense marital disputes can occur—for some couples, but of course, not ourselves—when memories of key events fail to jibe. It is clear that human memory is imperfect and, as time passes, events are subject to reinterpretation. This is especially the case if an individual feels pressured into responding to questions about the past. A client may be able to recall only a portion of a specific memory, but when the client is pressured to elaborate on that memory, confabulation can occur. Here is an example of confabulation on a simple test of remote memory.

**Interviewer:** "Okay, now I'm going to ask you a few questions to test your memory. Ready?"
**Client:** "Yeah, I guess."
**Interviewer:** "Name five men who have been president of the United States since 1950."
**Client:** "Right. There was, uh Truman . . . and Ronald Reagan . . . uh, yeah there's uh, Bush and Bush again. I've almost got another one . . . it's on the tip of my tongue."

**Interviewer:** "You're doing great. All you need is one more."
**Client:** "Yeah, I know. I can do it."
**Interviewer:** "Take your time."
**Client:** "Jefferson. That's it, William Jefferson."

In this case, the examiner is slightly pressuring the client by being enthusiastic and supportive. Based on what the examiner is saying, it sounds almost as if he is rooting for the client to pass this memory test. When pressuring occurs, through either positive or more coercive means, humans often tend to make something up to relieve the pressure and give the examiner what he or she wants.

The preceding example pertains to a client's memory for historical fact. In contrast, when interviewing clients about personal history, depending on the question, you may not be able to confirm or disconfirm the accuracy of the client's answer. For example, if a client claims to have been "abducted" as a child, it may be difficult to judge the accuracy of his or her claim.

In general, when clients respond to questions about their history, answers always contain some degree of inaccuracy or confabulation. It is the examiner's responsibility to determine the accuracy of a client's historical reports. Pursuing truth can be a challenging experience.

When confabulation or memory impairment is suspected, it may be helpful to ask clients about objective events that occurred during childhood or early adulthood. This usually involves inquiring about significant and memorable social or political events (e.g., Who was president when you were growing up? What countries were involved in World War II? What were some popular recreational activities during your high school years?). Of course, using social and political questions may be unfair to cultural minorities, so exercise caution when using such strategies.

If the accuracy of a client's historical report is questionable, it may be useful (or necessary) to call on friends or family of the client to confirm historical information. Such a procedure can be complicated because releases of information must be signed by all parties to ensure legal protection. In addition, friends and family members may not be honest with you or may themselves have impaired or confabulated memories. Consequently, although verification of client personal history is in some cases essential, it is by no means problem-free.

Clients may directly admit to memory problems. However, such an admission does not necessarily constitute evidence of memory impairment. In addition, a client's admission to memory problems does not indicate that the impairment has a neurological or organic component. In fact, clients with brain injury or damage are sometimes more likely to deny memory problems and try to cover them up through confabulation. Conversely, depressed clients often exaggerate the extent to which their cognitive skills have diminished, complaining to great lengths that something is wrong with their brain (Othmer & Othmer, 1994).

In fact, depressed clients' cognitive skills are sometimes impaired. This phenomenon is called *pseudodementia* (de Rosiers, 1992; B. Robinson, 1997). In other words, depressed clients may have no organic impairment but still suffer from emotionally based memory problems. In many cases, once the depression is alleviated, memory problems are also resolved.

Evaluating clients' recent and immediate memories is simpler than evaluating remote memory because experiences of the recent past are more easily verified. If the client has been hospitalized, questions can be asked pertaining to reasons for hospitalization, treatments received, and hospital personnel with whom the client had contact.

Clients may be asked what they ate for breakfast, what clothes they wore the day before, and whether they recall the weather of the prior week.

Immediate memory requires sustained attention, the ability to concentrate on cognitive input. There are several formal ways of evaluating client immediate memory. The most common of these are serial sevens, recall of brief stories, and digit span (Folstein, Folstein, & McHugh, 1975; Wechsler & Stone, 1945).

*Serial sevens* is administered by simply asking the client to "begin with 100 and count backwards by 7" (Folstein et al., 1975, p. 197). Clients who can sustain attention (and who have adequate cognitive ability) should be able to perform serial sevens without difficulty. However, excessive anxiety—sometimes associated with clients who have an anxiety disorder, but also associated with clients who have a history of difficulty with math or performance-based tasks—may interfere with concentration and impair performance. Clients of divergent cultural backgrounds also struggle with this task, partly because of their difficulty comprehending and lack of experience participating in such activities (Paniagua, 2001). Additionally, the research on using serial sevens to evaluate cognitive functioning is weak (C. Hughes, 1993). Consequently, anxiety level, cultural and educational background, distractibility, and potential invalidity of the procedure should all be considered when evaluating a client's memory using serial sevens.

*Digit span* is administered by saying, "I am going to say a series of numbers. When I am finished, repeat them to me in the same order." A series of numbers is then read clearly to the client, with about one-second intervals between numbers. Examiners begin with a short series of numbers they believe the client can accurately repeat and then proceed to longer lists. For example:

**Interviewer:** "I want to do a simple test with you to check your ability to concentrate. First, I'll say a series of numbers. Then, when I'm finished, you repeat them to me. Okay?

**Client:** "Okay."

**Interviewer:** "Here's the first series of numbers: 6–1–7–4.

**Client:** "6 . . . 1 . . . 7 . . . 4."

**Interviewer:** "Okay. Now try this one: 8–5–9–3–7.

**Client:** "Um . . . 8 . . . 5 . . . 9 . . . 7 . . . 3."

**Interviewer:** "Okay, here's another set: 2–6–1–3–9." (Notice that the examiner does not point out the client's incorrect response but simply provides another set of five numbers to give the client another opportunity to respond correctly. Usually, if a client gets one of two trials of a specific set of numbers correct, he or she can proceed to the next higher level, until both trials are completed incorrectly).

After completing digit span forward, it is common to administer digit span backward.

**Interviewer:** "Now I'm going to have you do something slightly different. Once again, I'll read a short list of numbers, but this time when I'm finished I'd like you to repeat them to me in reverse order. For example, if I said: 7–2–8, what would you say?"

**Client:** "Uh . . . 8 . . . 2 . . . 7. That's pretty hard. These better be real short lists of numbers."

**Interviewer:** "That's right, I think you've got it. Now try this: 4–2–5–8."

Clients may become especially sensitive about their performance on specific cognitive tasks. Their responses may range from overconfidence (not acknowledging the need to guess or their fears of poor performance), to excuse making (e.g., "Today's just not a good day for me!"), to open acknowledgment of performance concerns (e.g., "I'm afraid I got that one wrong, too. I'm just horrible at this."). The way clients respond to cognitive performance tests may reveal important clinical information, such as an inability to admit weaknesses, a style of rationalizing or making excuses for poor performance, or a tendency toward negative self-evaluation.

When clients are referred specifically because of memory problems, an initial mental status examination is appropriate, but should always be followed by further clinical assessment. In particular, especially in the early stages of memory assessment, it is imperative for examiners to interview knowledgeable family members to corroborate memory deficits reported by the patient and noted in the mental status exam. In particular, interviewers should ask family members specific questions pertaining to "the onset, duration, and severity of memory difficulties" (Steffens & Morgenlander, 1999, p. 72).

*Intelligence*

Evaluation of intellectual functioning is traditionally a controversial subject, perhaps especially so when the evaluation takes place during a brief clinical interview (Flanagan, Genshaft, & Harrison, 1997). Despite the potential of evaluation misuse, general statements about intellectual functioning are usually made following a mental status exam. However, we emphasize the importance of exercising caution when judging intelligence after the brief and limited contact typical of a mental status examination. Statements about intellectual functioning should be phrased in a tentative manner, especially when the statements are based on a brief clinical encounter.

Few people agree on a single definition of *intelligence.* Wechsler (1958) defined it as a person's "global capacity . . . to act purposefully, to think rationally, and to deal effectively with his environment" (p. 35). Though general, this definition is still useful. Put as a question, it might be "Is there evidence that the client is resourceful and consequently functions adequately in a number of life domains?" or "Does the client make mistakes in life that appear due to limited 'intellectual ability' rather than clinical psychopathology?" Although these questions are difficult, an answer should be attempted at the conclusion of a mental status examination.

Research suggests that it may be more reasonable to view intelligence as a composite of several specific abilities than as a general adaptive tendency (Sternberg, 1985; Sternberg & Wagner, 1986). Using this construct, an individual might be evaluated as having strong intellectual skills in one area but deficiencies in another.

Sternberg and Wagner (1986) refer to a triarchic theory of intelligence. They identify three forms of intelligence:

Academic problem solving
Practical intelligence
Creative intelligence

Using this concept of triarchic intelligence, a mental status examiner might conclude that a client has excellent practical and creative intellectual skills, as exemplified by social competence, good street survival skills, and the ability to come up with creative solutions to mechanical problems. However, the same individual might lack formal education and appear unintelligent if evaluated strictly from the perspective of academic problem-solving abilities.

H. Gardner's (1983, 1999) theory of multiple intelligences posits that human intelligence can be divided into seven or eight different forms. This perspective, although exceedingly popular among educators, has yet to accumulate substantial supporting research (Klein, 1997; Morgan, 1996). From an interviewer's perspective, Gardner's (1999) and Sternberg's (1985) theories are most relevant for reminding us that people can express their intellectual capacities in divergent ways. This reminder may prevent us from prematurely or inappropriately concluding that minority clients or clients from lower socioeconomic backgrounds are unintelligent based primarily on a single intellectual dimension (e.g., language/vocabulary use).

During a mental status exam, intelligence is usually measured using several methods. First, native intelligence is inferred from a client's education level. Obviously, this method overvalues academic intelligence (Gould, 1981). Second, intelligence is assessed by observing a client's language comprehension and use (i.e., vocabulary or verbal comprehension). It has been shown that vocabulary is the single strongest IQ predictor (Sattler, 1992). Again, this method is biased in favor of the formally educated over cultural minorities (Elliott, 1988). Third, intelligence is inferred from client responses to questions designed to determine fund of knowledge. Once again, fund of knowledge is often a by-product of a stimulating educational background, and questions used to assess knowledge are generally culturally biased. Fourth, intelligence is measured through client responses to questions designed to evaluate abstract thinking abilities. Fifth, questions designed to measure social judgment are used to evaluate intellectual functioning. (See Table 8.3 for sample questions that test fund of knowledge, abstract thinking, and social judgment.) Sixth, intelligence is inferred from observations of responses to tests of orientation, consciousness, and memory. Based on these procedures, statements about intellectual functioning should be phrased tentatively, especially when they pertain to minority clients.

## Reliability, Judgment, and Insight

### Reliability

*Reliability* refers to a client's credibility and trustworthiness. A reliable informant is one who is careful to present his or her life history and current personal information honestly and accurately. In contrast, some clients may be highly unreliable; for one reason or another, they distort, confabulate, or blatantly lie about their life circumstances and personal history.

It is often difficult to determine when a client is being untruthful during an interview. Even experienced interviewers can be deceived by their clients (Yalom, 1995). For example, in a case we worked with, a very depressed male client was admitted to a psychiatric hospital. When asked if he would like to participate in the hospital's recreational program, the client replied, "I'm too depressed to move." The next day, after being left unsupervised during the recreational outing, this same client managed to find the energy to run away from the hospital without medical approval. His report regarding his inability to move had been extremely unreliable.

Reliability may be estimated based on a number of observable factors. Clients with good attention to detail and who spontaneously elaborate to your questions are likely to be reliable informants. In contrast, clients who answer questions in a vague or defensive manner have a greater probability of being unreliable. In some cases, you will

**Table 8.3. Sample Mental Status Exam Questions Used to Assess Intelligence**

Many questions used to assess intelligence during a mental status exam are taken from standardized tests or are otherwise copyrighted, and therefore it is inappropriate to reproduce them here. The following questions are similar in content to typical questions used by mental status examiners.

*Fund of Knowledge*

Name six large U.S. cities.

What is the direction you go when traveling from New York to Rome?

Who was president of the United States during the Vietnam War?

Which president "freed the slaves"?

What poisonous chemical substance is in automobile emissions?

What is Stevie Wonder's profession?

*Abstract Thinking*

In what way are a pencil and a typewriter alike?

In what way are a whale and a dolphin alike?

What does this saying mean: People who live in glass houses shouldn't throw stones?

What does this saying mean: A bird in the hand is worth two in the bush?

*Judgment*

What would you do if you discovered a gun hidden in the bushes of a local park?

If you won a million dollars, how would you spend it?

How far would you say it is from Los Angeles to Chicago?

If you were stuck in a desert for 24 hours, what measures might you take to survive?

How would you handle it if you discovered that your best friend was having an affair with your boss's spouse?

Note: These items were developed for illustrative purposes. Interviewers should consult published, standardized testing materials when conducting formal evaluations of intelligence. It is inappropriate to make conclusive statements about client intellectual functioning based on just a few interview questions.

have a clear sense that clients are intentionally omitting or minimizing parts of their history.

When you suspect a client is unreliable, it is useful to contact family, employers, or other client associates to corroborate the client's story. This step can be problematic, but it is often necessary. If no one is available with whom you can discuss the client's story, it is advisable to proceed cautiously with your client's care while observing his or her behavior closely. You should also note reservations about the client's reliability in your mental status report.

*Judgment*

People with good judgment are able to consistently make constructive and adaptive decisions that affect their lives in a positive way. In the clinical setting, a client's judgment can be evaluated during an intake interview by exploring his or her activity, relationship, and vocational choices. Ask, for example, if your client regularly involves himself or herself in illegal activities or in relationships that seem destructive. Does he or she flirt with danger by engaging in potentially life-threatening activities? Obviously, consistent participation in illegal activities, destructive relationships, and life-threatening activities constitutes evidence that an individual is exercising poor judgment regarding relationship or activity choices.

Adolescent clients frequently exercise poor judgment. For example, a 17-year-old we worked with impulsively quit his job as a busboy at an expensive restaurant simply because he found out an hour before his shift that he was assigned to work with an employee whom he did not like and viewed as lazy. Six months later, still complaining about lack of money and looking for a job, he continued to defend his impulsive move, despite the fact that it obviously was an example of shortsightedness and poor judgment.

Some clients, especially impulsive adolescents or adults in the midst of a manic episode, may exhibit grossly impaired judgment. They may profoundly overestimate or underestimate their physical, mental, and social prowess. For example, manic patients often exhibit extremely poor judgment in their financial affairs, spending large amounts of money on sketchy business ventures or gambling schemes. Similarly, driving while intoxicated, engaging in promiscuous and unprotected sex, or participating in poorly planned criminal behavior are all behavior patterns usually considered as evidence of poor judgment.

In addition to evaluating judgment on the basis of clients' reports of specific behaviors, judgment is frequently assessed by having clients respond to hypothetical scenarios. Sample scenarios are provided in Table 8.3.

## Insight

*Insight* refers to clients' understanding of their problems. Take, for example, the case of a male client who presented with symptoms of exhaustion. During the interview, he was asked if he sometimes experienced anxiety and tension. He insisted, despite shallow breathing, flushing on the neck, and clenched fists, that he did not have any problems with tension and, therefore, learning to relax would be of no use to him. On further inquiry as to whether there might be, in some cases, a connection between his chronically high levels of tension and his reported exhaustion, his response was a terse "No, and anyway I told you I don't have a problem with tension." This client displayed absolutely no insight into a clear problem area.

Toward the mental status examination's end, it is useful to ask clients to speculate on the cause or causes of their symptoms. Some clients respond with powerfully insightful answers, while others immediately begin discussing a number of physical illnesses they may have contracted (e.g., "I don't know, maybe I have mono?"), and still others simply have no clue as to potential underlying causes or dynamics. Clients with high levels of insight are generally able to intelligently discuss the possibility of emotional or psychosocial factors contributing to their symptoms; they are, at least, open to considering and addressing nonbiological factors. In contrast, clients with little or no insight become defensive when faced with possible psychosocial or emotional explanations for their condition; in many cases, clients without insight blatantly deny they have any problems.

Mental status examiners usually describe degree of client insight by referring to one of four descriptors:

*Absent:* Clients who are labeled as having an absence of insight usually do not admit to having any problems. They may blame someone else for being referred for treatment or for being hospitalized. Obviously, these clients show no evidence of grasping a reasonable explanation for their symptoms because they deny that they have any problematic symptoms. If an interviewer suggests that a problem may exist, this type of client usually becomes very defensive.

*Poor:* Clients who admit to having a minor problem or some nuisance symptoms, but rely exclusively on physical, medical, or situational explanations for symptoms, are often referred to as having poor insight. There is resistance to accepting the fact that life situations or emotional states can contribute—at all—to personal problems or illnesses. These clients deny the existence of any personal responsibility or nonphysical factors contributing to their problems. If they admit a problem exists, they are likely to rely solely on medications, surgery, or getting away from people they blame for their problems, as treatment for their condition.

*Partial:* Clients who admit, more often than not, that they have a problem that may warrant treatment are considered as having partial insight; however, this insight can pass and such clients often leave treatment prematurely. These clients can occasionally articulate how situational or emotional factors contribute to their condition and how their own behavior may contribute to their problems. They are reluctant to focus on such factors, but gentle reminders motivate them to work with nonmedical treatment approaches.

*Good:* Clients who readily admit to having a problem for which an appropriate treatment is required are considered to have good insight. When appropriate, these clients take personal responsibility for modifying their life situation. They can articulate and use nonphysical treatment approaches with minimal help from the therapist. These clients may even be exceptionally creative in formulating ways to address their illness through nonmedical methods.

## WHEN TO USE MENTAL STATUS EXAMINATIONS

Formal mental status examinations are not appropriate for all clients. A good basic guideline is: Mental status examinations become more necessary as suspected level of client psychopathology increases. If clients appear well adjusted and you are not working in a medical setting, it is unlikely you will need to conduct a full mental status evaluation. However, if you have questions about diagnosis or client psychopathology and you are working in a medical setting, administration of a formal mental status examination is usually routine. R. Rosenthal and Akiskal (1985) state:

> Some individuals who present for outpatient psychotherapy or counseling can be viewed as having "problems of living." In such cases, the relevant mental status information can be largely gleaned from a well-conducted history-taking or intake interview . . . . On the other hand, if the patient appears to be suffering from significant disturbance of mood, perception, thinking, or memory, a formal Mental Status Examination is in order. (p. 25)

The primary exception to Rosenthal and Akiskal's (1985) advice is the multicultural client. Some practitioners suggest that it is nearly always inappropriate to use a traditional mental status examination with a multicultural client (Paniagua, 1998, 2001). Individual and Cultural Highlight 8.1 is designed to sensitize you to potentially invalid conclusions you might reach when using mental status exams with culturally diverse clients.

All evaluation procedures, including mental status examinations, are culturally biased in one way or another. Consequently, examiners must use caution when applying the procedures described in this chapter to clients from diverse cultural backgrounds.

---

### INDIVIDUAL AND CULTURAL HIGHLIGHT 8.1

## Cultural Differences in Mental Status

Cultural norms are very important to consider when evaluating mental status. For each category addressed in the traditional mental status examination, try to think of cultures that would behave very differently but still be within "normal" parameters for their cultural or racial group. Examples include differences in cultural manifestations of grief, stress, humiliation, or trauma. In addition, persons from minority cultures who have recently been displaced may display confusion, fear, or resistance that is entirely appropriate to the situation. Further, in traumatic or stressful situations, persons with disabilities may be misunderstood.

Work with a partner to generate multicultural mental status observations that might lead an interviewer to an inappropriate and invalid conclusion regarding client mental status. Use the mental status categories listed below:

| Category | Observation | Invalid Conclusion |
|---|---|---|
| Appearance: | | |
| Behavior/psychomotor activity: | | |
| Attitude toward examiner: | | |
| Affect and mood: | | |
| Speech and thought: | | |
| Perceptual disturbances: | | |
| Orientation and consciousness: | | |
| Memory and intelligence: | | |
| Reliability, judgment, and insight: | | |

---

Before applying mainstream mental status and diagnostic principles to minority populations, examiners should explore potential cultural explanations. As is the case with all interviewing procedures, respect for client individuality and cultural background should always be factored into interviewer conclusions. It is important for interviewers to be reminded of this fact, especially when engaging in objective assessment procedures.

## SUMMARY

Mental status examinations are a way of organizing clinical observations to maximize evaluation of current mental status. Administration of an examination is common in medical settings. Although mental status information is useful in the diagnostic process, mental status examinations are not primarily diagnostic procedures.

Complete mental status examinations require interviewers to observe and query client functioning in nine areas: appearance; behavior or psychomotor activity; attitude toward examiner (interviewer); affect and mood; speech and thought; perceptual disturbances; orientation and consciousness; memory and intelligence; and reliability, judgment, and insight. The validity of clinical observations in a mental status examination can be compromised when clients come from a divergent individual or cultural background.

*Appearance* refers to client physical and demographic characteristics, such as sex, age, and race. *Behavior or psychomotor activity* refers to physical movements made by clients during an interview. Movements may be excessive, limited, absent, or bizarre. Documentation of client movement during an interview is important evidence that may support your mental status conclusions.

Client attitude toward the evaluator is assessed primarily as interpersonal behavior toward the examiner or interview. Determination of client attitude may be affected by an interviewer's emotional reactions during an interview; therefore, interviewers should exercise caution when labeling client attitude.

*Affect* refers to the client's prevailing emotional tone as observed by an interviewer; *mood* refers to the client's self-reported emotional state. Affect may be described in terms of its content or type, range or variability, and duration, appropriateness, and depth or intensity. In contrast, mood consists simply of the client's response to the question, "How are you feeling today?"

Speech, thought, and perceptual disturbances are interrelated aspects of client functioning evaluated during a mental status examination. Evaluation of thought is divided into two categories: thought process and thought content. *Thought process* is defined as *how* a client thinks and includes process descriptors such as circumstantiality, flight of ideas, and loose association. In contrast, *thought content* is defined as *what* a client thinks and includes delusions and obsessions. Suicidal or homicidal thought content is also routinely noted on mental status examinations. Perceptual disturbances include hallucinations and illusions. *Hallucinations* are false or inaccurate perceptual experiences. *Illusions* are distorted perceptual disturbances.

Client orientation, consciousness, memory, and intelligence are cognitive functions evaluated during a mental status exam. Intellectual and memory assessments involve only surface evaluations during a mental status exam; more formalized assessments should follow if potential problems are identified. Interviewers should take care to avoid cultural biases when making such assessments.

Reliability, judgment, and insight are higher-level interpersonal/cognitive functions evaluated in the mental status exam. *Reliability* refers to the degree to which a client's reports about self and situation are believable and accurate. *Judgment* refers to the presence or absence of impulsive activities and poor decision making. *Insight* refers to the degree to which a client is aware of the emotional or psychological nature of his or her problems. Various procedures can be used to assess reliability, judgment, and insight.

Mental status examinations are usually administered in cases in which psychopathology is suspected. If clients are getting help on an outpatient basis for problems associated with daily living, mental status evaluation is less important. As in all evaluation procedures, client cultural background should be considered and integrated into any evaluation reports.

## SUGGESTED READINGS AND RESOURCES

Folstein, M. E., Folstein, S. E., & McHugh, P. R. (1975). "Mini-mental state": A practical method for grading the cognitive state of patients for the clinician. *Journal of Psychiatric Research, 12,* 189–198. This article presents a quick method for evaluating client mental state. The mini-mental state is a popular technique in psychiatric and geriatric settings.

Morrison, J. (1994). *The first interview: A guide for clinicians* (vol. 2., revised for the *DSM-IV*). New York: Guilford Press. This text includes two chapters discussing the mental status exam.

It is especially helpful in giving guidance regarding potential diagnostic labels associated with specific mental status symptoms.

Othmer, E., & Othmer, S. C. (1994). *The clinical interview using* DSM-IV-*R* (vol. 1., Fundamentals). Washington, DC: American Psychiatric Press. Chapter 4 of this text, "Three Methods to Assess Mental Status," is strongly recommended.

Paniagua, F. A. (2001). *Diagnosis in a multicultural context.* Thousand Oaks, CA: Sage Publications.

Polanski, P. J., & Hinkle, J. S. (2000). The mental status examination: Its use by professional counselors. *Journal of Counseling and Development, 78,* 357–364. This brief article, published in a major counseling journal, illustrates the central place mental status examinations have taken with regard to client assessment in all mental health professions.

Robinson, D. J. (2001). *Brain calipers: Descriptive psychopathology and the psychiatric mental status examination* (2nd ed.). Port Huron, MI: Rapid Psychler Press. This book provides an overview of the mental status examination (MSE) with examples, sample questions, and discussions of the relevance of particular findings. It uses an entertaining approach complete with illustrations, humor, mnemonics, and summary diagrams. It also has a helpful chapter on the Mini-Mental-State exam.

Strub, R. L., & Black, W. (1999). *The mental status examination in neurology* (4th ed.). Philadelphia: F. A. Davis. This is a very popular and classic mental status examination training text for medical students. It provides excellent practical and sensitive methods for determining client mental status along with some norms for evaluating patient performance on specific cognitive tasks.

Zuckerman, E. L. (2000). *Clinician's thesaurus: The guidebook for writing psychological reports* (5th ed.). New York: Guilford Press. This guidebook has a practical section on conducting and writing up the mental status evaluation. It also includes reproducible forms for documenting client mental status.

# Chapter 9

# *SUICIDE ASSESSMENT*

*There was no answer. The door of the lighthouse was ajar. They pushed it open and walked into a shuttered twilight. Through an archway on the further side of the room they could see the bottom of the staircase that led up to the higher floors. Just under the crown of the arch dangled a pair of feet.*

—Aldous Huxley, *Brave New World*

*There are two basic, albeit contradictory, truths about suicide: (a) Suicide should never be committed when one is depressed (or disturbed or constricted); and (b) almost every suicide is committed for reasons that make sense to the person who does it.*

—E. S. Shneidman, "Aphorisms of Suicide and Some Implications for Psychotherapy"

---

### CHAPTER OBJECTIVES

Suicide is an issue most people do not like to talk or think about. For better or for worse, talking and thinking about suicide is an important part of professional interviewing. In this chapter, we outline and discuss practical suggestions for conducting a complete suicide assessment interview. After reading this chapter, you will know:

- The importance of examining your own personal and philosophical reactions to suicide.
- Suicide statistics and common suicide myths and realities.
- Risk factors associated with suicide and procedures for conducting a suicide risk assessment.
- How to conduct a thorough suicide assessment interview, including an evaluation of client depression, suicide ideation, suicide plans, client self-control, and suicide intent.
- Methods for crisis intervention with suicidal clients, including empathic and relationship strategies with suicidal clients, identifying alternatives to suicide, separating the emotional pain from the self, establishing a suicide prevention contract, becoming directive, and making decisions about hospitalization and referral.
- Essential professional methods for working with suicidal clients, including self-reflection, consultation, documentation, and dealing with completed suicides.

---

Working with suicidal or homicidal clients constitutes one of the most stressful tasks mental health professionals face (Kleepsies, 1993). It does not take much imagination to conjure up a small dose of this tension. Just think of the following succinct and tragic scenario: *Your new client tells you of his plans to kill himself . . . and during the subsequent week, he follows through with it.* This sequence of events can be devastating both personally and professionally, which is one reason most mental health professionals dread working with suicidal clients.

As you read this chapter and face the possibility of interviewing a suicidal client, you may need to work on both your attitude and your anxiety (Herron, Ticehurst, Appleby, Perry, & Cordingley, 2001), because health professionals without suicide prevention experience sometimes hold negative attitudes toward suicidal individuals. It is simply impossible to ensure you will never interview a suicidal person. In fact, trying to do so would probably be unethical. Sometimes, clients do not even realize the depth of their suicidal impulses until they are sitting in the room talking with you.

When mental health professionals discover a client is a threat to self or someone else, the law is clear: Confidentiality must be broken. Our professional mandate is to side with life. When clients report suicidal or homicidal plans to mental health professionals, the professionals become legally responsible for initiating a series of communications to protect clients and/or potential victims (Costa & Altekruse, 1994; *Tarasoff v. Regents of the University of California,* 1974). Obviously, having responsibility for someone else's lethal impulses is both frightening and stressful.

Because it is not possible to know in advance whether a given client may be suicidal, even beginning students should prepare for the possibility of being face-to-face with a distressed suicidal client or an angry homicidal client (J. Sommers-Flanagan & Sommers-Flanagan, 1995a). Preparation for managing such clients should be a basic component of every human service training program (Bongar & Harmatz, 1989; Isaacs, 1997). In this chapter, we explore professional and personal issues you may grapple with when working with suicidal clients. We outline specific, state-of-the-art approaches to interviewing and evaluating suicidal clients that all prospective therapists should master.

## PERSONAL REACTIONS TO SUICIDE

Suicide as a concept and as an act evokes very strong feelings in many people. Even when it occurs from a distance, as in the much-publicized suicides of Vince Foster, Marilyn Monroe, and Kurt Cobain, people are affected so profoundly that suicide rates across the country or throughout the world usually increase (Knickmeyer, 1996; Mersky, 1996). Similarly, Dr. Kevorkian and his stance and actions in favor of assisted suicide have provoked philosophical and moral controversy throughout the United States. As you read this chapter and begin practicing the interview strategies we suggest, you may find some of your emotional buttons being pushed. This is especially likely if you have had someone close to you attempt or complete suicide, or if you, like many people, have contemplated suicide yourself at some point in your life. We recommend that you read this chapter with an awareness of your emotional reactions and that you discuss these reactions with colleagues and instructors. At the end of the chapter, we turn again to a discussion of suicide and its emotional ramifications for the interviewer.

## SUICIDE STATISTICS

The Centers for Disease Control reported that 30,810 Americans committed suicide in 1991. Each year since then, this number has changed only slightly, with a high of 31,284 completed suicides reported in 1995 and a low of 29,199 in 1999 (R. Anderson, 2001). However, because the U.S. population progressively increased from 1991 to 1999 (the last year reported at the time of this publication), suicide rates have fallen significantly. In 1991, the average suicide rate was 12.2 deaths per 100,000 people as compared to 11.91 deaths per 100,000 people in 1995 and under 10.0 deaths per 100,000 people in 1999. Overall, suicide is the 11th leading cause of death in the United States (it was the 9th leading cause of death in 1995, the latest figures available when the 2nd edition of this text went to press).

Though completed suicides are rare and difficult to predict, efforts to assess suicide risk during clinical interviews are justifiable on many grounds. First, suicide occurs much more frequently in a clinical population than in the general population (e.g., clients with clinical depression, panic disorder, alcoholism, and schizophrenia are at greater risk; Moscicki, 1997; Rossau & Mortensen, 1997). Second, suicide attempts occur about 20 times more frequently than completed suicides (about 1,900 adults attempt suicide in the United States each day; R. Anderson, Kochanek, & Murphy, 1997). The clinical interviewer's task is to try to reduce the incidence not only of completed suicides, but also of suicide attempts (especially severe suicide attempts, which seem to be associated with many of the same factors as completed suicides; Beautrais, 2001). Finally, clinically, ethically, and legally speaking, it is better to err in assuming a client may be suicidal and proceed with a thorough assessment than to err by assuming a suicidal client is not suicidal.

Despite the difficulty of suicide prediction, there exists an ethical and legal mandate for mental health professionals to conduct thorough suicide risk assessments with potentially suicidal clients (Ellison, 2001; Simon, 2000). Furthermore, accurate assessment constitutes one of the first steps in suicide prevention. Unless efforts are made to predict suicide, there will be less opportunity to prevent suicide attempts.

## CONSIDERING SUICIDE MYTHS

There are many unfounded myths about suicide. Perhaps the most dangerous myth is the belief that asking a person about suicide may cause that person to commit suicide. Pipes and Davenport (1999) offer the following reassurance:

> You can take solace in the fact that there is, as far as we know, consensus among experienced therapists that asking about suicide does not cause suicide. It is entirely possible that by not asking a client about suicidal thoughts you will lose an opportunity to help prevent suicide. (p. 113)

Therefore, if you have reason to believe your client might be thinking about suicide, the general rule for mental health professionals is to go ahead and inquire.

Before reading more about suicide myths, stop and think of what you believe about this topic and consider the sources of those beliefs. If someone threatens to commit suicide using an obviously nonlethal method (e.g., swallowing six aspirin), is he or she just playing games? Is suicide ultimately a manipulative expression of anger? Are women more likely to commit suicide using pills or poisons rather than firearms? What group constitutes the highest risk: the elderly, a particular ethnic or religious group, or teens?

---

**Putting It in Practice 9.1**

## A Suicide Quiz

Take the following true-false quiz to test your knowledge about suicide. Answers and explanations are in Putting It in Practice 9.5.

_____  1. About 25% to 50% of people who kill themselves have previously attempted to do so.

_____  2. People who talk about suicide won't commit suicide.

_____  3. Suicide happens without warning.

_____  4. If a parent of a child under five years of age commits suicide, the surviving child is many more times likely to grow up and commit suicide than a child who did not have that experience.

_____  5. Suicide attempters are more likely than other psychiatric patients to use substances in the 24 hours before admission to a hospital.

_____  6. Patients under a doctor's care are not at risk of suicide.

_____  7. Life stress factors are good predictors of suicide.

_____  8. More men commit suicide than women.

_____  9. In the United States, suicide is more prominent among Protestants than Catholics.

_____  10. A person who is very ill, perhaps even terminally ill, is not likely to commit suicide.

_____  11. When a suicidal patient begins to improve, it's usually a sign that the danger is over.

_____  12. A great deal of regional variation in suicide can be accounted for by weather variables such as temperature and precipitation.

_____  13. Improved standard of living is associated with higher rates of suicide and lower rates of homicide.

_____  14. The appearance of Halley's comet is associated with historical increases in the number of suicides.

_____  15. The most common means of suicide among women is firearms.

---

If you haven't yet done so, complete the suicide quiz as another means of exploring your beliefs in suicide myths (see Putting It in Practice 9.1).

Many misconceptions and fears are associated with suicide. Rather than taking a negative approach of systematically listing and dispelling every suicide myth in existence (and there are many), the next section focuses on suicide risk factors identified through scientific research.

## SUICIDE RISK FACTORS

Many specific risk factors are associated with suicide, but there is no single outstanding predictor of suicidal behavior. As Litman (1995) states:

At present it is impossible to predict accurately any person's suicide. Sophisticated statistical models . . . and experienced clinical judgments are equally unsuccessful. When I am asked why one depressed and suicidal patient commits suicide while nine other equally depressed and equally suicidal patients do not, I answer, "I don't know." (p. 135)

As you read about suicide risk factors, keep in mind that *an absence of these factors in an individual client is no guarantee that he or she is safe from suicidal impulses.* As a rule, in conducting suicide assessments, stay attuned to suicide possibilities, no matter how remote they seem. Closely observing for the following major suicide risk factors may alert you to suicide warning signs when particular clients have not directly talked about suicidal urges.

## Depression

The relationship between depression and suicidal behavior is well documented (Coppen, 1994; Roy, 1989). Some experts believe that depression before suicide is probably universal (C. Silverman, 1968). Support for this belief includes a study by Westefeld and Furr (1987) wherein every college student in their survey sample who had attempted suicide reported experiencing at least some depressive symptoms. This close association has led some writers and researchers to label depression a lethal disease (Coppen, 1994).

Suicide risk in depressed people is much greater than the risk in the general population. It has been estimated that 5% to 10% of all clinically depressed individuals will commit suicide (Litman, 1995). More specifically, suicidality among depressed people appears directly associated with severity of depression, with suicide prevalence among more mildly depressed inpatient/outpatient populations only around 2% (Bostwick & Pankratz, 2000).

Although not all depressed people are suicidal, the presence of depression is probably one of the best general suicide predictors; it is also a predictor that can be reliably evaluated in a clinical interview (Hamilton, 1967). Interviewing strategies for assessing depression are directly addressed later in this chapter.

Research has identified six variables frequently associated with suicidal behavior among depressed clients (Fawcett et al., 1990):

1. Severe psychic anxiety (general thoughts and feelings of anxiety).
2. Panic attacks (specific bouts of anxiety, including physical symptoms of panic).
3. Anhedonia (loss of pleasure when engaging in usually pleasurable activities).
4. Alcohol abuse (increased alcohol consumption during the depressive episode).
5. Decreased ability to concentrate (high distractibility).
6. Global insomnia (difficulty falling asleep, intermittent awakening, and early morning awakening).

Similarly, in a recent study of 100 patients who made severe suicide attempts, the best predictors included: (a) severe anxiety; (b) panic attacks; (c) depressed mood; (d) diagnosis of depression; (e) recent loss of an interpersonal relationship; (f) recent alcohol or substance abuse coupled with feelings of hopelessness, helplessness, worthlessness; (g) anhedonia; (h) inability to maintain employment; and (i) recent onset of impulsive behavior (R. Hall, Platt, & Hall, 1999). In this study, the preceding variables (notably consistent with the Fawcett et al., 1990, list) were better predictors than the existence of a specific suicide plan or suicide note.

Overall, general and severe distress—referred to by some as *psychic pain* (Shneidman, 1996) and often described as depression—is a very significant predictor of suicide. Additionally, specific negative cognitive appraisal of a person's life, such as feelings of *hopelessness* and *helplessness,* are important predictors of suicide among both depressed and nondepressed clients (Beck, Brown, & Steer, 1989).

## Age

Suicide rates vary among different age groups. Based on statistics released by the Centers for Disease Control (R. Anderson et al., 1997), suicide is most likely to occur among individuals 70 years and older. There is also a slight increase in suicide rates among young adults, ages 20 to 24. In contrast, suicide is unusual among 10- to 14-year-olds and rare in children under 10. Generally, age by itself is a fairly poor suicide predictor. However, several age groups are traditionally seen as having an increased risk of suicide. These groups include adolescents, college students, and the elderly.

Among adolescents 15 to 19 years old, suicide rates have increased dramatically (200% to 300%) over the past several decades. Essentially, this increased risk has brought the likelihood of adolescent suicide up from far less than the national average to near the national average (Berman & Jobes, 1996); suicide ranks as the third leading cause of death among 15- to 24-year-olds, just behind "accidents and adverse events" and "homicide and legal intervention" (R. Anderson, 2001, p. 26). In addition, it is likely that many lethal accidents may actually be suicides concealed by friends, relatives, and attending physicians because of the stigma associated with suicide.

Suicide rates among college students are approximately 50% higher than the general population (McIntosh, 1991). Suicide risk among college students is linked to alcohol use, depression, and academic or relationship problems. Several theorists speculate that college students have higher suicide rates because they're trying to escape from a difficult, pressure-filled situation (Dean, Range, & Goggin, 1996).

As an age group, older Americans constitute the highest suicide risk in the United States. Overall, elderly Americans tend to use lethal weapons more frequently and complete suicides more frequently than the young. They also communicate their suicidal intent less often. Generally, suicide risk rises after age 45 for men and after age 55 for women (Florio et al., 1997). However, among American Indians and Alaskan natives, suicide rates decrease with age.

## Sex

Statistics on suicide generally indicate that three times more women than men attempt suicide, but men actually complete suicide four times more frequently than women (R. Anderson et al., 1997). In later life, the disparity of male/female rates becomes even more marked.

An explanation often given for this disparity is that men usually choose more lethal methods, such as guns; and women choose less lethal methods, such as poison or pills. Approximately 73% of males and 31% of females choose firearms to kill themselves, making firearms the most commonly chosen method for committing suicide by both sexes. Obviously, firearm lethality is closely associated with suicide completion, which partly accounts for the greater ratio of completions to attempts among males (Evans & Farberow, 1988; Moscicki, 1997). Overall, males in general and older White males in particular are at significantly greater risk for completed suicide than females (R. Anderson, 2001).

## Race and Ethnic Background

Whites are significantly more likely to complete suicide than African Americans and Hispanics. Only among White males does the suicide rate increase throughout the life cycle.

Suicide rates among American Indians and Alaskan Natives who reside on or near reservations were systematically studied by the Centers for Disease Control from 1979 to 1992. Results of this study were reported in the *Violence Surveillance Summary Series* (Kachur, Potter, James, & Powell, 1995). During this 14-year period, American Indians and Alaskan Natives committed suicide at a rate approximately 1.5 times more often than the general U.S. population. Overall, the highest suicide rates were reported among Natives living in the Southwestern United States, northern Rocky Mountain and Plains states, and Alaska. It was also noted that patterns and rates of suicide varied widely among geographic regions and that age distribution of suicide rates among Indians and Alaskan Natives were quite different from the general U.S. population (i.e., among these populations, there are higher rates among young adults and lower rates among the elderly).

Suicide rates among African Americans have traditionally been only about 60% to 70% of rates among Whites. Rates are especially low among African American women (R. Anderson, 2001; J. Gibbs, 1997). These significant differences in suicidal behaviors among cultural groups suggest that different assessment approaches should be used depending on the cultural/ethnic group with whom you are working (see Individual and Cultural Highlight 9.1).

## Religion

Among the major religious groups in the United States, rates for Catholics have historically been slightly lower than the rates for Protestants and Jews. However, it appears

---

**INDIVIDUAL AND CULTURAL HIGHLIGHT 9.1**

### Interviewing Clients from Different Cultural Groups about Suicide

When working with potentially suicidal clients from different cultural groups, it's important to be aware of the fact that some general risk factors and interviewing strategies do not apply. A few of the differences to think about and consider integrating into your suicide assessment procedures follow:

- Among American Indian populations, generally, suicide risk does not increase with age; instead, suicide risk is highest among adolescents and young adults.
- Minority clients often are less likely than White clients to disclose suicidal ideation; this means you may need to rely more heavily on suicide risk factor assessment.
- African Americans are more likely to cite moral objections to suicide and specific reasons for living than White clients; this may be one reason that African Americans are less likely to commit suicide than White clients.
- In one research study contrasting Whites and African Americans, Whites tended to have a wide range of different suicide predictors, while for African Americans, only "use of mental health services" was identified as a useful risk factor.

that rather than religious denomination, degree of religious affiliation or degree of or-thodoxy is a more decisive factor in determining an individual's risk (Neeleman, Wes-sely, & Lewis, 1998; Resnik, 1980); more extensive religious affiliation seems to be as-sociated with lower suicide rates, although there are certainly many exceptions to this rule. Overall, there are no consistent data available that identify religion as a major vari-able in predicting an individual's suicide potential (Lester, 1996), although some re-searchers have speculated that increased suicide rates among our nation's White and African American youth may be associated with "rapid secularization of the young in the U.S." (Neeleman et al., 1998, p. 12).

## Marital Status

Divorced, widowed, and separated people are in a higher risk category for suicide (R. Anderson et al., 1997; M. T. Lambert & Fowler, 1997). Single, never-married indi-viduals have a suicide rate nearly double the rate of married individuals. Among di-vorced people, men in general and White men in particular have higher suicide rates than women. Marriage, especially when reinforced by children, appears to act as a buffer against suicide. However, as noted previously, suicide rates climb as people age, and this is true even of married people. Being unmarried may compound the suicide po-tential of single males over 70 years old, contributing to the fact that they have the high-est per capita suicide rate of any group. Interestingly, it appears that widowhood is not associated with an increase in suicide rates among women (Brockington, 2001).

## Employment Status

Unemployed and retired individuals are at a higher risk for suicide (Kposowa, 2001). Loss of employment can produce emotional distress for people of any age, sex, or eth-nic background; emotional distress as a contributor to suicidal behavior has been closely linked to substance abuse and depression (Overholser, Freiheit, & DiFilippo, 1997). Individuals who have retired sometimes report experiencing a loss of personal identity, meaningfulness, and self-esteem, which may be related to the increase in sui-cide after age 60.

## Socioeconomic Status

Higher suicide rates exist at both socioeconomic extremes, with lower rates for mem-bers of the middle class. Historically, poverty or economic disadvantage has sometimes been associated with higher suicide rates (Winslow, 1895); however, currently, lower economic status is associated with higher rates of death by homicide, and higher eco-nomic status is more often associated with suicide. It appears that when individuals of higher economic status commit suicide, they often are also suffering from severe psy-chiatric disorders (Agerbo, Mortensen, Eriksson, Qin, & Westergaard-Nielsen, 2001; Timonen et al., 2001).

## Physical Health

The majority of research on suicide rates among hospital patients has focused on psy-chiatric patients; however, suicide occurs among patients in medical and surgical sec-tions of hospitals as well. Researchers have linked the following factors to increased risk: frequent major surgery, depression related to chronic pain and altered body functions, fears of death and suffering, incapacitation, stroke, rheumatoid arthritis, and loss of social support. Hemodialysis and HIV patients have been identified as special risk groups; but overall, severity of physical illness, physical pain, and prognoses seem most likely to contribute to suicidal behavior, regardless of specific diagnosis (Bellini & Bruschi, 1996). Similar to previously hospitalized psychiatric patients, medical patients also exhibit higher suicidal behavior shortly after hospital discharge (McKenzie & Wurr, 2001).

One problem with studying the relationship between physical illness and suicide is the overlap between depressive symptoms and physical symptoms. Research by J. Brown, Henteleff, Barakat, and Rowe (1986) indicates that suicidal thoughts and the desire for death are linked exclusively to depressive symptoms. These authors suggest that physicians may fail to recognize and treat the depression, which points again to the importance of the depression factor in suicide. Additional research suggests that physical infirmity in itself may or may not present a higher risk for suicide, but that social isolation and depression associated with physical illness significantly increase suicide risk (Kishi, Robinson, & Kosier, 2001).

## Social and Personal Factors

The role of social and personal resources in suicide potential should not be underestimated. Such factors include: (a) food, shelter, clothing, and transportation; (b) adequate health care; (c) physical and mental strength; (d) productive and meaningful activities to pursue; and (e) significant and supportive relationships with others. The more of these basic resources available to the individual, the lower the suicide risk (M. T. Lambert & Fowler, 1997).

Living alone generally increases suicide risk. However, feelings of isolation and loneliness can be severe even for a person who lives with a group, and a person living alone may have a rewarding and satisfying support system available. The *feeling* of being isolated and socially detached is more important than the person's living situation, but obviously, both should be evaluated during a suicide assessment procedure.

Individuals who have suffered a recent, significant loss should be considered higher suicide risks (R. Hall et al., 1999). Such losses may take many forms, including (a) job loss, (b) status loss, (c) loss of a loved one, and (d) loss of physical health or physical mobility. Even the loss of a pet can increase risk among certain individuals.

## Substance Abuse

Research is unequivocal in placing alcoholics and other substance abusers in a high-risk category (Fawcett et al., 1990; R. Hall et al., 1999; G. Murphy & Wetzel, 1990; Ohberg, Vuori, Ojanpera, & Loenngvist, 1996). The problems of suicide and substance abuse are closely linked. Abuse of alcohol and other substances places individuals at risk for suicide, especially if such abuse is associated with depression, social isolation, and other suicide risk factors.

One way alcohol and drug use increases suicide risk is by decreasing inhibition. People act more impulsively when in chemically altered states and suicide is usually considered an impulsive act. No matter how much planning has preceded a suicide act, at the moment the pills are taken, the trigger is pulled, or the wrist is slit, most theorists believe that, in most cases, some form of disinhibition has occurred (Shneidman, 1996). Alcohol and drug use may give people who are afraid to commit suicide the courage (or foolhardiness) required to carry out the plan.

## Mental Disorders and Psychiatric Treatment

Most suicides are associated with a relatively small number of mental disorders or conditions. Patients with affective disorders (depression and bipolar disorder) and schizophrenia are at higher risk for suicide (Rossau & Mortensen, 1997; Roy, 1989). Thought disorders such as a paranoid delusional system or auditory hallucinations that tell a person to kill himself or herself or a loved one, especially when combined with depressed mood, put the sufferer at high risk (Resnik, 1980). Individuals with psychotic depressive reactions are at especially high risk for suicide.

On the other hand, completed suicides are less often associated with histrionic or antisocial personality types and various paraphilias, although suicide attempts in these groups are not uncommon (Robins, 1985). Even when a suicidal gesture appears manipulative, as is frequently found with personality-disordered individuals, the gesture should be taken seriously. Unfortunately, feigned suicide attempts may have fatal consequences.

For individuals admitted to hospitals because of a mental disorder, the period immediately following discharge carries increased risk for suicide. This is particularly true of individuals who also:

- Have attempted suicide previously.
- Suffer from a chronic mental disorder.
- Were admitted to the hospital recently.
- Live alone.
- Are unemployed.
- Are unmarried.
- Are vulnerable to depression. (Roy, 1989)

Furthermore, in a large-scale study of schizophrenic patients, suicide risk was identified as particularly high in the first five days after discharge (Rossau & Mortensen, 1997).

There have been some reports in the literature that administration of some serotonin-specific reuptake inhibitors (SSRIs; e.g., Prozac, Zoloft) to nonsuicidal adults may cause disinhibition and agitation leading to increased suicidality (Healy, 2000; King et al., 1991; Teicher, Glod, & Cole, 1990). Although this finding is preliminary, psychiatric practice parameters recommend careful monitoring of patients taking SSRIs to ensure that disinhibition, agitation, or increased suicidal impulses are identified and documented when present (*Journal for the American Academy of Child and Adolescent Psychiatry*, 2001).

## Sexual Orientation

There has been some controversy over whether gay and lesbian youth are at greater risk for suicide than heterosexual youth (Gibson, 1994; Muehrer, 1995). Nonetheless, overall, the research suggests that when young clients are struggling with sexual identity issues, they should be considered a higher than average suicide risk (McDaniel, Purcell, & D'Augelli, 2001; Russell & Joyner, 2001). Among gay and lesbian youth, as well as among the general population, suicide risk greatly increases with substance abuse and dependence and psychopathology (McDaniel et al., 2001).

## Trauma and Abuse History

Recent research indicates a strong link between child sexual abuse and client trauma with suicidality. Specifically, in a file review of 200 outpatients, child sexual abuse was a better predictor of suicidality than depression (Read, Agar, Barker-Collo, Davies, & Moskowitz, 2001). Similarly, data from the National Comorbidity Survey ($N = 5,877$) showed that women who were sexually abused as children were 2 to 4 times more likely to attempt suicide, and sexually abused men were 4 to 11 times more likely to attempt suicide (Molnar, Berkman, & Buka, 2001). Current physical or sexual abuse also can contribute to suicidal impulses (Thompson et al., 1999).

## Integrating Risk Factors

Risk factors do not add up neatly. You cannot automatically rest assured when a client has a low total number of risk factors nor routinely hospitalize clients with a high total number of risk factors. As described by numerous researchers, the prototypical suicide-prone individual is a depressed, alcohol abusing, socially isolated, elderly White male with physical health problems and access to firearms (Florio et al., 1997; M. T. Lambert & Fowler, 1997). However, in real life, prototypes don't usually exist, and, as discussed earlier, suicide prediction is never easy. Because of the large number of risk factors discussed, a comprehensive suicide assessment checklist is provided in Putting It in Practice 9.2.

## CONDUCTING A THOROUGH SUICIDE ASSESSMENT

Nearly all of us think about suicide at some point in our lives. For some, it is merely a fleeting thought countered by other thoughts about all the positive reasons for living, but for others, suicide is a very serious consideration. For a few, it becomes a preoccupation. In some cases, repeated suicide gestures are more cries for help or attention than a serious wish to die. In other cases, the opposite is true: Life has become so full of dissatisfaction, disappointment, or pain that death has become preferable. It is the mental health professional's responsibility to determine whether a given client is experiencing transient suicidal thoughts or severe suicidal preoccupations. Although a number of standardized assessment tools for measuring suicidality exist, the following discussion focuses on using a clinical interview for evaluating client suicide risk.

In addition to identifying relevant risk factors (as reviewed in the previous section), thorough suicide assessment interviews include detailed coverage of five major areas: (a) assessment of depression, (b) presence of suicidal thoughts, (c) exploration of suicide plans, (d) assessment of client self-control, and (e) a determination of whether the client *intends* to commit suicide.

## Assessing Client Depression

A complete suicide assessment interview includes a thorough depression assessment. Depression is both a significant suicide predictor and strongly associated with other suicide risk factors (e.g., substance abuse, poor health).

According to the *DSM-IV-TR,* there are two primary forms of depression:

- Major depression (a more acute and severe depression).
- Dysthymic disorder (a more chronic and usually milder form of depression).

=== **Putting It in Practice 9.2** ===

## Using a Comprehensive Checklist for a Thorough Suicide Assessment

After practicing and gaining familiarity with risk factors, the following checklist can be used in practice sessions and role plays to help you conduct a thorough suicide assessment in almost any circumstance. It is important to practice actually obtaining the information from different types of clients because the energy, setting, time allotted, and so forth, can make for interesting challenges when it comes to getting this information.

Either in pairs in class or with a willing friend or colleague, set up a suicide assessment role play. Using the following checklist, identify which risk factors fit your client. It might also be helpful to try role plays without the list in front of you to see how many you remember on your own.

**General Suicide Assessment Risk Factor Checklist**

_____ 1. The client is in a vulnerable group because of age/sex characteristics.

_____ 2. The client has made a previous suicide attempt.

_____ 3. The client is using alcohol/drugs excessively or abusively.

_____ 4. The client meets *DSM-IV* diagnostic criteria for a specific mental disorder.

_____ 5. The client is unemployed.

_____ 6. The client is unmarried, alone, or isolated.

_____ 7. The client is experiencing physical health problems.

_____ 8. The client recently experienced a significant personal loss (of ability, objects, or persons).

_____ 9. The client is a youth and is struggling with sexuality issues.

_____ 10. The client was a victim of childhood sexual abuse or is a current physical or sexual abuse victim.

_____ 11. The client meets diagnostic criteria for depression.

_____ 12. If depressed, the client also is experiencing one or more of the following symptoms:

Panic attacks

General psychic anxiety

Lack of interest or pleasure in usually pleasurable activities

Alcohol abuse increase during depressive episodes

Diminished concentration

Global insomnia

_____ 13. The client reports significant hopelessness, helplessness, or excessive guilt.

_____ 14. The client reports presence of suicidal thoughts.

*(continued)*

---

**Putting It in Practice 9.2 (continued)**

Note in your evaluation:

Frequency of thoughts (How often do these thoughts occur?)

Duration of thoughts (Once they begin, how long do the thoughts persist?)

Intensity of thoughts (On a scale of 1 to 10, how compelling are the thoughts?)

_____ 15. The client reports presence of a suicide plan.

_____ 16. The client reports a specific plan.

_____ 17. The client reports a lethal or highly lethal plan.

_____ 18. The client reports availability of the means to carry out the suicide plan.

_____ 19. The client does not have social support nearby.

_____ 20. The client reports little self-control.

_____ 21. The client has a history of impulsive behavior.

_____ 22. The client has a history of overcontrolled behavior or presents as emotionally constricted.

_____ 23. The client reports a moderate to high intent to kill self (or has made a previous lethal attempt).

_____ 24. The client was recently discharged from a psychiatric facility after apparent improvement.

_____ 25. The client was recently prescribed an SSRI and has associated disinhibition or agitation.

---

*Note.* Adapted from "Intake Interviewing with Suicidal Patients: A Systematic Approach," by J. Sommers-Flanagan and R. Sommers-Flanagan, 1995, *Professional Psychology: Research and Practice, 26,* 41–47. Adapted with permission of the authors.

---

To receive a diagnosis of major depression or dysthymic disorder, specific criteria must be met. For the purposes of our discussion here, we focus less on the specific diagnostic criteria and more on the general symptoms usually indicative of depression.

Overall, the *DSM* includes three major categories of depressive symptoms, plus one associated depressive symptom pertinent to our discussion:

- Mood-Related Symptoms
- Physical or Vegetative Symptoms
- Cognitive Symptoms
- Social/Interpersonal Symptoms

## Mood-Related Symptoms

Because depression is classified in *DSM-IV-TR* as a mood disorder, it makes perfect sense to begin a depression assessment by using mood questions derived from the mental status examination. For example, questions such as: "How have you been feeling lately?" or "Would you describe your mood for me?" constitute a good beginning. Listen for the client's quality of mood. Then, use a paraphrase to make sure you have heard the client correctly (e.g., "It sounds like you're feeling pretty sad and hopeless right now").

Clients won't be aware of the fact that in the *DSM-IV-TR*, a *depressed mood* is defined as: "A depressed mood most of the day, nearly every day, as indicated by either subjective report (e.g., feels sad or empty) or observation made by others (e.g., appears tearful). Note: In children and adolescents, can be irritable mood" (American Psychiatric Association, 2000, p. 327). Consequently, rather than reporting "sadness, emptiness, or irritability (in young clients)" your client may say something like "I've just been feeling really very shitty lately." If that's the case, respond initially using language similar to your client's (instead of the *DSM*'s) in your paraphrase. Later, you can begin using *DSM* diagnostic language in your interview.

After you obtain a sense of the *quality* of your client's mood, then you can move to assessing the *quantity* of his or her mood. It can be helpful to get a mood rating. For example:

> **Interviewer:** "You said you've been feeling really shitty. What I want to know next is how 'shitty' or how bad you're feeling right now, how you usually feel, and how bad you feel when you're at your very worst. So, on a scale of 1 to 10, with 1 being the worst you could possibly feel and with 10 being total and absolute perfect happiness, how would you rate how sad or how shitty you're feeling right now?"
>
> **Client:** "I don't know. I guess I'm at about a 3."
>
> **Interviewer:** "Okay, now how about recently, for the past two weeks or so, on that same scale, what's the very worst you've felt?"
>
> **Client:** "I think last weekend I was at about a 2. That was the worst I've ever felt."
>
> **Interviewer:** "That sounds pretty horrible. How about your normal mood, when you're not feeling down or depressed, what rating would you give your normal mood?"
>
> **Client:** "Usually I'm a pretty happy person. I think my normal mood is about a 6 or 7."

In this exchange, the interviewer has obtained valuable assessment information. Using a quantitative scale, she now has a rating of her client's subjective distress. Although this is not the level of statistical analysis we recommend for research reports or dissertation defenses, it is a very effective approach for quantifying your client's subjective distress.

According to the *DSM*, major depressive disorder in adults can be characterized by one of two primary mood symptoms. As noted, one of the mood symptoms is the existence of a sad or depressed mood. However, even if a sad or depressed mood is not present, adult clients may qualify for depression if they are experiencing the second mood symptom: a loss of interest or pleasure in usually pleasurable activities.

When clients, sometimes suddenly, no longer experience joy, interest, or pleasure, it is not surprising that life can begin to seem much less valuable. This mood symptom, also known as anhedonia, is frequently a specific depressive symptom that increases suicide potential. Consequently, suicide assessment interviewers should always check to see if clients are obtaining personal gratification from their usual social, recreational, sexual, or other usual pleasurable activities.

Lack of reactivity of mood is another mood-related symptom that may help distinguish between types of depression. Although this mood symptom is similar to anhedonia, it is slightly different and is usually evaluated via direct observation, rather than direct questioning. Specifically, when interviewing depressed clients, observe whether their mood seems to brighten when they discuss positive experiences. Alternatively, when you interject hope or other positive factors into a session, clients without a reactive mood do not smile or otherwise exhibit a brighter mood.

Guilt and hopelessness are also emotional states associated with depression. However, rather than discuss them here, we have included them in the section on cognitive symptoms, because these particular emotional states are often generated or moderated by specific and powerful cognitions (see later section).

### Physical or Vegetative Symptoms

Depressed clients frequently experience physical symptoms as a part of their depression. Psychiatrists often refer to these symptoms as vegetative or neurovegetative signs and consider them cardinal features of true biological depression (Morrison, 1993). Perhaps what is most fascinating about these physical signs/symptoms of depression is that most of them are bidirectional; in other words, clients may experience them on one end of a continuum or the other. Clients suffering from depression often report:

- Significant unintentional weight loss *or* weight gain.
- A decrease *or* increase in appetite nearly every day.
- Insomnia *or* hypersomnia nearly every day.
- Symptoms of agitation (excessive and unnecessary movement) *or* psychomotor retardation (less movement than usual).

The first three of these physical symptoms can usually be assessed by directly questioning clients about their weight loss/gain patterns, appetite, and sleep patterns. In contrast, although direct questioning about psychomotor agitation/retardation is also possible, as noted in the mental status examination chapter, this symptom is also evaluated via direct observation of client behavior.

Another important physical symptom of depression is fatigue. Depressed clients commonly experience diminished energy levels, sometimes staying in bed all or most of the day because of persistent fatigue. Again, this symptom is generally assessed via direct questioning, with a particular emphasis on whether client energy levels have changed from a previously higher level. On a related note, sexual disinterest, often considered a symptom of anhedonia, may be caused or exacerbated by client fatigue.

### Cognitive Symptoms

When clients are depressed, they frequently experience a wide range of negative cognitions. Although some theorists believe that client cognitions cause the depression, others emphasize that client thoughts are a by-product or secondary depressive feature. When it comes to accurately detecting depressive disorders, whether the cognitive features are primary or secondary in nature matters very little because everyone, including the compilers of the *DSM,* acknowledges that the presence of particular cognitive factors may signal depression.

The most common cognitive factors are worthlessness, guilt, and hopelessness. Worthlessness, or thoughts and feelings of inadequacy, should be evaluated directly. Some potentially useful questions include:

- How are you feeling about yourself?
- Tell me about a time recently when you were feeling particularly good about yourself.

- Lately, do you find yourself thinking a lot about your personal defects or deficiencies?

A key issue associated with cognitive features of depression is the concept of *preoccupation.* Depressed clients often become preoccupied or mentally consumed by negative thoughts. This is certainly true with regard to worthlessness, but is especially the case when it comes to guilt or remorse. Certain depressed clients have difficulty thinking of anything but whatever they feel guilty about. As an interviewer, you can almost observe the guilt process directly, as clients often look downward and seem stuck processing and reprocessing a past event where they disappointed themselves or a loved one.

"Normal" or transient sad feelings are unlikely to include extreme, persistent, or recurrent thoughts and feelings of worthlessness or guilt. In contrast, moderately or severely depressed clients may report they feel unworthy or burdened with guilt from some real, exaggerated, or imagined sin or transgression.

Depending on your affinity for numbers and your client's responsivity to the rating task (as previously described in the mood-related symptoms section), you may want to obtain additional ratings at some point in your depression assessment. One especially important cognitive symptom often linked with suicidality is hopelessness. You could repeat the rating task by asking:

"On that same scale from 1 to 10 that we talked about before, this time with 1 meaning you have no hope at all that your life will improve and 10 being you're totally full of hope that things in your life will improve and you'll start feeling better, what rating would you give?"

Getting a sense of your client's hopelessness is a good idea because believing the future is hopeless may be a more accurate indicator of suicide risk than overall level of depression (Beck et al., 1989). Suicide is less likely when a client believes there is hope for the future, and usually clients who express an interest in their personal short- and long-term life plans have a lower suicide risk than clients who indicate they have few interesting hopes, plans, or dreams.

Hopelessness may be expressed in a variety of statements, such as "I don't see how things will ever be any different" or "I've felt like this for as long as I can remember and I'll probably always feel this way." Conversely, the client's ability to project into the future and make constructive or pleasurable plans is an important gauge of hopefulness and is more likely in clients who are not severely depressed. Obviously, future-oriented questions are helpful when evaluating hopefulness.

- What plans do you have for tomorrow?
- What do you think you'll be doing five years from now?
- Do you think you'll start feeling better soon . . . or ever?

Another important feature associated with depressive thinking is helplessness. From the clients' perspective, helplessness may indicate a feeling or belief that they are incapable of making any changes necessary to feel better on their own. When they express helplessness, it may be an indirect request for help from the interviewer. They may believe that, though they are unable to effect change in their life, you may be able to do so.

Depressed clients also exhibit additional cognitive symptoms, including: (a) difficulty concentrating, (b) recurrent thoughts about death or suicide, (c) difficulty making decisions and/or problem solving, and (d) mental constriction (an inability to see alternative solutions).

### Social/Interpersonal Symptoms

The most common interpersonal manifestation of depression is withdrawal from friends, family, and usual social activities. Listen for signs of such emotional withdrawal because, at times, depressed persons are not fully aware of their isolation. If you have reason to believe you do not have the full picture, you may need to obtain information from others who know the client. Such informants might describe their depressed friends or family members as changed, distant, hard-to-reach, despondent, or exceptionally touchy or irritable.

## Exploring Suicidal Ideation

After you have evaluated client risk factors and depression and if you are concerned your client may be at risk for suicide, you should directly and calmly ask him or her about the presence or absence of suicidal thoughts. This may be difficult. Graduate interviewers often tell us that the most difficult areas to ask about are suicide and sex. Learning to ask difficult questions in a deliberate, compassionate, professional, and calm manner requires practice for most people (so go ahead and practice saying the words *sex* and *suicide* with your colleagues). It also may help to know that in a study by Hahn and Marks (1996), 97% of previously suicidal clients were either receptive or neutral about discussing previous suicide attempts with their interviewers during intake sessions.

One way to overcome the awkwardness of asking about suicidal thoughts is to develop a standard question using words you are comfortable with. We recommend a question that includes some kind of empathic paraphrase, such as "Well, Jane, you've really got a lot to deal with right now. And you don't have the energy you used to, and sometimes you feel pretty hopeless. Do you ever find yourself feeling suicidal?" A common fear is that asking directly about suicide will put ideas in the person's head. There is no clinical evidence to suggest this occurs (Pipes & Davenport, 1999). Instead, most clients are relieved to talk about their suicidal thoughts (Hahn & Marks, 1996). In addition, the invitation to share self-destructive thoughts reassures the client that you are comfortable with the subject, in control of the situation, and capable of dealing with the problem.

Most, but not all, suicidal clients readily admit self-destructive thoughts when asked about them. Some deny such thoughts, perhaps in an attempt to reaffirm their self-control. If denial occurs, do not just heave a sigh of relief and immediately drop the subject. Try to make it easier for the person to admit such thoughts. Wollersheim (1974) provides this example:

> Well, I asked this question since almost all people at one time or another during their lives have thought about suicide. There is nothing abnormal about the thought. In fact it is very normal when one feels so down in the dumps. The thought itself is not harmful. However, if we find ourselves thinking about suicide rather intently or frequently, it is a cue that all is not well, and we should start making some efforts to make life more satisfactory. (p. 223)

When a client admits to suicidal ideation, the onset, frequency, antecedents, intensity, and duration of suicidal thoughts should be explored. Exploring suicidal thoughts should always lead to evaluating whether your client has a suicide plan.

## Assessing Suicide Plans

Once rapport is established with an interviewer, most clients give at least some details of their suicide plans. It is useful to begin exploration of your client's plan with a paraphrase and a question, such as:

> "You've talked about how you sometimes think it would be better for everyone if you were dead. Have you planned how you would kill yourself if you decided to follow through on your thoughts?"

Many clients respond to questions about suicide plans with reassurance that indeed they're not really contemplating taking action on their suicidal thoughts. They may cite religion, fear, children, or other reasons for staying alive. Typically, they indicate "Oh yeah, I think about suicide sometimes, but I'd never do it." After hearing a client's reasons for living, you may be adequately reassured and decide you don't need to further assess his or her suicide plan. However, if a client identifies a potential suicide plan, further exploration of that plan is essential.

When exploring and evaluating a client's suicide plan, assess the following four areas (M. Miller, 1985): (a) *specificity* of the plan; (b) *lethality* of the method; (c) *availability* of the proposed method; and (d) *proximity* of social or helping resources. Notice that these four areas of inquiry can be easily recalled with the acronym SLAP.

### Specificity

*Specificity* refers to the details of a client's suicide plan. Has the person thought through the details necessary to complete a suicide? Ordinarily, the more specific the plan, the higher the suicide risk. Some clients clearly outline a suicide method. Others avoid the question, and still others state something like, "Oh, I think about how things might be easier if I were dead, but I don't really have a plan." At this point, it is up to your clinical judgment to determine how hard to push the client for the specifics of his or her plan. Again, we recommend following Wollersheim's (1974) advice in most cases by normalizing and making it easy for the client to answer in the affirmative, if such is the case:

> "You know, most people who have thought about suicide have at least had passing thoughts about how they might do it. What kinds of thoughts have you had about how you would commit suicide if you decided to do so?" (p. 223)

This way of inquiring accomplishes two important objectives. First, the statement reassures the client that it is not unusual to have thoughts about a suicide plan. Second, the question assumes the client has had thoughts about a plan and inquires about them.

### Lethality

*Lethality* refers to the speed with which enactment of a suicide plan could produce death. The greater the lethality, the higher the suicide risk. Lethality varies depending on the way a particular method is used. If you believe your client is a very high suicide risk, you should inquire not simply about your client's general method (e.g., firearms, toxic overdose, razor blade), but also about the way the method will be employed. For example, does your client plan to shoot himself or herself in the stomach, temple, or mouth? Does he or she plan to use aspirin or cyanide? Is the plan to slash his or her wrists or throat with a razor blade? In each of these examples, the latter alternative is, of course, more lethal.

*Availability*

*Availability* refers to how readily a client could implement a suicide plan. Are the means available for immediate implementation of the plan? If the client plans to overdose with a particular medication, check whether that medication is available. (Keep in mind this cheery thought: Most people keep more than enough substances in their home medicine cabinets to complete a suicide.) To overstate the obvious, if the client is considering committing suicide by driving a car off a cliff and has neither car nor cliff available, the immediate risk is lower than, for example, the person who plans to shoot himself or herself and has a loaded gun in the bedroom.

*Proximity*

*Proximity* refers to the proximity of social support. How nearby are helping resources? Are other individuals available who could intervene and rescue the client if an attempt is made? Does the client live with family or roommates? Does the client live alone with no friends or neighbors nearby? Is the client's day spent mostly alone or around people? Generally, the further a client is from helping resources, the greater the suicide risk.

If you are working on an ongoing basis with a client, check in periodically regarding his or her plan. Suicide plans can change; monitoring such changes keeps you up-to-date regarding suicide risk and client progress.

## Assessing Client Self-Control and Past or Familial Attempts

When assessing suicide risk, you should also evaluate the client's belief in his or her own self-control. Individuals who fear losing control and committing suicide are at high risk. Asking directly about the client's sense of self-control is important. You can ask: "Do you ever feel worried that you might lose control and try to kill yourself, even though you might not want to do it right now?" You can also inquire as to the client's general level of self-control and ask about recent changes in this area. If the client admits fearing a loss of control, suicide risk is increased. It may be necessary to consider hospitalization or other changes so that external control is available until the client feels more internal control.

Thoroughly explore client self-control. If a client has had suicidal thoughts in the past, ask what has kept him or her from losing control and committing suicide. This information may become a valuable therapeutic ally. What has worked in the past stands a chance of working again. For instance, you may find the client states something like the following:

**Client:** "Yes, I often fear losing control late at night."
**Interviewer:** "Sounds like night is the roughest time."
**Client:** "I hate midnight."
**Interviewer:** "So, late at night, especially around midnight, you're sometimes afraid you'll lose control and kill yourself. But, so far, something has kept you from doing it."
**Client:** "Yeah. I think of the way my kids would feel when they couldn't get me to wake up in the morning. I just start bawling my head off at the thought. It always keeps me from really doing it."

A brief verbal exchange, such as the previous, should never be considered sufficient to make a determination that a client is safe *nor* that the client needs hospitalization. However, strong mitigating factors, such as this client's love for her children, will work against a loss of self-control.

Determining if your client has a history of impulse-control problems can aid you in deciding whether he or she is likely to lose control and make a suicide attempt. For instance, if the client has a tendency toward explosive verbal outbursts or physical altercations, it may indicate a problem with impulse control and increased suicide risk. In addition, clients who are emotionally overcontrolled most of the time but who, on rare occasions, *completely* lose control may be at greater risk. Because making this kind of judgment call is very stressful, when you have a client who reports fear of losing control, you should seek immediate supervision or consultation.

Finally, always ask if the client has threatened or attempted suicide in the past, or if close friends or family members have attempted or committed suicide. Nearly three-fourths of people who ultimately commit suicide have a history of previous attempts (Resnik, 1980); and the greater the lethality of previous attempts, the higher the present risk. Additionally, for complex reasons, past suicide attempts or completions among a client's friends or family members are associated with increased loss of control and suicidal behavior.

## Assessing Suicidal Intent

Another component of suicide risk assessment involves determining clients' suicidal intent. Intent to commit suicide may be established through self-report, peer or family report, or behavioral observation. Essentially, assessing intent involves determining whether clients are talking or acting in ways suggesting they intend to kill themselves.

Some clients are persistent and creative in their efforts to kill themselves. We know of clients who have swallowed needles, razor blades, and virtually any dangerous substance they could locate (e.g., Drano and Campho Phenique). Some have run nude onto busy freeways or thrown themselves into large bodies of water in efforts to drown themselves. Others manage to hang themselves with pillowcases or slash their wrists with the top of soda bottles or cans. These clients may or may not have had carefully developed plans for how they were going to kill themselves; instead, they were ready to take advantage of any means through which they could end their lives. It is an understatement to suggest that such clients *intend* to kill themselves; they are desperately seeking self-destruction.

Intent can be rated as absent, low, moderate, or high. However, unlike the subjective rating of mood or hopelessness discussed earlier, it is usually not helpful to ask clients to rate their intent. If their intent is high, they are probably not going to admit it, as they are likely aware you would hospitalize them to keep them alive. Instead, intent must be indirectly assessed, or inferred, based on client plan, past suicide attempts, and overall demeanor. The greater the intent, the greater the suicide risk (see Table 9.1 for a sum-

**Table 9.1.   Assessing Suicide Intent**

*Nonexistent:* No suicidal ideation or plans exist.

*Mild:* Suicidal ideation but no specific or concrete plans exist. Few risk factors are present.

*Moderate:* Suicidal ideation and a general plan exist. Self-control is intact; client knows several "reasons to live," and client does not "intend" to kill self. Some risk factors are present.

*Severe:* Suicide ideation is frequent and intense. Plan is specific and lethal, means are available, and nearby helping resources are few. Self-control is questionable, but the client does not really "want" to kill self; intent appears low. Many risk factors may be present.

*Extreme:* Same description as Severe, except that client expresses a clear intent to kill self as soon as the opportunity presents itself. Many risk factors are usually present.

mary of suicide intent levels and Putting It in Practice 9.2 for a comprehensive suicide assessment checklist).

## CRISIS INTERVENTION WITH SUICIDAL CLIENTS

The following guidelines, although not foolproof, provide basic ideas about how to handle yourself and your client during a suicide crisis. They are consistent with Shneidman's (1996) advice for therapists working with suicidal clients: "Reduce the pain; remove the blinders; lighten the pressure—all three, even just a little bit" (p. 139).

### Listening and Being Empathic

The first rule of working therapeutically with suicidal clients is to listen closely to their thoughts and feelings. Often, suicidal clients feel isolated, and, therefore, it is imperative to establish an empathic connection with them. They may have never openly discussed their depressive or suicidal thoughts and feelings with another person. Consequently, let them know you truly hear how miserable and desperate they are feeling (Shneidman, 1980, 1996).

Obviously, when clients begin discussing suicide, expressions of shock or surprise should be avoided. This is easier said than done, but you must deal with clients' thoughts and feelings in a matter-of-fact manner; this suggests to clients that you have dealt with such issues previously, and reassures them that their experiences are not completely unusual. In some situations, you may want to be openly reassuring and supportive, even acknowledging that suicidal urges are sometimes a natural response, by saying something like the following:

> "You've told me about some of the difficult experiences you've had recently-losing your wife, your job, and your good health. It's not unusual for you to consider killing yourself. Many people you're your situation might think about whether life is still worth living."

### Establishing a Therapeutic Relationship

As you make efforts to empathize with your client, you also should work on establishing a therapeutic relationship. As a professional, it's your job to side with life. Continue to be empathic, but also let your client know your professional stance:

> "Right now it probably doesn't feel like your life is worth much, but I want to let you know that things can, and probably will, get much better for you. It's a fact that just about everyone who gets depressed also gets over it and then feels much better. And you can accelerate the 'getting better' process by involving yourself in therapy."

Research indicates that people who are depressed or in a mood characterized by psychological or emotional discomfort have difficulty remembering positive events or emotions (Blaney, 1986; E. Clark & Teasdale, 1982; Eich, 1989). You can help clients focus on positive events and past positive emotional experiences, but also remain empathic with the fact that it is not easy for most depressed and suicidal clients to recall anything positive.

On the other hand, too often interviewers become uniformly negative and problem-focused when working with depressed and suicidal clients (J. Sommers-Flanagan, Rothman, & Schwenkler, 2000). This makes it all the more important for interviewers to weave comments about current resources, strengths, and reasons for living into interviews with suicidal clients. If nothing else, you will be able to further assess your client's level of depression and suicidality by observing his or her responses to your efforts to integrate positive content into the interview.

Finally, suicidal clients may find it difficult to attend to what you are saying. Speak slowly and clearly, occasionally repeating key messages, when working with clients who are depressed and suicidal.

## Identifying Alternatives to Suicide

The primary thought disorder in suicide is that of a pathological narrowing of the mind's focus, called constriction, which takes the form of seeing only two choices; either something painfully unsatisfactory or cessation of life. (Shneidman, 1984, pp. 320–321)

Suicide is, in fact, a possible alternative to life. It is fruitless to debate with clients about whether suicide is a philosophically acceptable course of action. (We've tried that ourselves.) Instead of arguing with clients about whether they should commit suicide, help them identify options *in addition to* suicide.

Encourage suicidal clients to examine the question "Why commit suicide now?" Talk about the fact that there's no rush. An individual can always commit suicide later, after other life options have been explored. In fact, because suicide is a permanent choice, all other options should be explored first. The key here is that if you get your clients reinvolved with life, they often reap natural rewards and gratifications that eventually reduce the desire to commit suicide.

Usually, suicidal clients suffer from mental constriction; they are unable to identify options to suicide. As Shneidman (1980, p. 310) suggests, help your clients "widen" their view of life options. They need to take off their mental blinders and see that suicide is not the only alternative.

Shneidman (1980) writes of a case in which he goes through a list of alternatives with a pregnant suicidal teenager in an effort to remove her mental blinders. This is a practical and concrete approach that can be used with clients to enhance the working relationship and at the same time open their minds to constructive alternatives. Get out a pencil and paper to brainstorm alternative actions with regard to a specific life dilemma. Encourage clients to contribute to the list, but have plenty of your own to offer. After all alternatives are listed, ask your clients to rank the alternatives in order of preference. There is always the possibility that clients will decide suicide is the best choice (at which point you have obtained very important assessment information). On the other hand, it is surprising how often suicidal clients discover other, more preferable, options through Shneidman's method.

## Separating the Psychic Pain from the Self

Rosenberg (1999, 2000) described a helpful cognitive reframe intervention for use with suicidal clients. Specifically, she states: "The therapist can help the client understand that what she or he really desires is to eradicate the feelings of intolerable pain rather than to eradicate the self" (p. 86). This technique can help suicidal clients because it provides much needed empathy for the clients' psychic pain, while at the same time helping them see that they wish for the pain to stop existing, not for the self to stop existing.

Similarly, Rosenberg (1999) recommends that therapists help clients reframe what is usually meant by the phrase "feeling suicidal." She notes that clients benefit from seeing their suicidal thoughts and impulses as a communication about their depth of feeling, rather than an "actual *intent to take action*" (p. 86). Once again, this approach to intervening with suicidal clients can decrease clients' needs to act, partly because of the elegant cognitive reframe and partly because of the empathic message by the therapist.

## Establishing Suicide-Prevention Contracts

Many writers and clinicians recommend establishing suicide-prevention contracts (Davidson, Wagner, & Range, 1995; Drye, Goulding, & Goulding, 1973). Although most clinicians we know use verbal suicide-prevention contracts, contracts may be formally written as well. The typical contract is a verbal agreement between client and therapist (or interviewer), sometimes sealed with a handshake. The agreement often sounds something like this:

**Interviewer:** "You've said that sometimes you feel an urge to kill yourself. The possibility of your taking your own life during an especially bad moment concerns me. Can you promise me that if the urge to kill yourself wells up inside you, and you're afraid you're going to lose control, you'll call me first? We can talk things over and hopefully you'll be able to regain control."
**Client:** "Okay. Yeah, I can call you if I start to feel out of control."
**Interviewer:** "Fine, then. Let's set up your next appointment time."

Before reading on, stop and reread the previous suicide-prevention contract statement. Think about what is wrong with this agreement where the therapist tells the client to "call me first" in case of strong suicidal impulses. First, although as a professional helper you may feel completely committed to your clients, you may not want to deal with client crises at any time, night or day. But that is exactly what might happen with the preceding offer. Second, you may not be able to respond to your client immediately. For example, you may not be home, or you may be at home dealing with a smaller crisis of your own. Therefore, if you enter into a suicide contract like the one described, be sure to provide your client with alternative telephone numbers (e.g., the local suicide hotline) in case you are unavailable when the suicidal urges occur. Third, what if your client simply calls you as his or her final act? For example:

"Doc, I was calling because you said to call if I felt out of control. Well, I just wanted to say good-bye; I promised I would. Don't feel bad. You're a good counselor, but I gotta do this. No other way. Good-bye."

Instead of the traditional "call me if you feel out of control" contract, Mahoney (1990) recommends making an agreement with clients to meet face-to-face before following through with suicide impulses. Although this approach has several advantages, it also may be difficult for severely suicidal clients to honestly agree to such a contract. To avoid having clients feel pressured into establishing a suicide-prevention contract with you, give them an opportunity to decline your contract offer (e.g., "I want you to agree to this contract only if you really believe you can follow through with it."). In addition, when establishing a suicide contract with clients, be sure to acknowledge that you cannot always be available to them.

Suicide-prevention contracts (even contracts that specify only telephone contact) probably decrease suicide risk in most cases because they constitute a lifeline between client and interviewer. Consequently, to be most effective, you should establish a solid therapeutic relationship before entering into a suicide-prevention contract. In many cases, even a single interview can be adequate for establishing the type of relationship necessary to make a suicide-prevention contract effective. If it does not seem you are relating well enough to a particular client to establish a suicide contract, it may mean the client is severely suicidal and that more immediate intervention is warranted.

Suicide-prevention contracts also help evaluators assess client self-control and intent. If clients agree to a suicide-prevention contract, they probably have some control and have only low to moderate intent. Clients with low self-control or high intent often will not agree to a suicide contract. However, as emphasized by Simon (1999, 2000), in terms of liability, a suicide prevention contract is not an adequate substitute for a comprehensive suicide risk assessment.

### Becoming Directive and Responsible

When clients are a clear danger to themselves, in our culture and by our laws, it becomes the interviewer's responsibility to intervene and provide protection. For many counselors and psychotherapists, this means taking a much more directive role than usual. You may have to directly tell the client what to do, where to go, whom to call, and so forth. It also may involve prescriptive therapeutic interventions, such as strongly urging the client to get involved in daily exercise, consistent recreational activity, church activities, or whatever seems preventative based on the individual client's needs.

Clients who are severely or extremely suicidal (see Table 9.1) may require hospitalization. If you have such a client, be positive and direct regarding the need for and potential benefit of hospitalization. Clients may have stereotyped views of what life is like inside a psychiatric hospital. Statements similar to the following may help you begin the discussion.

> "I wonder how you feel (or what you think) about the possibility of staying in a hospital for a while, until you feel safer and more in control?"

> "I think being in the hospital may be just the right thing for you. You can rest and work on feeling better. And the staff members at the hospital are great. They'll be there to talk with you, but they'll also leave you alone and let you rest."

> "Some people feel uncomfortable about staying in a hospital. I think you should give it a try and see if it helps. If it doesn't help, you can check out in a few days or a week. My opinion is that life can be better for you, but that you need to take some steps to help make that happen. Going into the hospital is one of those steps: It's a chance to be in a safe place while you focus on yourself and how you can feel better."

Linehan (1993, 1999) has discussed a number of directive approaches for reducing suicide behaviors based on her dialectical behavior therapy work with chronically parasuicidal borderline clients. For example, she advocates:

- Emphatically instructing the client not to commit suicide.
- Repeatedly informing the client that suicide is not a good solution and that a better one will be found.
- Giving advice and telling the client what to do when/if he or she is frozen and unable to construct a positive action plan.

## Making Decisions about Hospitalization and Referral

When using interview methods to conduct a suicide assessment, most professionals follow procedures similar to those described in this chapter. However, once the assessment is completed, there is still the question of how to proceed with the client's professional care.

The first question to be addressed in the decision-making process is: How suicidal is the client? Suicidality can be measured along a continuum from nonexistent to extreme. Clients with mild to moderate suicide potential can usually be managed on an outpatient basis. Obviously, the more frequent and intense the ideation and the more clear the plan (assess using SLAP), the more closely the client should be monitored. We recommend making verbal suicide-prevention contracts with clients who are a mild to moderate suicide risk. We also recommend discussing suicide as one of many alternatives. However, we are less directive with and take less responsibility for mild to moderately suicidal clients than for severely to extremely suicidal clients.

If moderately suicidal clients fit into several important high-risk categories, we sometimes treat them as severely suicidal. For example, imagine a 55-year-old depressed male who presents with a consistent suicide ideation and a vague plan. The man is socially isolated and has increased alcohol use since the onset of his depression. Depending on a number of clinical issues, this client might be a good candidate for psychiatric hospitalization (a strategy usually reserved for severely or extremely suicidal clients). This would especially be true if he had made a previous suicide attempt.

Severely and extremely suicidal clients warrant swift and directive intervention. If possible, such clients should not be left alone while you consider intervention options. Instead, inform them in a supportive but directive manner that it is your professional responsibility to ensure their safety. Such actions may include contacting the police or a county or municipal mental health professional. Unless you have special training and it is the policy of your agency, *never* transport a severely or extremely suicidal client to a psychiatric facility on your own. Suicidal clients have jumped from moving vehicles, attempted to drown themselves in rivers, and thrown themselves into freeway traffic to avoid hospitalization and accomplish their suicidal goal. Regardless of whether they succeed during such an attempt, the attempt itself is traumatic to both client and interviewer.

There are several reasons why hospitalization may not be the best option for moderately or severely suicidal clients (although it is probably always the best option for extremely suicidal clients). For some clients, hospitalization itself is traumatic. They experience deflated self-esteem and may regress to lower functioning, becoming cut off from more socially acceptable support networks. Severely suicidal clients who are employed and have adequate social support networks may, in some instances, be better off without hospitalization. In such cases, you might increase client contact, perhaps even meeting for brief sessions every working day.

Regardless of how suicidal a client seems on a given day, interviewers and therapists should consistently check with clients to determine whether suicidal status has changed. Do not assume that because your client was only mildly suicidal yesterday, he or she is still only mildly suicidal today.

## PROFESSIONAL ISSUES

When working with suicidal clients, it is your responsibility to be a competent and caring professional who lives up to professional standards of practice. Meeting professional standards makes your practice more effective and helps protect you if one of your clients actually completes a suicide (Moris, 1990; J. Sommers-Flanagan & Sommers-Flanagan, 1995a).

Many important professional issues are associated with suicide assessment. Some of these issues are personal; others emphasize professional or legal issues. It is sometimes difficult to disentangle the personal from the professional-legal. These issues are discussed briefly in the following section.

## Can You Work with Suicidal Clients?

Some interviewers are not well-suited to working with suicidal clients. Depressed and suicidal clients are often angry and hostile toward those who try to help them. However, it remains your responsibility to maintain rapport and not become too irritated, even with hostile clients. Avoid taking the comments of irate or suicidal clients personally.

If you are prone to depression and suicidal thoughts yourself, it is wise to avoid regular work with suicidal clients. Working with suicidal clients may trigger your depressive thoughts and add to your tendency to become depressed and/or suicidal.

Strong values about suicide, too, can be an important professional consideration. Some people strongly believe that suicide is a viable life choice and that clients should not be prevented from committing suicide if they truly want to (Szasz, 1986):

> All this points toward the desirability of according suicide the status of a basic human right (in its strict, political-philosophical sense). I do not mean that killing oneself is always good or praiseworthy; I mean only that the power of the state should not be legitimately invoked or deployed to prohibit or prevent persons from killing themselves. (p. 811)

On the other hand, Shneidman (1981) believes the inherent psychological and emotional states of suicidal people make it so suicide should not be considered a right: "Suicide is not a 'right' anymore than is the 'right to belch.' If the individual feels forced to do it, he will do it" (p. 322).

If you have strong philosophical or religious beliefs either for or against suicide, these beliefs could impede your ability to be objective and helpful when working with suicidal clients. You may still be able to conduct initial interviews and must strive to do so professionally and supportively. However, if your beliefs predispose you to negatively judge clients, consider referring suicidal clients to other professionals who can work more neutrally and effectively with them. It is not a failure to have certain groups of people or problem areas that you do not want to work with. It *is* a failure to have such areas and not recognize them or the harm done to clients because of them.

## Consultation

As mental health professionals and instructors, we believe ongoing peer consultation is essential to competent, ethical practice. Consultation with peers and supervisors serves a dual purpose. First, it provides interviewers with much-needed professional support; dealing with suicidal clients is difficult and stressful, and input from other professionals is helpful. As we have stated elsewhere: "For the sake of their health and sanity, suicide assessors should not work in isolation" (J. Sommers-Flanagan & Sommers-Flanagan, 1997, p. 12).

Second, consultation also provides interviewers with feedback regarding appropriate practice standards in each individual case. When it comes to defending your actions (or lack thereof) during a postsuicide trial, you will need to demonstrate that you have functioned in the usual and customary manner with regard to professional standards; consultation is one way to review your professional competency.

## Documentation

Professional interviewers should always document contact with clients (Soisson, VandeCreek, & Knapp, 1987; Wiger, 1999). It is especially important when working with suicidal clients to document the rationale underlying your clinical decisions (Bongar, 1991; Jobes & Berman, 1993). For example, if you are working with a severely or extremely suicidal client and decide against hospitalization, outline in writing exactly why you made that decision. You might be justified choosing not to hospitalize your client if a suicide-prevention contract has been established and your client has good social support resources (e.g., family or employment).

When you work with suicidal clients, keep documentation to show that you:

1. Conducted a thorough suicide risk assessment.
2. Obtained adequate historical information.
3. Obtained records regarding previous treatment.
4. Asked directly about suicidal thoughts and impulses.
5. Consulted with one or more professionals.
6. Discussed limits of confidentiality.
7. Implemented suicide interventions.
8. Gave resources (e.g., telephone numbers) to the client.

Remember, the legal bottom line with regard to documentation is that if an event was not documented, it did not happen (see Putting It in Practice 9.3; and Wiger, 1999 for additional information).

## Dealing with Completed Suicides

In the unfortunate event that one of your clients completes a suicide, be aware of several personal and legal issues. First, seek professional and personal support. Sometimes, therapists need psychotherapy or counseling to deal with their feelings of grief and guilt. In other cases, postsuicide discussion with supportive colleagues is sufficient. Some professionals conduct "psychological autopsies" in an effort to identify factors that contributed to the suicide (Conwell et al., 1996). Psychological autopsies are especially helpful for professionals who regularly work with suicidal clients; autopsies may help prevent suicides in future situations (Kaye & Soreff, 1991).

Second, consult an attorney immediately. You need to know the nature of your legal situation and how to best protect yourself (Jobes & Berman, 1993).

Unless your attorney is adamantly against it, you probably should be available to your deceased client's family. They may want to meet with you personally or simply discuss their loss over the telephone. At the legal level, if you refuse to discuss the situation with a client's family, you risk their anger; angry families are more likely to prosecute than are families who feel you have been open and fair (Moris, 1990). Realize that anything you say to a deceased client's family can be used against you. Therefore, continue

```
╔══════════════════════════════════════════════════════════════╗
║                   Putting It in Practice 9.3                   ║
```

## Assessing Your Assessment Procedures: Documentation Guidelines

For this exercise, have two brave individuals volunteer to role-play a suicide assessment in front of the class, using the instruments from the earlier exercises. Have the entire class observe and evaluate the assessment, including the following important aspects.

**Suicide Assessment Documentation Checklist**

Check off the following items to ensure that your suicide assessment documentation is up to professional standards.

_____ 1. The limits of confidentiality and informed consent were discussed.

_____ 2. A thorough suicide assessment was conducted, including:

_____ Risk factor assessment.

_____ Suicide assessment instruments or questionnaires.

_____ Assessment of suicidal thoughts, plan, client self-control, and suicidal intent.

_____3. Relevant historical information from the client regarding suicidal behavior (e.g., suicidal behaviors by family members, previous attempts, lethality of previous attempts, etc.) was obtained.

_____4. Previous treatment records were requested/obtained.

_____5. Consultation with one or more licensed mental health professionals was sought.

_____6. An appropriate no-suicide contract was established.

_____7. The patient was provided with information regarding emergency/crisis resources.

_____8. In cases of high suicide risk, appropriate and relevant authority figures (police officers) and/or family members were contacted.

_____

*Note:* From *Tough Kids, Cool Counseling: User-Friendly Approaches with Challenging Youth,* by J. Sommers-Flanagan and R. Sommers-Flanagan, 1997, p. 200. Alexandria, VA: American Counseling Association. Adapted with permission of the authors.

to consult with your attorney regarding what you can discuss with them. Your attitude toward the family may be more important than what you disclose about your client's case. Avoid saying, "My attorney recommended that I not answer that question." Make efforts to be open about your own sadness regarding the client's death, but avoid talking about your guilt (e.g., don't say, "Oh, I only wish I had decided to hospitalize him after our last session."). At the therapeutic level, talking with the family can be important for both them and you. In most cases, they will regard you as someone who was trying to help their loved one get better. They will appreciate all that you tried to do and will expect that, to some degree, you share their grief and loss. Each case is different, but do not allow legal fears to overcome your professional concern and your humanity.

## Concluding Comments

Suicide is a common topic during intake interviews and ongoing therapy. Even beginning interviewers should not sit down in a room with a client unless they understand how to competently conduct a suicide assessment. Dealing with suicidal clients without adequate preparation is not only anxiety-provoking, but risky and unprofessional as well. Similarly, although homicidal or violent clients are much more rare, especially for beginning interviewers, we recommend reviewing the material in Putting It in Practice 9.4 to enhance your awareness of violence assessment strategies.

There is no replacement for direct practice in conducting suicide assessment interviews. Repeated practice increases the likelihood that you can conduct suicide assessment interviews competently and without excessive anxiety.

We also encourage you to repeatedly test yourself regarding risk factors and other interview information covered in this chapter. If someone asks you to assess a potentially suicidal client, you should immediately think: risk factors, depression, thoughts, plan, control, intent, intervention, consultation, and documentation. Several checklists are included in this chapter to assist you in remembering these key suicide assessment inter-

---

### Putting It in Practice 9.4

### Assessment and Prediction of Dangerousness

Stop and think about how you might discern if someone is contemplating a violent or dangerous act. Ethical and legal guidelines for mental health professionals are clear: If you have good reason to suspect that someone plans to do violence to another person, you are required to contact the police and warn the potential victim. The part that is much less clear is this: How will you know whether to suspect your client is considering violent or dangerous behavior?

Legally, to justify reporting potential violence, you must hear (or read about) a specific threat to a specific person or place. Therefore, the first and most important guideline in violence assessment is simple: Did your client make a specific threat? If so, and if you consider the threat serious, then it is your responsibility to gather the information needed to warn the potential victim.

In class, or with a study partner, review the following questions that to consider when assessing for possible violent behavior. Generate ideas about how, as an interviewer, you might obtain answers for these questions.

1. Is there a prior instance or pattern of violent or dangerous behavior?
2. Is the situation similar to his or her previous violent incidents? Is his or her psychological state similar to the previous incidents?
3. Is your client experiencing significant family or relationship distress or discord?
4. Was your client a previous victim of abuse or violence?
5. Is your client abusing substances?
6. Is your client male (about 89% of violent crime is committed by males)?

In his book *The Gift of Fear* (1997), Gavin de Becker emphasizes the importance of using intuition to predict dangerousness. Discuss in your class or with a partner the pros and cons of using intuition to predict potential violence.

---

**Putting It in Practice 9.5**

## Suicide Quiz Answers and Explanations

___T___  1. *About 25% to 50% of people who kill themselves have previously attempted to do so.* Previous suicide attempts constitute one of the better predictors of further attempts and possible suicide completion.

___F___  2. *People who talk about suicide won't commit suicide.* People who eventually commit suicide often have tried to communicate their despair to others in a number of ways. All comments even vaguely associated with suicide or death, such as "Life just doesn't seem worthwhile anymore" or "I wish I were dead," should be considered attempts at communicating despair.

___F___  3. *Suicide happens without warning.* Suicidal people usually leave clues or give warnings either verbally or through their behavior. For example, appearing depressed or apathetic is a potential clue that an individual is considering suicide.

___T___  4. *If a parent of a child under five years of age commits suicide, the surviving child is many more times likely to grow up and commit suicide than a child who did not have that experience.* One research study showed that such children are nine times more likely to commit suicide when they grow up (Birtchnell, 1973).

___T___  5. *Suicide attempters are more likely than other psychiatric patients to use substances in the 24 hours before admission to a hospital.* Ingestion of disinhibiting substances can help people "get up the nerve" to follow through on thoughts about suicide. The final act of attempting suicide, although perhaps preceded by detailed planning, requires strong uninhibited impulses (which are more likely to occur after ingestion of substances).

___F___  6. *Patients under a doctor's care are not at risk of suicide.* Medical patients are often depressed because of their pain or prognosis. They may feel life isn't worth living anymore.

___F___  7. *Life stress factors are good predictors of suicide.* This is false for two reasons. First, there are no "good" predictors of suicide. Second, many people with huge amounts of "life stress" are not the least bit suicidal.

___T___  8. *More men commit suicide than women.* Most reports suggest that men are about four times more likely to complete suicide than women. Women are about three times more likely to attempt suicide than men.

___T___  9. *In the United States, suicide is more prominent among Protestants than Catholics.* There is some evidence that predominantly Catholic countries, such as Italy and Spain, have lower suicide rates than predominantly Protestant countries. However, in countries with heterogeneous religious compositions, the data are inconclusive.

*(continued)*

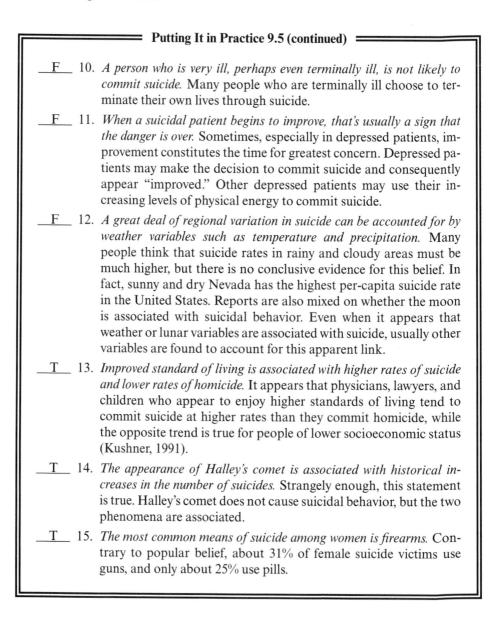

**Putting It in Practice 9.5 (continued)**

_F_  10. *A person who is very ill, perhaps even terminally ill, is not likely to commit suicide.* Many people who are terminally ill choose to terminate their own lives through suicide.

_F_  11. *When a suicidal patient begins to improve, that's usually a sign that the danger is over.* Sometimes, especially in depressed patients, improvement constitutes the time for greatest concern. Depressed patients may make the decision to commit suicide and consequently appear "improved." Other depressed patients may use their increasing levels of physical energy to commit suicide.

_F_  12. *A great deal of regional variation in suicide can be accounted for by weather variables such as temperature and precipitation.* Many people think that suicide rates in rainy and cloudy areas must be much higher, but there is no conclusive evidence for this belief. In fact, sunny and dry Nevada has the highest per-capita suicide rate in the United States. Reports are also mixed on whether the moon is associated with suicidal behavior. Even when it appears that weather or lunar variables are associated with suicide, usually other variables are found to account for this apparent link.

_T_  13. *Improved standard of living is associated with higher rates of suicide and lower rates of homicide.* It appears that physicians, lawyers, and children who appear to enjoy higher standards of living tend to commit suicide at higher rates than they commit homicide, while the opposite trend is true for people of lower socioeconomic status (Kushner, 1991).

_T_  14. *The appearance of Halley's comet is associated with historical increases in the number of suicides.* Strangely enough, this statement is true. Halley's comet does not cause suicidal behavior, but the two phenomena are associated.

_T_  15. *The most common means of suicide among women is firearms.* Contrary to popular belief, about 31% of female suicide victims use guns, and only about 25% use pills.

viewing ingredients. We also recommend strongly that you explore some of the suggested readings at the end of this chapter to further expand your knowledge about suicide and its assessment. Proceeding with knowledge and caution, obtaining supervision, developing a norm of consulting with colleagues, and documenting factors contributing to your clinical decision are the basic rules for handling this area of mental health care.

Finally, in this chapter we have focused exclusively on using clinical interviews to evaluate clients' suicidality. There are many standardized measures of depression, hope, and suicidal impulses available in the literature. Additionally, research has shown that sometimes clients are more likely to disclose suicide ideation on a self-report form than with a clinician during a face-to-face interview (Kaplan et al., 1994). For this reason, we recommend that agencies and private practitioners routinely consider including a suicide ideation query on their intake forms.

At this point, if you have not already done so, take time to grade yourself on the Suicide Quiz (see Putting It in Practice 9.5).

# SUMMARY

Suicide is a significant social problem and, theoretically, a preventable cause of death. There are many myths regarding suicide; this may be partly because many different risk factors are associated with suicidal behavior. Prominent risk factors include depression, hopelessness, age, sex, race, marital status, employment status, physical health, substance abuse, history of previous suicide attempt, and presence of a mental disorder.

Conducting a suicide risk assessment involves several important steps. First, you should know and inquire about risk factors commonly associated with suicide. Second, you should explore the extent of the client's depression. Third, evaluate the frequency, duration, and intensity of the client's suicidal thoughts (suicide ideation). Fourth, clarify whether the client has a suicide plan. Fifth, if appropriate, evaluate the client's suicide plan in terms of SLAP-specificity of the plan, lethality and availability of the means, and proximity of supportive resources. Sixth, assess client self-control by asking about it directly, identifying reasons for living, and exploring the client's history of impulsive behavior. Seventh, evaluate whether your client intends to kill himself or herself.

When working with suicidal clients, it is important to establish rapport and a therapeutic relationship through effective listening strategies. Supportive empathy is crucial. Suicidal clients may not have informed anyone previously of suicidal thoughts and wishes. Let them know you hear their pain and misery, but at the same time, help them begin to see that there are good reasons to be hopeful; most depressed and suicidal clients improve and begin to feel life is worth living again.

Avoid arguing with clients about whether suicide is a viable life option. Instead, focus on widening the client's view of personal options by emphasizing that suicide is only one of many life options. Help clients understand that because suicide is a permanent choice, all other options should be explored first. Try to reinvolve clients in reinforcing life activities.

Many interviewers establish suicide-prevention contracts with suicidal clients. Mahoney (1990) recommends requiring that the client commit to a face-to-face session before attempting suicide. Client willingness to establish contract usually indicates that client self-control is adequate and suicide intent is low. Sometimes, interviewers must become very directive and take action when working with suicidal clients.

Deciding whether a client's suicidal impulses warrant immediate hospitalization is difficult. A client's suicide risk can be rated to help facilitate decision making, but there is no foolproof formula available to help interviewers decide how to most effectively manage each suicidal case. Ratings of suicidality range from nonexistent, mild, moderate, severe, to extreme. Clients who are mildly or moderately suicidal can normally be managed in an outpatient setting. Severely and extremely suicidal clients usually require hospitalization.

Interviewers should know and adhere to professional standards when working with suicidal clients. When possible, interviewers should consult with other professionals about suicidal clients. Clearly document all professional decisions. In the unfortunate event of a client's actually committing suicide, interviewers are advised to follow several key steps.

# SUGGESTED READINGS AND RESOURCES

## Professional Books and Articles

Bennett, B. E., Bryant, B. K., VandenBos, G. R., & Greenwood, A. (1990). *Professional liability and risk management.* Washington, DC: American Psychological Association. This text provides excellent guidelines for therapists who want to avoid professional liability in this age of frequent litigation.

Ellison, J. M. (2001). *Treatment of suicidal patients in managed care.* Washington, DC: American Psychiatric Press. This book outlines the essentials of treating suicidal patients within a managed care setting. It includes information on brief hospitalization, alternatives to hospitalization, pharmacotherapy, and methods for formulating suicide risk.

Healy, D. (2000). Antidepressant induced suicidality. *Primary Care in Psychiatry, 6,* 23–28. This article focuses on ways in which serotonin-specific reuptake inhibitors may, in some cases, increase client suicidality.

Jacobs, D. G. (1999). *The Harvard Medical School guide to suicide assessment and intervention.* San Francisco: Jossey-Bass. This volume of over 700 pages details a distinctly psychiatric-medical perspective on suicide assessment and intervention.

Jobes, D. A., & Berman, A. L. (1993). Suicide and malpractice liability: Assessing and revising policies, procedures, and practice in outpatient settings. *Professional Psychology: Research and Practice, 24,* 91–99. This is a practical article that includes helpful guidelines for agencies or clinics that work with potentially suicidal clients. Its appendices provide administrative forms and procedures.

Juhnke, G. A. (1996). The adapted-SAD PERSONS: A suicide assessment scale designed for use with children. *Elementary School Guidance & Counseling, 30,* 252–258. This short article discusses the adaptation of Patterson et al.'s (1983; see next item) SAD PERSONS scale for evaluating school-aged children. It is a handy approach for therapists who plan to work with children.

Patterson, W. M., Dohn, H. H., Bird, J., & Patterson, G. A. (1983). Evaluation of suicidal patients: The SAD PERSONS scale. *Psychosomatics, 24,* 343–349. This is a useful article that provides an acronym to help clinicians recall suicide predictor variables.

Shea, S. C. (1999). *The practical art of suicide assessment: A guide for mental health professionals and substance abuse counselors.* New York: John Wiley & Sons. This entire book focuses primarily on interview methods for uncovering suicide ideation and intent in clients.

Shneidman, E. S. (1996). *The suicidal mind.* New York: Oxford University Press. In this powerful book, the most renowned suicidologist in the world reviews three cases that illustrate the psychological pain associated with suicidal impulses. It is a must read for those who work with highly suicidal populations.

Szasz, T. S. (1986). The case against suicide prevention. *American Psychologist, 41,* 806–812. In this article, Szasz outlines his provocative belief that coercive suicide-prevention efforts violate individual human rights.

Wollersheim, J. P. (1974). The assessment of suicide potential via interview methods. *Psychotherapy: Theory, Research and Practice, 11,* 222–225. Wollersheim's article focuses on assessing suicidal clients exclusively through interview procedures.

## Self-Help for Suicidal People and Violence Prediction

de Becker, G. (1997). *The gift of fear.* Boston: Little, Brown, & Co. Having grown up in a violent family, worked as a consultant for many government agencies, and been a three-time presidential appointee gives de Becker a unique perspective on predicting violent behavior. His main message is clear: Often, our intuition informs us of potentially dangerous situations when our rational minds are still searching for concrete explanations for our fear.

Ellis, T. E., & Newman, C. F. (1996). *Choosing to live: How to defeat suicide through cognitive therapy.* Oakland, CA: New Harbinger. Based on principles of cognitive therapy, this self-help book is designed to help suicidal people work through their psychological pain and depression and choose life.

Heckler, R. A. (1996). *Waking up alive: The descent, the suicide attempt, and the return to life.* New York: Ballentine. In this unique book, the author examines the process and depression, suicide attempts, and survival. It includes information from 50 individuals who attempted suicide and survived.

## Suicide Support Organizations and Web Sites

American Foundation for Suicide Prevention, 120 Wall Street, 22nd Floor, New York, NY 10005. Phone: 888-333-AFSP or 212-363-3500. www.afsp.org

American Association of Suicidology, Alan L. Berman, Ph.D., Executive Director, 4201 Connecticut Avenue, N.W., Suite 310, Washington, DC 20008. Phone: 202-237-2280. www .suicidology.org

National Crisis Hotline: 888-284-2433 or 888-suicide.

National Youth Crisis Hotline: 888-999-9999.

National Organization for People of Color Against Suicide, P.O. Box 125, San Marcos, TX 78667 830-625-3576. E-mail: db31#swt.edu.

Suicide Prevent Triangle: SuicidePreventTriangle.org. Lists support groups, suicide self-assessment procedures, software, and educational/resource information on suicide.

## Video and Film

American Foundation for Suicide Prevention. (1997). *Fatal Mistakes: Families Shattered by Suicide.* New York: Author. This is an inexpensive video for professional groups who work with suicidal individuals. It can be ordered through the American Foundation for Suicide Prevention (see entry under Suicide Support Organizations).

On occasion, feature films include themes of suicide or extreme self-destructive behavior. Three interesting and provocative films include *Ordinary People, Leaving Las Vegas,* and *Dead Poets Society.*

# Chapter 10

# DIAGNOSIS AND TREATMENT PLANNING

*We propose to group those who receive psychotherapy into five rough categories: the psychotic, the neurotic or persistently disturbed, the shaken, the misbehaving, and the discontented.*

—J. Frank and J. Frank, *Persuasion and Healing*

---

**CHAPTER OBJECTIVES**

From the perspective of the medical model, the primary—and sometimes only—purpose of a clinical interview is to identify the appropriate diagnosis and treatment plan for a client. In this chapter, we look at philosophical and practical aspects of diagnosis; we also review several approaches for establishing treatment plans for clients who are beginning counseling or psychotherapy. After reading this chapter, you will know:

- Basic principles of psychiatric diagnosis, including the definition of mental disorders according to the *Diagnostic and Statistical Manual of Mental Disorders, 4th Edition, Text Revision (DSM-IV-TR; American Psychiatric Association, 2000)*.
- Common problems associated with assessment and diagnosis.
- Methods and procedures for diagnostic assessment.
- A balanced approach for conducting diagnostic clinical interviews.
- An integrated or biopsychosocial approach to treatment planning.
- How to identify client problems, associated goals, and establish a treatment plan to guide the therapy process.
- The importance of matching client resources with specific approaches to clinical treatment.

---

## PRINCIPLES OF PSYCHIATRIC DIAGNOSIS

Numerous formal and informal systems exist for categorizing the distress experienced by individuals seeking mental health treatment. These systems may be as simple and intuitive as the one in the opening quote or as complex as the Diagnostic and Statistical Manual of Mental Disorders *(DSM)*, which now includes over 300 mental disorders in its 943 pages (American Psychiatric Association, 2000). The *DSM* is generally considered the authoritative diagnostic guide for North American mental health profession-als. The first edition was published in 1952; the second, in 1968; the third, in 1980; a re-vision of the third edition, in 1987; and the fourth edition, in 1994. In 2000, the text re-vision of *DSM-IV* was published *(DSM-IV-TR)*. Even with so many editions and such lengthy coverage, as Widiger and Clark (2000) state, psychiatric diagnosis remains con-troversial: "There might not in fact be one sentence within *DSM-IV* for which well-meaning clinicians, theorists, and researchers could not find some basis for fault" (p. 946).

Disputes surrounding psychiatric diagnosis and the concept of mental disorders run so deep that the *DSM-IV-TR* contains a brief but articulate section titled "Definition of Mental Disorder." In this section, the *DSM* authors clearly admit they have pro-duced a manual for diagnosing a concept that lacks an adequate operational definition:

> . . . although this manual provides a classification of mental disorders, it must be admitted
> that no definition adequately specifies precise boundaries for the concept of "mental dis-
> order." The concept of mental disorder, like many other concepts in medicine and science,
> lacks a consistent operational definition that covers all situations. (American Psychiatric
> Association, 2000, p. xxx)

So, as we discuss diagnostic strategies in the following pages, be forewarned that you are venturing into only partially charted waters. Nonetheless, as scientists and profes-sionals, we believe it is a fascinating journey, filled with adventure, intrigue, and more than an occasional unresolved dispute.

## Defining Mental Disorders

As you probably already realize from your own experience, it is often difficult to draw a clear line between mental and physical disorders. Sometimes, when you become phys-ically ill, it is obvious that your stress level or mental state has contributed to your ill-ness. On the other hand, when you're emotionally or psychologically distressed, your physical condition (perhaps physical pain or illness) frequently and sometimes pro-foundly contributes to your disturbed emotional state and thinking processes (Witvliet, Ludwig, & Vander Laan, 2001). The difficulty distinguishing between mental and phys-ical problems is acknowledged by *DSM*'s authors:

> A compelling literature documents that there is much "physical" in "mental" disorders
> and much "mental" in "physical" disorders. The problem raised by the term "mental" dis-
> orders has been much clearer than its solution, and, unfortunately, the term persists in the
> title of DSM-IV because we have not found an appropriate substitute. (American Psychi-
> atric Association, 2000, p. xxx)

Despite ongoing quandaries over what to call mental disorders, and whether mind or body is the primary contributor to such disorders, it is safe to say that the *DSM-IV-TR* authors and others have identified numerous important cognitive, emotional, and behavioral problems or deviances that exist in many people throughout the world. These mental conditions or mental disorders produce immeasurable suffering, conflict, and distress in the lives of millions of people. Without a doubt, and no matter what we call them, mental disorders are frequently identifiable and have clear and adverse ef-fects on individuals, couples, families, and communities.

In its introduction, the *DSM-IV-TR* offers a general definition of *mental disorder* us-ing the following criteria:

1. a clinically significant behavioral or psychological syndrome or pattern
2. that occurs in an individual
3. and that is associated with
   (a) present distress (e.g., a painful symptom) or
   (b) disability (i.e., impairment in one or more important areas of functioning) or
   (c) a significantly increased risk of suffering death, pain, disability, or
   (d) an important loss of freedom.

Specific criteria are provided to help mental health professionals exclude particular symptoms or conditions from being considered mental disorders. The *DSM-IV-TR* provides examples and criteria for what *should not be* considered a mental disorder:

> . . . this syndrome or pattern must not be merely an expectable and culturally sanctioned response to a particular event, for example, the death of a loved one. Whatever its original cause, it must currently be considered a manifestation of a behavioral, psychological, or biological dysfunction in the individual. Neither deviant behavior (e.g., political, religious, or sexual) nor conflicts that are primarily between the individual and society are mental disorders unless the deviance or conflict is a symptom of a dysfunction in the individual. . . . (American Psychiatric Association, 2000, p. xxxi)

Not surprisingly, significant vagueness in the *DSM-IV-TR* general definition of *mental disorder* remains. There is room for debate regarding what constitutes "a clinically significant behavioral or psychological syndrome or pattern." Further, the manual recognizes that "culturally sanctioned" behavioral responses may not be a mental disorder, but notes the inverse; that is, deviant or culturally unsanctioned behaviors may not, in and of themselves, be considered a mental disorder. This vagueness and subjectivity in defining mental disorders is another area where the *DSM* has received criticism (Halling & Goldfarb, 1996; Szasz, 1961, 1970; Wakefield, 1997). For example, Szasz (1970) states:

> Which kinds of social deviance are regarded as mental illnesses? The answer is, those that entail personal conduct not conforming to psychiatrically defined and enforced rules of mental health. If narcotics-avoidance is a rule of mental health, narcotics ingestion will be a sign of mental illness; if even-temperedness is a rule of mental health, depression and elation will be signs of mental illness; and so forth. (p. xxvi)

Szasz's point is well taken. After all is said and done, *DSM*'s general definition of *mental disorder* and the criteria for each individual mental disorder consist of carefully studied and meticulously outlined subjective judgments.

## Why Diagnose?

Like Szasz (1970), many of our students want to reject the entire concept of diagnosis. They are critical of and cynical about the *DSM-IV-TR,* or they believe that applying diagnoses dehumanizes clients by affixing a label to them and then ignoring their individual qualities, what Morrison (1993) refers to as *pigeonholing* (p. 200). Whatever their arguments, our position regarding diagnosis remains consistent. We empathize with our students' complaints, commiserate about problems associated with diagnosing unique individuals, and then move on to teaching diagnostic assessment strategies and procedures, justifying ourselves with both philosophical and practical arguments.

## Philosophical Support

No matter what we call them, mental disorders exist. As far as we know, emotional distress, mental suffering, character pathology, and suicidal behavior have existed since humans have existed. Psychiatric diagnosis is designed to classify or categorize mental disorders based on their defining characteristics. Knowledge about mental disorders, their similarities, differences, usual course and prognosis, prevalence, and so on, helps us provide more appropriate and more effective treatments. Such knowledge is reassuring and empowering to mental health professionals who want to help their clients. Additionally, such knowledge can assist in preventing mental disorders.

## Practical Support

There are a number of positive practical outcomes of accurate diagnosis. A *diagnosis* is a consolidated, organized description of symptoms or distresses experienced by clients. Arriving at this shorthand description requires careful observation and inquiry. After the best diagnosis is obtained, the practitioner can communicate with other professionals, insurance or managed care companies, and other interested parties.

At best, a diagnosis is a working hypothesis. It forces interviewers to bring together disparate pieces of the puzzle and tentatively name a specific relationship among the various symptoms and problem areas. It then suggests a general course of action that, if pursued, should yield a somewhat predictable set of responses. It lays the groundwork for planned interventions and informed use of theory and technique.

In addition to enabling professional communication and hypothesis testing, a final positive and practical aspect of diagnosing is this: Sometimes, a label is a huge relief for clients. Clients come for help with a confusing and frightening set of problems, distresses, or symptoms. They may feel alone and uniquely troubled. They may feel no one else in the world has ever been quite so dysfunctional, quite so odd, quite so anxious, or quite so "flipped out." It can be quite a relief to be *diagnosed,* to have your problems named, categorized, and defined. It can be comforting to realize that others—many others—have reacted to trauma in similar ways, experienced depression in similar ways, or even developed similar maladaptive coping strategies (such as irrational thoughts or damaging compulsions). The wise clinician realizes there can be hope implied in a diagnosis and hope instilled or enhanced in an interactive diagnostic process (Frank & Frank, 1991).

## Specific Diagnostic Criteria

In contrast to establishing a satisfactory definition for mental disorders, identifying a *DSM* diagnosis for a particular client may seem, on the surface, rather simple and straightforward. After all, accurate diagnosis is based on determining the presence or absence of various symptom clusters or patterns (i.e., syndromes). In most cases, *DSM-IV-TR* provides specific, somewhat measurable criteria for its diagnoses. Typically, *DSM* diagnoses are characterized by a list of symptoms for defining the condition accompanied by a few factors that, if present, would rule out the condition in question. For example, to qualify for the *DSM*'s generalized anxiety disorder, individuals must meet the criteria in Table 10.1.

The diagnostic criteria for generalized anxiety disorder illustrate tasks associated with accurate diagnosis. First, based on criterion A, diagnostic interviewers must establish whether a given client is experiencing "excessive" anxiety and worry, how frequently the anxiety is occurring, how long the anxiety has been occurring, and how

**Table 10.1.   Diagnostic Criteria for Generalized Anxiety Disorder (*DSM-IV-TR:* 300.02)**

A. Excessive anxiety and worry (apprehensive expectation), occurring more days than not for at least 6 months, about a number of events or activities (such as work or school performance).

B. The person finds it difficult to control the worry.

C. The anxiety and worry are associated with three (or more) of the following six symptoms (with at least some symptoms present for more days than not for the past 6 months). *Note:* Only one item is required in children.

   (1) restlessness or feeling keyed up or on edge

   (2) being easily fatigued

   (3) difficulty concentrating or mind going blank

   (4) irritability

   (5) muscle tension

   (6) sleep disturbance (difficulty falling or staying asleep, or restless unsatisfying sleep)

D. The focus of the anxiety and worry is not confined to features of an Axis I disorder, e.g., the anxiety or worry is not about having a Panic Attack (as in Panic Disorder), being embarrassed in public (as in Social Phobia), being contaminated (as in Obsessive-Compulsive Disorder), being away from home or close relatives (as in Separation Anxiety Disorder), gaining weight (as in Anorexia Nervosa), having multiple physical complaints (as in Somatization Disorder), or having a serious illness (as in Hypochondriasis), and the anxiety and worry do not occur exclusively during Posttraumatic Stress Disorder.

E. The anxiety, worry, or physical symptoms cause clinically significant distress or impairment in social, occupational, or other important areas of functioning.

F. The disturbance is not due to the direct physiological effects of a substance (e.g., a drug of abuse, a medication) or a general medical condition (e.g., hyperthyroidism) and does not occur exclusively during a Mood Disorder, a Psychotic Disorder, or a Pervasive Developmental Disorder.

Note: *DSM-IV-TR* diagnostic criteria are reprinted here with permission from the American Psychiatric Association.

many events or activities the individual is anxious or worried about. This information (recall Chapter 6 and our descriptions involving assessment of symptom frequency, duration, and intensity) relies on both the interviewer's ability to gather appropriate symptom-related information and the client's ability to articulately report symptom-related information. In addition, obtaining information required by criterion A involves interviewer and client subjectivity (i.e., determinations of what constitutes "excessive").

Second, under criterion B, the interviewer must assess how difficult the client finds it to control the worry. This information compels the interviewer to evaluate client coping skills and efforts, which essentially involves asking questions about what the client has tried to do to quell his or her anxiety and how well these coping efforts have worked in the past.

Third, and perhaps the most straightforward diagnostic task, the interviewer must identify whether the client is experiencing a range of specific anxiety-related symptoms. Unfortunately, even this apparently straightforward task is fraught with complications, especially in cases where clients are motivated to either overreport or underreport symptoms. For example, clients seeking disability payments for an anxiety disorder may be motivated to exaggerate their symptoms, and clients who desperately want to remain in the workplace may minimize their symptoms. Consequently, along with questioning about these specific anxiety symptoms, the interviewer must stay alert to the validity and reliability of the client's self-reported symptoms (J. Sommers-Flanagan & Sommers-Flanagan, 1998).

Fourth, to label an individual as having *generalized anxiety disorder,* an interviewer needs considerable knowledge of other *DSM* diagnostic criteria. Eight other diagnoses that may need to be ruled out are listed in the generalized anxiety disorder criterion D. An interviewer needs to have working knowledge of diagnostic criteria associated with posttraumatic stress disorder, somatization disorder, obsessive-compulsive disorder, and so on. Obviously, this is no small task; it requires lengthy education, training, and supervision.

Fifth, criterion E requires the interviewer to determine whether the reported anxiety symptoms cause "clinically significant distress or impairment in social, occupational, or other important areas of functioning." Criterion E is the distress and impairment criterion (Widiger, 1997). Although this criterion is essential to diagnostic labeling, it is also inherently subjective: ". . . nowhere in *DSM-IV* is a clinically significant impairment defined, not even within the section of the manual identified by the heading 'Criteria for Clinical Significance'" (p. 6).

Sixth, based on criterion F, before establishing a definitive diagnosis, interviewers need to determine whether their client's anxiety symptoms may be caused by exposure to or intake of a substance or general medical condition. Take note that substances and medical conditions need to be ruled out as causal factors in virtually every *DSM-IV-TR* diagnostic category.

Overall, the generalized anxiety disorder example illustrates a range of tasks and issues with which diagnostic interviewers must grapple. Unfortunately, when it comes to developing diagnostic interviewing acumen, it may be appropriate to borrow a phrase that we often use with new clients: Although it is good to have hope about learning diagnostic interviewing procedures, sometimes the confusion associated with identifying a correct diagnosis gets worse before it gets better.

## Assessment and Diagnosis Problems

To competently determine that a client meets the diagnostic criteria for generalized anxiety disorder, an interviewer must determine, by collecting assessment data, whether the client has three of six symptoms from criterion C. Given this fact, it may be sufficient (and justifiable) to directly ask the client a series of specific *DSM-IV-TR*–generated questions pertaining to generalized anxiety disorder. For example, the following questions could be directed to the client:

1. Over the past six months or more, have you felt restless, keyed up, or on edge for more days than not?
2. Over the past six months, have you felt easily fatigued more often than not?
3. Over the past six months, have you noticed, on most days, that you have difficulty concentrating or that your mind keeps going blank?
4. Over the past six months, have you felt irritable at some point on most days?
5. Over the past six months, have you found yourself troubled by muscle tension more often than not?
6. Over the past six months, have you had difficulty falling asleep, or have you found that you regularly experience restless or unsatisfying sleep?

Using this simple and straightforward diagnostic approach may, in some circumstances, produce an accurate diagnosis. However, in reality, accurate diagnostic assessment is considerably more complex. As we have discussed elsewhere:

> Like many mental disorders described in the *DSM-IV,* accurate detection . . . is not as simple as it may seem after a quick perusal of the . . . criterion behaviors . . . . It can be surprisingly difficult to accurately obtain information necessary to determine whether a particular . . . client meets the diagnostic criteria. (J. Sommers-Flanagan & Sommers-Flanagan, 1998, p. 189)

Furthermore, in *DSM-IV-TR*'s introduction section, its authors emphasize that diagnostic criteria should not be applied mechanically by untrained individuals: "The specific diagnostic criteria included in *DSM-IV* are meant to serve as guidelines to be informed by clinical judgment and are not meant to be used in a cookbook fashion" (American Psychiatric Association, 2000, p. xxxii).

Before moving on to a detailed description of diagnostic assessment strategies and procedures, we identify several additional problems associated with establishing an accurate diagnostic label for individual clients:

*Client deceit or misinformation:* Clients may not be straightforward or honest in their symptom descriptions (Noshpitz, 1994). Even in cases when they are honest, they may have difficulty accurately describing their symptoms in ways that match *DSM* criteria. In addition, if you gather information from individuals other than the client (e.g., from teachers, parents, romantic partners), you may obtain invalid information for many reasons beyond your control. In fact, research indicates that when children, parents, teachers, and others rate the same individual, their interrater agreement is generally low (Kazdin, 1995). Despite this fact, it is essential, especially when working with children and adolescents, that interviewers obtain diagnostic-related information from parents and other available informants.

*Interviewer countertransference:* As an interviewer, you may lose your objectivity and/or distort information provided to you by the client. This may occur partly because of countertransference (Sarles, 1994). For example, if a client produces a negative reaction in you, you may feel an impulse to "punish" the client by giving a more severe diagnostic label. Similarly, you may minimize psychopathology and associated diagnoses if you like your client.

*Diagnostic comorbidity:* In many cases, clients qualify for more than one *DSM* diagnosis. In fact, with regard to children, diagnostic comorbidity occurs more often than not (Harrington, 1993). This comorbidity problem makes sorting out appropriate diagnostic labels even more difficult.

*Differential diagnosis:* Although some clients report symptoms consistent with more than one diagnostic entity and are appropriately assigned two or more diagnostic labels, other clients report confusing symptom clusters requiring extensive questioning for diagnostic clarity. For example, it is notoriously difficult, albeit important, to discriminate some diagnoses from others (e.g., mood disorder with psychotic features versus schizoaffective disorder versus schizophrenia versus delusional disorder; American Psychiatric Association, 2000; Sheitman, Lee, Strauss, & Lieberman, 1997; Weiner, 1966/1997). Despite the difficulty of sorting out these various disorders, diagnostic specificity is very important because of treatment implications (i.e., medication type, treatment approach, hospitalization, prognosis).

*Confounding cultural or situational factors:* DSM-IV-TR (American Psychiatric Association, 2000) indicates that some specific diagnoses should be applied only ". . . when the behavior in question is symptomatic of an underlying dysfunction within the individual and not simply a reaction to the immediate social context" (p. 96). Consequently, your diagnostic task includes a consideration of your clients' individual social, cultural, and situational contexts when providing diagnoses, which is not always an easy task (North, Smith, & Spitznagel, 1993).

Given these problems in obtaining accurate diagnostic information, many therapists and researchers, including ourselves, advise using what has been referred to as "multimethod, multirater, multisetting assessment procedures" (J. Sommers-Flanagan & Sommers-Flanagan, 1998, p. 191). This means that, under ideal circumstances, diagnosticians gather a broad spectrum of diagnostic-related information from: (a) various assessment methods (e.g., clinical interview, behavior rating scales, projective assessments), (b) various raters (e.g., parents, teachers, clinicians, and/or romantic partners), and (c) various settings (e.g., school, home, clinician's office, work).

## DIAGNOSTIC ASSESSMENT: METHODS AND PROCEDURES

After this brief taste of diagnostic interviewing problems and tasks, you may feel a little overwhelmed. Learning diagnostic interviewing assessment procedures is a formidable challenge. However, amazingly, many mental health professionals manage the *DSM-IV-TR*'s 943 pages with sensitivity, precision, and grace. In some ways, learning to use the *DSM-IV-TR* is like learning a new language. You just have to take it one step at a time.

A number of methods are available for gathering diagnostic-relevant information, including diagnostic interviews, social/developmental history, questionnaires and rating scales, physical examinations, behavioral observations, projective techniques, and performance-based testing. Because this book focuses on interviewing-based approaches, we limit our discussion primarily to diagnostic interviewing.

### Diagnostic Interviewing

Structured and semistructured diagnostic interviews consist of a systematic series of specific questions to evaluate clients' diagnosis-related behavior patterns, thoughts, and feelings. Many published diagnostic interviewing procedures exist, most of which are based on the *DSM-III-R* or *DSM-IV* diagnostic criteria. The determination of an appropriate diagnostic label is the primary or exclusive goal of these procedures. Diagnostic interviews can be administered by counselors, social workers, psychologists, physicians, or technicians with specific training in administering a particular diagnostic interview (R. Rogers, 2001; Vacc & Juhnke, 1997). In some cases, the training required for an individual to administer a particular diagnostic interview is rather extensive (Kronenberger & Meyer, 1996). Specific diagnostic interviews are usually aimed at either adult or child client populations.

*Adult Diagnostic Interviewing*

Numerous adult diagnostic interviewing schedules exist. Some schedules are broad spectrum, in that they assess for a wide range of *DSM-IV-TR* disorders (e.g., Structured Clinical Interview for Axis I *DSM-IV* Disorders; First, Spitzer, Gibbon, & Williams, 1995). Other schedules are more specific and circumscribed in their goals; for example, some structured and semistructured interview schedules evaluate specifically for substance disorders (Psychiatric Research Interview for Substance and Mental Disorders; Hasin et al., 1998), anxiety disorders (Anxiety Disorders Interview Schedule; T. Brown, Atony, & Barlow, 1995), depressive disorders (Diagnostic Interview for Depressive Personality; Gunderson, Phillips, Triebwaser, & Hirschfeld, 1994), and more. Common adult diagnostic interviews are reviewed and described by Vacc and Juhnke (1997), Kronenberger and Meyer (1996), and R. Rogers, (2001).

## Child Diagnostic Interviewing

There are also numerous child diagnostic interviewing schedules. Again, these can be classified as either broad spectrum (e.g., The Child Assessment Schedule; Hodges, 1985) or circumscribed (e.g., Anxiety Disorders Interview Schedule for Children; W. Silverman, 1987). Common diagnostic interviews for children and adolescents also are reviewed and briefly described in recent publications (Kronenberger & Meyer, 1996; R. Rogers, 2001; Vacc & Juhnke, 1997).

## Advantages Associated with Structured Diagnostic Interviewing

Advantages associated with structured diagnostic interviewing include the following:

1. Structured diagnostic interview schedules are standardized and straightforward to administer. Technicians can ask clients specific diagnostic-relevant questions.
2. Diagnostic interview schedules generally produce a *DSM-III-R* or *DSM-IV-TR* diagnosis, consequently relieving clinicians of subjectively weighing many alternative diagnoses.
3. Diagnostic interview schedules generally exhibit greater interrater reliability than clinical interviewers functioning without such schedules. This means that two interviewers using the same structured interview protocol come up with the same diagnosis for the same client more often than two interviewers who are relying on less structured diagnostic interview procedures.
4. Diagnostic interviews are well-suited for scientific research. It is imperative that researchers obtain valid and reliable diagnoses to effectively study the nature, course, prognosis, and treatment responsiveness of particular disorders.

## Disadvantages Associated with Diagnostic Interviewing

There are also numerous disadvantages are associated with diagnostic interviewing:

1. Many diagnostic interviews require considerable time for administration. For example, the Schedule for Affective Disorders and Schizophrenia for School-Age Children (Kiddie-SADS or K-SADS; Puig-Antich, Chambers, & Tabrizi, 1983) may take one to four hours to administer, depending on whether both parent and child are interviewed. Most diagnostic interviews require training for therapists who use them, which makes them even more time-consuming.
2. Diagnostic interviews do not allow experienced diagnosticians to take shortcuts. This is cumbersome because experts in psychiatric diagnosis require far less information to accurately diagnose clients than beginning interviewers (Schmidt, Norman, & Boshuizen, 1990).

3. Some clinicians complain that diagnostic interviews are too structured and rigid, deemphasizing rapport-building and basic interpersonal communication between client and therapist (Bögels, 1994). Extensive structure and rigor may not be acceptable for practitioners who prefer relying on their intuition and relationship development for establishing treatment procedures.

4. Although structured diagnostic interviews have demonstrated reliability, some clinicians question their validity. For example, there are no interview schedules that assess for every *DSM-IV-TR* diagnostic label available. Diagnostic interviews must leave out important information about client personal history, personality style, and more (Bögels, 1994). Therefore, critics contend that two different interviewers may administer the same interview schedule and consistently come up with the same incorrect or inadequate diagnosis.

Because of the preceding disadvantages, formal diagnostic interviewing procedures are rarely used in actual clinical practice (Kronenberger & Meyer, 1996). Given their time-intensive requirements in combination with mental health provider needs for time-efficient evaluation and treatment, it is not surprising that diagnostic interviewing procedures are underutilized and sometimes unutilized in clinical practice. In reality, researchers and academicians studying the prevalence, course, prognosis, and treatment of mental disorders use these procedures almost exclusively.

## THE SCIENCE OF CLINICAL INTERVIEWING, PART II: DIAGNOSTIC RELIABILITY AND VALIDITY

As suggested in Chapter 6, the clinical interview is the cornerstone of diagnostic assessment. To put it bluntly, no self-respecting (or ethical) mental health professional would ever consider diagnosing a client without conducting a clinical interview. Nevertheless, the scientific question remains: Does a diagnostic interview provide reliable and valid diagnostic data and thereby conclusions?

In terms of judging the psychometric qualities of a given procedure, *reliability* refers to replicability and stability. If a procedure, such as a diagnostic interview, is reliable, it consistently produces the same result; two interviewers, interviewing the same client, would come up with the same clinical data and therefore the same diagnosis. Statistically speaking, it is a commonly agreed-on fact that an instrument or procedure must be reliable (it must produce reproducible results) for it to have a chance at being valid (producing a correct or truthful result). It is also possible for a diagnostic interview procedure to be highly reliable but invalid—as in the case where two or more interviewers consistently agree on diagnoses, but the diagnoses are incorrect.

In 1980, along with the publication of the *DSM-III,* many mental health professionals, especially psychiatrists, breathed a collective sigh of relief. Finally, after nearly 30 years of rampant subjectivity in diagnosis, there was a comprehensive and atheoretical system for objectively determining whether an individual suffered from a mental disorder. Even more importantly, there was now a clear system, complete with specific diagnostic criteria, for determining exactly what type of mental disorder an individual was suffering from. Shortly before and after its publication, the *DSM-III* was showered with praise. The reliability problem (the problem articulated by the fact that two different psychiatrists, seeing the same patient in a brief period of time, often disagreed about the proper diagnosis) was finally addressed; and in the minds of some mental health professionals, the reliability problem was solved (Klerman, 1984; Matarazzo, 1983; Spitzer, Forman, & Nee, 1979).

Unfortunately, as it turns out, *DSM*'s diagnostic reliability problem is far from solved. In their scathing critique of contemporary diagnosis, Kutchins and Kirk (1997) state:

> Twenty years after the reliability problem became the central scientific focus of *DSM*, there is still not a single major study showing that *DSM* (any version) is routinely used with high reliability by regular mental health clinicians. Nor is there any credible evidence that any version of the manual has greatly increased its reliability beyond the previous version. The *DSM* revolution in reliability has been a revolution in rhetoric, not in reality. (p. 53)

Granted, the position of Kutchins and Kirk (1997) is somewhat radical. However, even if we discount their arguments as the rantings of radical malcontents, we are still faced with the fact that mainstream and conservative researchers consistently question the reliability and validity of the *DSM* system. For example, in his review of *DSM* reliability studies, Segal (1997) reports on a number of studies that show both acceptable and marginal reliability. Keep in mind that these studies were designed and conducted for the sole purpose of demonstrating the diagnostic reliability of several different interview procedures (hardly any of which are ever really used by practicing clinicians). In the end, Segal does conclude that the "reliability rates" of diagnostic interviews are "now more acceptable" (p. 52). However, he also notes "that no 'quick fix' is currently available to ameliorate our currently severe validity problems" and ". . . for validity, structured interviews are tied to specific diagnostic criteria. Unfortunately, these interviews do not provide an estimate of how good the criteria actually are, and no diagnostic assessment device can compensate for poor criteria" (p. 28–29).

Overall, we can offer you the following scientifically supported conclusions:

- Generally, the diagnostic criteria for *DSM-IV* have more potential and, in many cases, have demonstrated higher levels of reliability than previous diagnostic nomenclatures.
- The more closely you stick to the *DSM* diagnostic criteria, the more likely you can produce reliable diagnoses, but even so, reliability among clinical practitioners is likely to be only moderate at best.
- The more formal training you receive in a specific diagnostic interviewing procedure, the more likely you are to produce reliable diagnoses.

There is, unfortunately, no gold standard in science for determining, in the end, that a particular diagnosis is valid.

## A BALANCED APPROACH TO CONDUCTING DIAGNOSTIC CLINICAL INTERVIEWS

Our position on diagnostic interviewing procedures should not be particularly surprising. We advocate a middle ground, recognizing that some interviewing texts and practitioners prefer to ignore or minimize the entire issue of diagnosis (Martin & Moore, 1995), whereas others promote diagnostic interviewing as the "main assessment tool in mental health care" (Bögels, 1994). As numerous authors and researchers have concluded, a basic understanding of diagnostic skills is part of standard practice for counselors, social workers, psychologists, and psychiatrists (Kronenberger & Meyer, 1996; Mead, Hohenshil, & Singh, 1997; J. Sommers-Flanagan & Sommers-Flanagan, 1998). On the other hand, paying too much attention to diagnosis risks losing track of our clients' unique, human qualities. A balanced diagnostic interview contains the following components:

1. An introduction characterized by warmth, role induction, and active listening. During this introduction, review of standardized questionnaires and intake/ referral information may occur.
2. An extensive review of client problems, associated goals, and a detailed analysis of the client's primary problem and goal. This should include questions about the client's symptoms, using the *DSM-IV-TR* as a guide.
3. A brief discussion of client personal experiences (personal history) relevant to the client's primary problem. This should include a history of the presenting problem if such a history has not already been conducted.
4. A brief mental status examination.
5. A review of client's current situation, including his or her social support network, coping skills, physical health, and personal strengths.

## Introduction and Role Induction

All clients should be greeted with warmth and compassion. The fact that our goal is to arrive at a diagnosis and devise a treatment plan should not change our interest in the client as a unique individual.

After reviewing confidentiality limits, skillful interviewers introduce the nature of a diagnostic interview to the client using a statement similar to the following:

"Today, we'll be working together to thoroughly understand whatever's been troubling you. This means I want you to talk freely with me, but also, I'll be asking lots of questions to clarify as precisely as possible what you've been experiencing. The better we're able to identify your main concerns, the better we'll be able to come up with a plan for resolving them. Does that sound okay to you?"

This statement emphasizes collaboration and deemphasizes pathology. The language "thoroughly understand" and "main concerns" are client-friendly ways of talking about diagnostic issues. The statement is a role induction wherein clients are educated regarding their responsibilities during the clinical interview. When clients understand what is expected of them, they are more helpful in allowing you to accomplish your interviewing goals. In addition, clients usually become engaged in the interviewing process when asked "Does that sound okay to you?" Rarely do clients respond to this collaborative question with "No! It doesn't sound okay to me!" If they do, you have instantly obtained important diagnostic information.

Throughout the interview, do not forget about using your active listening skills. As Shea and Mezzich (1988) have noted, interviewers in training often become too structured, thus almost excluding client spontaneity, or too unstructured, allowing the client to ramble. Remember to integrate listening and diagnostic questioning throughout the diagnostic interviewing process.

## Reviewing Client Problems

Although we covered client problem conceptualization systems in Chapter 7, we would like to reiterate a few basic issues in the diagnostic interviewing context. At minimum, a diagnostic interview should include an extensive review of client problems (and questioning about symptoms based on *DSM* diagnostic criteria), associated goals, and a detailed analysis of the client's primary problem and goal. While reviewing these areas with clients, there are several issues to consider and some to avoid.

### *Do Not Automatically Accept Your Client's Self-Diagnosis as Valid*

Many clients tell you about their symptoms by using a diagnostic label. For example:

> "Over the past three months, I've been so depressed. This depression has really been getting to me."
>
> "I just get these compulsive behaviors that I can't stop. I have no control over them."
>
> "Really, my main problem is panic. Whenever I'm out in public, I just freeze."

Some diagnostic terminology has been so popularized that it has lost its specificity. This is especially the case with regard to the term *depression.* Many people now use the word to describe themselves whenever feeling down or sad. The astute diagnostician recognizes that depression is a syndrome and not a mood state. In the preceding example, further questioning about sleep dysfunction, appetite or weight changes, concentration problems, and so on are necessary before concluding that a depressive syndrome is present.

Similarly, the lay public overuses the terms *compulsive* and *panic.* In diagnostic circles, compulsive behavior generally alerts the clinician to symptoms associated with either obsessive-compulsive disorder or obsessive-compulsive personality disorder. In contrast, many individuals with eating disorders and substance abuse disorders refer to their behaviors as *compulsive.* Once again, further questioning is needed before assuming that the client is suffering from a compulsive disorder. Finally, panic disorder is a very specific syndrome in *DSM-IV-TR.* However, many individuals with social phobias, agoraphobia, or public speaking anxiety talk about being frozen with panic. Therefore, although client use of the word *panic* should alert the interviewer to the possibility of an anxiety disorder, the appropriate diagnosis may not be panic disorder.

### *Keep Diagnostic Checklists Available*

When questioning clients about problems, it is crucial to keep *DSM-IV-TR* diagnostic criteria in the forefront of your mind. Unfortunately, few of us have a memory that allows for instant recall of diagnostic criteria. We recommend that you design checklists to aid in recalling specific *DSM-IV-TR* diagnostic criteria. Using homemade diagnostic checklists can help you become familiar with key diagnostic criteria, without necessarily committing them to memory. This simple procedure relieves you of the burden of memorizing 943 pages of diagnostic information.

### *Accept the Fact That You May Not Be Able to Accurately Diagnose after a Single Interview*

Sometimes, it is good to have high expectations and lofty goals. However, as cognitive theory and therapy has shown, unreasonably high expectations can set us up for frustration and disappointment (Blatt, Zuroff, Bondi, Sanislow, & Pitkonis, 1998; Norman, Davies, Nicholson, Cortese, & Malla, 1998). As a diagnostic interviewer, your job is to do the best you can to identify appropriate diagnostic labels. You will be aided in your task if you doggedly pursue and analyze your clients' problem-related symptoms. However, in many cases, partly because of inexperience and partly because of diagnostic complexity, you will be unable to assign an accurate diagnosis to a client after a single interview. In fact, you may leave the first interview more confused than when you began it. Fear not. The *DSM-IV-TR* provides practitioners with procedures for handling diagnostic uncertainty (see American Psychiatric Association, 2000, pp. 4–5). These procedures include:

*V codes: DSM-IV*-TR includes a number of V codes for indicating that the practitioner has insufficient information for identifying a mental disorder or indicating that the treatment is focusing on a problem that does not meet diagnostic criteria for a mental disorder. Examples include V61.20 (parent-child relational problem) and V62.82 (bereavement).

*Code 799.9:* This code may be used on either Axis I or Axis II and is labeled *Diagnosis or Condition Deferred.* It is used when information is inadequate to make any judgment about a diagnosis or condition.

*Code 300.9:* This code refers to *Unspecified Mental Disorder (nonpsychotic).* It is used when the diagnostician believes a nonpsychotic mental disorder is present, but does not have enough information to be more specific.

*Provisional diagnosis:* When a diagnostician provides a specific diagnosis followed by the word *provisional* in parentheses, it communicates a degree of uncertainty. A provisional diagnosis is a working diagnosis, indicating that additional information may modify the diagnosis.

## Client Personal History

At least a minimal social or developmental history information is necessary for accurate diagnosis. Take the assessment of clinical depression as an example. Currently, *DSM-IV-TR* lists numerous disorders that have depressive symptoms as one of their primary features, including (a) dysthymic disorder, (b) major depression, (c) adjustment disorder with mixed anxiety and depression, (d) adjustment disorder with depressed mood, (e) bipolar I disorder, (f) bipolar II disorder, and (g) cyclothymic disorder. Additionally, there are a number of disorders outside the general mood disorder category that include depressive-like symptoms or that are commonly comorbid with one of the previously listed depressive disorders. These include, but are not limited to: (a) posttraumatic stress disorder, (b) generalized anxiety disorder, (c) anorexia nervosa, (d) bulimia nervosa, and (e) conduct disorder. As you may have already concluded from this rather formidable list, the question is not necessarily whether depressive symptoms exist in a particular client, but rather, which depressive symptoms exist, in what context, and for how long? Without adequate historical information, interviewers are unable to discriminate between various depressive disorders and comorbid conditions.

Social and developmental history content areas are listed in Table 7.2 (see Chapter 7). It is up to the interviewer to select the areas to emphasize from this rather comprehensive list. Clients have different presenting problems and should be questioned primarily in areas relevant to their problems. Some practitioners have clients or parents of clients complete a developmental history questionnaire before or during the initial appointment.

Often, it is difficult to sift through massive amounts of client personal history information. Determining what information is important and which questions to ask is a daunting task. Putting It in Practice 10.1 includes a case conceptualization that may assist you in organizing your thinking about what client information is relevant to treatment.

---

**Putting It in Practice 10.1**

## Case Conceptualization and Theoretical Orientation

One of the guiding forces determining what information is valued by interviewers and counselors is theoretical orientation. Although it may be too soon for you to identify your theoretical orientation, you may find yourself having particular leanings. The following questions are designed to help you explore your theoretical perspective, and at the same time, develop greater focus during your interviewing assessments and treatment planning. While answering the questions, keep in mind a few cases with which you have worked or cases that have been discussed in class.

1. How would you define your theory of therapy? In other words, what processes do you believe must occur for people to change? As you think of a particular case, how would your theory of therapy influence the information you want to obtain from your client?
2. Given your response to question 1, what is your theory of etiology? In other words, what causes or contributes to individuals' personal problems? Again, what information does this make you to want to obtain from your client?
3. What factors do you believe play a strong role in symptom maintenance? What client information do you need to have to understand symptom maintenance?
4. Given your theoretical perspective, what are your usual treatment goals and plans for your individual client?
5. What intuitive reactions do you have when imagining yourself working with this particular case? How would you let your intuition guide or influence your assessment and treatment plan?

---

### Mental Status Examination

As emphasized in Chapter 8, mental status examinations are not the same as diagnostic interviews and should not be considered a diagnostic procedure per se. However, a review of client current mental state provides information crucial to accurate diagnosis. In particular, mental status exam information can help you determine whether substance use is an immediate factor affecting client consciousness and functioning. Mental status examinations also inform you of client thinking and perceptual processes that may be associated with particular diagnostic conditions.

### Current Situation

As discussed in Chapter 7, obtaining information about a client's current functioning is a standard part of the intake interview. With regard to diagnostic interviewing, a few significant issues should be reviewed and emphasized.

A detailed review of your client's current situation includes an evaluation of his or her social support network, coping skills, physical health (if this area has not been covered during a medical history), and personal strengths. Each of these areas may provide information crucial to the diagnostic process.

## Client Social Support Network

Sometimes, it is critical to obtain diagnostic information from people other than the client, especially when interviewing children and adolescents. In such cases, parents are often interviewed as part of the diagnostic work-up (see Chapter 11 for more detailed information regarding interviewing young clients and their parents). However, even when interviewing adults, it may be necessary to obtain outside information to substantiate diagnostic impressions. To rely exclusively on a single clinical interview to establish a diagnosis may be inappropriate and unprofessional. As Morrison (1993) has stated:

> Adults can also be unaware of their family histories or details about their own development. Patients with psychosis or personality disorder may not have enough perspective to judge accurately many of their own symptoms. In any of these situations, the history you obtain from people who know your patient well may strongly influence your diagnosis. (p. 203)

Information obtained from people other than your client is often referred to as *information from collateral informants.*

## Client Coping Skills Assessment

Assessing client coping skills provides an excellent opportunity for determining what approaches clients have used to manage their personal distress or personal problems. For example, clients with anxiety disorders frequently use avoidance strategies to reduce their anxiety (e.g., agoraphobics do not leave their homes; individuals with claustrophobia stay away from stuffy rooms or enclosed spaces). In contrast, clients with dissociative disorders are likely to completely block out their painful emotional experiences. It is important to examine whether clients are coping with their problems and moving toward mastery or simply reacting to their problems and thereby exacerbating their symptoms and/or restricting themselves from social or vocational activities.

Coping skills also may be assessed by using projective techniques or behavior observation. Projective techniques are employed when interviewers have their clients imagine a particular stressful scenario (sometimes referred to as a simulation), and behavioral observations may be collected either in an interviewer office or in some outside setting (e.g., school, home, workplace). As noted previously, collateral informants may provide important information regarding how clients cope when outside your office.

## Physical Examination

In virtually every case, a conclusive psychiatric diagnosis cannot be achieved without at least a cursory medical examination. Interviewers should always inquire about most recent physical examination results when interviewing new clients. Some therapists inquire about most recent physical examination results on their intake form.

Physical and mental states often have powerful and reciprocal influences on each other. Consider the following options when completing a diagnostic work-up:

1. Gathering information about physical examination results.
2. Consulting with the client's primary care physician.
3. Referring clients for a physical examination.

It is our professional obligation to make sure potential medical or physical causes or contributors to mental disorders are adequately investigated.

### Client Strengths

Clients who come for professional assistance often have lost sight of their personal strengths and positive qualities. Furthermore, after experiencing an hour-long diagnostic interview, clients may feel sad or demoralized. It is important to ask clients to identify and comment on some of their positive personal qualities throughout the interview, but especially toward the end of an assessment/diagnostic process. For example:

> "Throughout this interview today, we've been talking mostly about your problems and symptoms. Obviously, talking about these problems tells me a lot about your suffering, but it doesn't tell me much about your personal strengths. So, before we finish today, tell me about some of your good qualities . . . things you like about yourself."

Exploring client strengths provides important diagnostic information. Clients who are more depressed and demoralized have trouble with this question and may not be able to identify any personal strengths. Be sure to provide support, reassurance, and positive feedback. In addition, as the solution-oriented theorists emphasize, do not forget that diagnosis and assessment procedures can—and should—include a consistent orientation toward the positive. For example, Bertolino and O'Hanlon (2002) state:

> Formal assessment procedures are often viewed solely as a means of uncovering and discovering deficiencies and deviancies with clients and their lives. However, as we've learned, they can assist with learning about clients' abilities, strength, and resources, and in searching for exceptions and differences. (p. 79)

Effective diagnostic interviewing is not necessarily an exclusively fact-finding, impersonal process. Throughout the interview, skilled diagnosticians express compassion and support for a fellow human being in distress (Othmer & Othmer, 1994). The purpose of diagnostic interviewing goes beyond simply establishing a diagnosis or "pigeonhole" for our client. Instead, it is an initial step in developing an individualized treatment plan for a person in need.

## TREATMENT PLANNING

*Treatment planning* refers to a procedure outlining therapeutic techniques and processes as they are applied to individual clients. Developing a treatment plan involves deciding which therapy techniques to use to accomplish a specific set of treatment goals and objectives. Not surprisingly, as managed care approaches to mental health treatment have increased in popularity and therapists have greater accountability for treatment outcomes, careful planning and problem delineation have become increasingly central psychological treatment components (Jongsma & Peterson, 1995).

The purpose of this section is to introduce beginning mental health therapists to approaches for developing treatment plans for (and with) clients. Before conducting clinical interviews and beginning mental health treatment with clients, try to become familiar with treatment planning models and methodologies. Your theoretical orientation and treatment planning preferences, along with the client's needs and presenting problem(s), will very much influence your first contact with clients.

## Treating Client Problems versus Treating Client Diagnoses

Although there are many approaches to developing and formulating client treatment plans, two contrasting models are important to understand.

### Psychosocial Treatment Planning

The first approach focuses on identifying client problems or symptoms and consequently developing treatment strategies for helping clients resolve identified problems. To accomplish this task, therapists conduct a problem-focused initial intake interview. The intake interview follows the model described in Chapter 7, wherein client and interviewer collaboratively explore: (a) what brings the client to therapy (presenting problem and initial goals), (b) the client's personality style and personal history (the person), and (c) the client's current life circumstances (the situation). After exploring these fundamental issues, therapy goals are established interactively with the client and a plan for goal attainment is developed. This approach is characterized by a greater emphasis on collaborative identification of client problems and a lesser emphasis on establishing a definitive psychiatric diagnosis. As such, we refer to this approach as the *psychosocial treatment planning model.* This particular treatment planning model can also be modified to focus primarily on solutions and goals, rather than problems (McNeilly, 2000).

### Medical Treatment Planning

The medical or psychiatric approach to conceptualizing client problems and identifying client treatments has increased in popularity in recent years (Eagen, 1994; Kramer, 1993; Sanua, 1996). This approach involves interviewers performing diagnostic assessments on their clients and then recommending specific treatment interventions based on diagnostic assessment results. In this second approach, the interviewer is the expert who knows *DSM-IV-TR* diagnostic criteria and related efficacy research and applies this knowledge or expertise accordingly. This approach emphasizes accurate diagnostic labeling, a primary purpose of which is to assist in identification of possible medications for treatment. Because of the strong emphasis on biological/medical issues, we refer to this approach as the *medical treatment planning model* (E. L. Zuckerman, 2000).

In practice, most therapists recognize that integrating psychosocial and biological treatment planning approaches is useful and do so to some extent. However, many practitioners lean toward one approach or the other. The key difference is whether client-identified problems or therapist-identified diagnoses primarily influence treatment planning. Either approach is acceptable, depending on your setting. As Jongsma and Peterson (1995) have noted, sometimes managed care companies are more interested in behavioral problem indices than in diagnoses. However, when working with insurance companies or managed care organizations, treatment plans that emphasize psychosocial problems and goals must also provide diagnostic labels. A recent survey confirms that most counselors consider diagnostic labeling as especially important for both insurance billing and treatment planning (Mead et al., 1997).

## AN INTEGRATED (BIOPSYCHOSOCIAL) APPROACH TO TREATMENT PLANNING

The treatment planning approach that follows is an integrated or biopsychosocial treatment planning model. With this model, our goal is to respect the reality and utility of diagnoses, while at the same time respecting clients' unique personal experiences. The model draws from previous writing and research on treatment planning (i.e., Jongsma & Peterson, 1995; Jongsma, Peterson, & McInnis, 1996; L. Seligman, 1996).

### Determining Appropriate Treatments

The process of identifying appropriate treatments requires that interviewers consider the following information:

*Client problem and empirical research:* Depending on client problems and diagnosis, there may be published outcome research outlining effective treatment approaches. Unfortunately, in most cases, research does not definitively indicate which treatment approach is most effective with specific client problems (Castonguay, 2000; M. E. P. Seligman & Levant, 1998). Although some guidelines are available (e.g., cognitive therapy for bulimia and panic disorder; behavior therapy and medications for agoraphobia; interpersonal therapy, cognitive-behavioral therapy, and medications for unipolar depression), clear empirical treatment mandates have yet to be established for most mental disorders.

*Client problem and treatment literature:* Reputable scholarly journals and treatment books in clinical psychology, clinical social work, counseling, and psychiatry provide important treatment information in the form of case studies, short reports, outcome studies, and reasoned theoretical discussions regarding treatment choices.

*Therapist skill or expertise:* The treatment plan must use an approach in which the therapist has education, training, experience, and previous or current supervision. For example, if the therapist has no training or experience in a particular treatment technique (e.g., hypnosis or eye movement desensitization reprocessing), that technique should not be employed.

*Therapist preference:* Mental health professionals vary in their theoretical orientations. Some adhere to psychoanalytic treatment formulations; others are behavioral in their approach to treatment. Although it may be inappropriate at times, clients are sometimes offered whatever treatment approach a given therapist prefers.

*Client preference:* Given the choice, clients may prefer one form of treatment over another. For example, some clients struggling with maladaptive habits prefer short-term, specific behavioral therapy to successfully change the habit. Others prefer depth work, seeking understanding of the purpose the habit served in their lives, while still others prefer medication treatment. Client treatment preference can have a strong influence on client cooperation or compliance with treatment.

### Designing a Treatment Plan

Subsequent to a reasonably thorough diagnostic assessment, interviewers should outline, based on the assessment data obtained, an individualized client treatment plan. As noted by Jongsma and Peterson (1995), assessment data form the foundation of treatment plans: "The foundation of any effective treatment plan is the data gathered in a thorough biopsychosocial assessment" (p. 3). This fact is not likely to be disputed. After gathering a plethora of assessment data, the challenging question is: On what part of the assessment data shall we base our treatment plan?

There are many answers to this question. As we reviewed earlier in this text, Lazarus (1976) might suggest that we organize our treatment plan along the lines of his BASIC ID multimodal therapeutic formulation. Linda Seligman (1996) suggests the acronym DO A CLIENT MAP, which captures the major elements of her formulation of an adequate treatment plan (see Table 10.2). A third approach to treatment planning is presented by Jongsma and Peterson (1995) in their psychotherapy treatment planner for adults. They include the following treatment planning steps:

*Problem selection:* Selecting a problem, or perhaps two or three problems, collaboratively with the client, to focus on in counseling is essential. Although many problems may exist at the outset of counseling, clear choices must be made regarding treatment focus. A good treatment plan always includes a clearly stated problem.

*Problem definition:* Jongsma and Peterson (1995) include numerous behavioral definitions for 34 different problems in their treatment planner. Their approach emphasizes establishing an operational or behavioral definition for each problem listed in the treatment plan. Operational definitions, especially when linked with *DSM-IV-TR* diagnostic criteria, are used to help move therapy toward a definable and measurable outcome.

*Goal development:* In the context of this approach, long-term goals can be global descriptions of positive outcomes. For example, Jongsma and Peterson (1995) list the problem (e.g., impulse control disorder), a problem definition ("Pattern of impulsively pulling out hair leading to significant hair loss"; p. 72), and then a long-term goal ("Establish the ability to effectively channel impulses"; p. 73).

*Objective construction:* Objectives are short-term goals, cast in behaviorally measurable language. From the preceding example, objectives could include "Decrease the overall frequency of impulsive actions" or "Increase the ability for self-observation" (Jongsma & Peterson, 1995, p. 73). For managed care or insurance

**Table 10.2.   DO A CLIENT MAP Treatment Planning Model**

*Diagnosis*

*Objectives* of treatment

*Assessments* needed (e.g., neurological or personality tests)

*Clinician* characteristics viewed as therapeutic

*Location of treatment* (e.g., hospital or outpatient setting)

*Interventions* to be used

*Emphasis* of treatment (level of directiveness; level of supportiveness; cognitive, behavioral or affective emphasis)

*Nature* of treatment (individual, couple, family, or group)

*Timing* (frequency, pacing, duration)

*Medications* that may be needed

*Adjunct* services (e.g., support groups, legal advice, or education)

*Prognosis*

*Note.* From L. Seligman (1996), *Diagnosis and Treatment Planning in Counseling* (2nd ed.), New York: Plenum Press. Reprinted with permission.

providers, it is essential to have measurable objectives to justify continued treatment or treatment termination.

*Intervention creation:* The authors recommend including at least one intervention for each treatment objective. An intervention related to the previous goal and objectives might involve the client's using self-monitoring strategies to identify when hair-pulling impulses arise and repeated rehearsal and practice of more adaptive behavioral alternatives.

*Diagnosis determination:* While addressing diagnosis, this treatment planning guide leans toward the psychosocial model referred to earlier in this chapter. Diagnosis is seen as an important step, but is less influential in treatment planning than problem identification and selection. In the example we have been discussing, an appropriate diagnostic label is *DSM-IV-TR Axis I: 312.39 trichotillomania.*

Most treatment planning approaches are useful because they provide an organizing framework for the material you and your client must consider in charting a course for your work together. In addition, The Complete Psychotherapy Treatment Planner (Jongsma & Peterson, 1995), from which the previously described steps were taken, gives you a valuable way to make sure you have covered the basics likely to be required by managed care companies, even if the actual chosen treatment includes components not mentioned in the planner. Jongsma and Peterson's model has the advantage of being simple, straightforward, and relatively easy to learn. Putting It in Practice 10.2 includes a case example for rehearsing your treatment planning skills.

Our own amalgamation of these various treatment planning aids follows:

---

**Putting It in Practice 10.2**

## Treatment Planning: Application

You are working with Michael, a 26-year-old African American male. He is single, has a bachelor's degree in business management, and is employed as a manager at a local appliance store. He reports a history of hypertension (high blood pressure), which is well-managed using medication. During the session, he complains that although he can work with his employee team effectively and regularly meet individual and team sales goals, he has a long history of heterosexual social anxiety. He also claims he can socialize outside work without significant problems. When asked what he would like to accomplish in counseling, he states, "I want to have a date at least a couple times a month, and I want to ask the person out on the date without feeling like I'm going to have a heart attack every time I start to approach her." Michael also reports intermittent insomnia, muscular tension, and increased irritability, all three of which worsened after his mother passed away nine months ago. Develop a treatment plan for Michael using Jongsma and Peterson's (1995) model. *Note:* You may target one or more problems for Michael's treatment.

Step 1    Problem Selection:

Step 2    Problem Definition:

Step 3    Goal Development:

Step 4    Objective Construction:

Step 5    Intervention Creation:

Step 6    Diagnosis Determination:

1. Gain the most complete understanding of client problem(s) possible, given the limits of time; client expressive abilities; and client awareness. Use Lazarus's (1976) BASIC ID or some other guide to remind you of the many complex aspects of a client in need of assistance. Often, we use a model that includes a review of (a) social, (b) cognitive, (c) emotional, (d) physical, (e) behavioral, and (f) cultural aspects of the individual's functioning.

2. Gain the most complete understanding of your client's goal(s) that you can. Ask clients what their life would look like if things were better. What would be a tolerable outcome? What would be the best imaginable outcome? Sometimes, projective questions such as de Shazer's (1985) "miracle question" help clients articulate their goals (i.e., "Imagine tonight while you sleep, a miracle happens and your problem is solved. What will be happening the next day, and how will you know that your problem is solved?").

3. Do your homework, part one: Go over what you know about your clients and their problems. Ask yourself what you still need to know to fill in any crucial gaps and make every effort to obtain this information. If you have time limits regarding when you must have your treatment plan completed (e.g., after session one), you may need to ask clients to wait for a minute or two as you sort through the information they have given you. Then, moving back to a collaborative mode, summarize your thoughts about primary and secondary problems and establish a provisional treatment plan.

4. Do your homework, part two: After the session, review a short list of viable treatment options, given what you know from your problem conceptualization and client goal statements. If you are unable to identify clear and appropriate treatment interventions, read, consult, and, if needed, obtain supervision. At that point, you can rank-order the intervention alternatives and present them to your client during session two.

5. Develop meaningful objectives that help both you and your client know if you are moving toward the goal(s). Do this collaboratively with your client.

6. Frequently check in with clients regarding how therapy is progressing. Even if one of your central objectives is simply developing a healthy working alliance, check with clients regarding their perception of your work together. Clients are empowered by being asked if things are moving in the direction they imagined, hoped for, or need. Research supports the importance of an ongoing working alliance for treatment success (Gaston, 1990; Hubble et al., 1999; Raue et al., 1997).

7. Plan for termination at the outset of treatment. If a specified number of sessions are available, note this and use it constructively in all phases of your therapy work together. Research indicates that having a time limit can sometimes help clients reach their therapy goals (Barkham et al., 1996; Steenbarger, 1994). Regardless, termination is an important aspect of mental health work and should be addressed throughout the counseling relationship.

8. When termination occurs, follow a model for appropriate therapeutic termination (see Barnett, 1998; J. Sommers-Flanagan & Sommers-Flanagan, 1997, for termination guidelines).

## Treatment Planning R & R

Absent from most standard models for treatment planning are two very important dimensions that ethical mental health professionals must keep in mind as the treatment plan takes form. Although it would be nice if our R & R acronym represented Rest & Relaxation, both of which are essential for clinical interviewers, such is not the case. When we refer to *treatment planning R & R,* we are referring to *Resources and Relationship.*

On the surface, the *resources* dimension of our R & R formula is very pragmatic and is simply a fact of life in current medical and social policies and practices. It can be a delicate matter in some cases and an ethical matter in others, but it is fairly easy to assess. The *relationship* dimension is maddeningly difficult to measure, control, or define, and yet it plays an enormous role in treatment choice and outcome.

### Resources

Counseling, therapy, psychotherapy, psychoanalysis, and/or psychiatric consultation each cost a significant amount of money. Some clients have insurance. Some have health management organizations, preferred provider plans, Medicaid, Medicare, employee assistance programs, and so on. Each of these health care programs has specific benefits for mental health care coverage and specific limitations. The client's health care coverage and the resources available after the coverage runs out are important practical and ethical considerations in charting a treatment plan.

Some may assume that the fastest possible course for specific symptom alleviation or relief is the best, most ethical choice, no matter what the client's resources. However, as with everything else in mental health work, the bottom line is complex. Efficacy and consumer research clearly indicate that therapy is mostly a good thing (M. Seligman, 1995; M. Smith et al., 1980): It can help with simple problems in living; and it can help with deeper, more entrenched, and disturbing behaviors. Except in involuntary clients, people generally report that being in counseling is beneficial (Herman, 1998; M. Seligman, 1995; Yu & Watkins, 1996). It seems safe to speculate that at least some clients, and perhaps many, would stay in counseling and benefit from doing so for much longer than their financial or health care resources allow (M. Seligman, 1995). Therefore, resources simply must be considered and, as such, they must in part guide problem-selection and goal-setting processes.

Unfortunately, considering available resources does not mean simply picking a problem that fits into the number of paid sessions available or the number of sessions a client can budget from private funds. Certainly, it is important to clarify primary and secondary problems (Jongsma & Peterson, 1995) and to recognize that, quite often, not all problems can be addressed in a given course of treatment. Ethically, the counselor is bound to choose effective treatment and to see the client through to some kind of responsible closure or transfer (ACA, 1995; American Psychological Association, 1992). Therefore, in agreeing to a course of treatment, you must assess your own resources as well, including availability, willingness to reduce fees, adequate referral network, appropriate supervision, and access to collateral professionals (attorneys, medical personnel, etc.).

Besides the resources represented in finances and insurance benefits, and the resources represented in the person and practice of the professional, there are other resources to be considered in treatment planning. These include client motivation, ego strength, and psychological mindedness of the client. It is your duty to assess, either formally or informally, each client's capacity to engage in treatment.

## CASE EXAMPLE

*Opal, a 63-year-old Caucasian woman, was referred for counseling by her family practice physician. She was referred because of repeated panic attacks. Her life history was rich and varied in many fascinating respects. The biggest trauma she disclosed was the death of her oldest daughter to breast cancer two years earlier. This daughter, Emily, had been a strong, feminist woman with a successful career who had often chided her mother for her "old-fashioned, subservient ways." Opal was married to her third husband, a farmer named Jeff. Jeff was quite wealthy and very traditional in his views of marriage. Opal's job was to keep the house clean, prepare meals that met with Jeff's approval, and "keep herself presentable." Her panic attacks began about six months before the referral and, at first, happened exclusively outside grocery stores as Opal was preparing to buy the week's groceries. Opal was forced to seek a neighbor's assistance in obtaining groceries because Jeff refused to be seen in a grocery store.*

*After three sessions devoted primarily to assessment and preliminary psychoeducational work regarding panic attack management, the counselor developed enough of a relationship with Opal to suspect that she would not do well with depth work regarding her grief, her conflicts over her marital role, and other related issues. However, it seemed important to involve Opal in this treatment determination. The counselor explained two treatment options: (a) continue training to manage the panic attacks with behavioral strategies, imagery, and medication or (b) begin more depth work, exploring the meaning of the panic attacks and their possible linkage to role conflicts, and perhaps even looking at Opal's deep and mostly buried grief and anger over losing her daughter. Without hesitation, Opal indicated she had no interest in any depth work unless it was absolutely necessary.*

*The treatment plan continued along cognitive-behavioral lines. After eight more sessions, Opal resumed grocery shopping on her own. She left therapy feeling a sense of accomplishment and closure. She assured the counselor she would be back if "things didn't hang together in her head."*

As this case illustrates, mental problems, disorders, and disturbances in living are multilayered and complex. The people involved have varying levels of potential and motivation for psychological insight and depth. These issues must be taken into consideration in treatment planning.

Finally, with regard to resources, the pressure to efficiently and quickly treat presenting problems must be mitigated by professional commitment to our clients' welfare and our professional integrity. Sometimes, the stated, initial problem suggests a straightforward treatment that, if implemented and held to, would miss a major portion of the "real" problem.

## CASE EXAMPLE

*Jane came to see a counselor because she was worrying excessively about her 3-year-old daughter, Kate. Jane had picked Kate up from day care approximately a month earlier, and Kate had said, "Mommy, I hate it when they stick yucky things in my mouth." Jane experienced a rush of fear and carefully questioned Kate, afraid that someone at the day care had abused or violated Kate. Kate, clearly alarmed by her mother's reaction, refused to talk about day care. This interaction unleashed all sorts of worries for Jane. She found that she could no longer leave Kate at day care and was paying for an in-home nanny. Finances were strained. In addition, Jane would no longer allow Kate to play with her boy cousins or her older half-brother. This was causing marital strain. Finally, Jane was having trouble allowing Kate to be out of her sight, which was, as Jane said, "making everyone totally crazy."*

*Directly addressing Jane's behavior by pointing out the irrational nature of her fears and urging her to create a chart and reward herself for leaving Kate for longer and longer periods were treatment options in this case. In addition, these options might stand a good chance of changing Jane's presenting problem. However, as many astute readers might have guessed, Jane's sudden inordinate attention to her daughter and her self-declared overreactions were clues to an important unaddressed life experience of Jane's. Jane had been sexually molested by her uncle at age 4. She remembered the uncle kissing her and fondling her, often forcing his tongue down her throat, but she had never told anyone about her experiences, including her husband.*

*Jane was able to access community support groups for adults who had been molested as children. She used her therapy time carefully, exploring her tendencies to ignore her own pain and put up tough, hard-driving defenses. Although it may have helped in the short run, addressing Jane's surface wish to leave her daughter alone for longer periods would have blatantly missed Jane's more pressing needs.*

The two case examples illustrate the complexities of assessing client resources and preferences as they relate to treatment planning. However, such assessment must be based on information that comes from the working alliance, or therapeutic relationship, between the people involved. This important fact brings us to the other *R* in the treatment planning R & R. A multicultural case example is provided in Individual and Cultural Highlight 10.1.

## Relationship

The *C* in L. Seligman's (1996) mnemonic DO A CLIENT MAP (see Table 10.2) represents "Clinician characteristics viewed as therapeutic." This is as close to swinging the spotlight on the therapist as most treatment planning models get. Seligman consistently focuses on professional and personality attributes of the clinician that are necessary in a well-developed treatment plan in her book *Selecting Effective Treatments* (1998). To be comprehensive, treatment planning must include the person of the therapist in the equation. For example, when you use bibliotherapy as a treatment adjunct, the books you recommend should be books you have read yourself and can personally or professionally endorse. Also, the techniques you use must feel authentic and helpful, not contrived or simplistic. The homework you assign should be in the realm of something you would consider doing yourself, if you were faced with a problem similar to your client's. If this is not the case, and you find yourself willing merely to match a set of techniques with a set of problems, you are violating not only your client's humanity—you are violating your own. Just as the treatment plan must strive to include all relevant aspects of the client, the treatment plan equation must include you as a caring, informed professional. If it does not, your clients sense it, and the working alliance never develops to any significant extent.

In case we have not made our biases and values clear, consider this: Even with respect to diagnosis and treatment planning, mental health work is about human relationships. If, in the process of diagnosing or formulating, planning, and goal setting, we lose contact with our clients as unique human beings, we risk missing their real needs and causing damage. If, in this same process, we lose contact with ourselves as unique, complex human beings as well as professionals, we diminish our work and the potential of our profession.

========= INDIVIDUAL AND CULTURAL HIGHLIGHT 10.1 =========

## Cultural Issues in Treatment Planning: A Case Example

Often, client cultural issues take center stage in treatment planning. The following very brief example is adapted and summarized from "The Case of Dolores" (R. Sommers-Flanagan, 2001, in Paniagua, 2001).

Dolores, a 43-year-old American Indian woman, came to counseling because she was suffering from sadness, inability to concentrate, insomnia, and anhedonia. These depressive symptoms were associated with two major concerns. First, Dolores was very upset because her husband of 23 years, Gabe, was suffering from a serious gambling addiction but was refusing to go to treatment. Second, Dolores was worried that, because of her diminished functioning and her husband's gambling, she might lose custody of her adopted daughter, Sage.

Even with the minimal information provided in this example, several cultural issues rise to the fore. Specifically, because Dolores's major concerns center around family issues, it is important to explore the onset and duration of her concerns in the context of familism—as Dolores's symptoms might be more directly associated with her family identity than with her "self." Additionally, it could be that the decision to come to counseling was producing nearly as much stress as her family situation because some American Indian tribes consider it disloyal to say negative things about other family members. Consequently, Dolores's feelings about counseling and what it says about her Indian identity (or about her losing her Indian identity) may be a major focus of treatment—especially if she is seeing a counselor from the dominant culture.

Dolores's fears of losing her adopted daughter also bring up cultural issues. In this case, the adoption was an informal tribal arrangement, and she may need to consult with legal professionals and her tribe to determine if the adoption is binding. It is likely that the U.S. government would support the adoption placement under the Indian Child Welfare Act (O'Brien, 1989); therefore, communication with her tribe is probably more important than exposing Dolores to the U.S. legal system. Finally, although to some counselors it may seem that Dolores's anxiety about losing her child is overblown, historically, American Indians have experienced intergenerational trauma when children are taken from families. Hence, Dolores's feelings about those historical facts (and personal experiences) should be evaluated before effort to reduce her anxiety proceeds.

In summary, for American Indian and other multicultural clients, treatment planning should be culture specific and culture sensitive. For example, the following treatment planning statements might be formulated:

- Explore Dolores's feelings about pursuing counseling.
- Explore what Dolores is thinking and feeling when she makes negative statements about her family members.
- Educate Dolores regarding the Indian Child Welfare Act.
- Encourage Dolores to discuss her custody fears with members of her tribe and possibly a tribal lawyer.
- Discuss Dolores's fears of losing her daughter in the context of multigenerational trauma.

## SUMMARY

This chapter addresses the basics of diagnosing mental disorders. Controversies regarding this process abound, but there are important reasons for all mental health professionals to develop their diagnostic skills. A diagnosis can serve an organizing function and thereby facilitate treatment planning and treatment process. It can be seen as a working hypothesis and can offer clients relief by assuring them that others suffer with similar reactions, struggles, and complaints.

Interviewers should use a balanced approach to conducting diagnostic interviews, including (a) a warm introduction to diagnostic assessment with an explanation of what the client should expect; (b) an extensive review of client problems and associated goals; (c) a brief review of client personal history, especially those historical experiences closely associated with the client's primary problem; (d) a brief mental status examination; and (e) a review of the client's current situation, including social supports, coping skills, physical health, and personal strengths. In the diagnostic interviewing context, no one can be expected to keep all diagnostic parameters in mind. Interviewers are encouraged to purchase or develop their own abbreviated diagnostic checklists so they can adequately address the specific domains in question for a certain diagnostic inquiry.

Treatment planning flows directly from diagnosis or problem analysis. Professionals can use psychosocial approaches to treatment planning, wherein the problem complex is the guide for treatment goals and objectives; or they can use the medical or biological approach, wherein symptoms are categorized into a diagnosis, which then dictates treatment choice. It is also possible to combine these two and use a biopsychosocial approach, which includes diagnosis but also addresses specific symptoms and problems interactively with the client.

Treatment planning involves identifying reasonable goals and objectives to be pursued in therapy. Choosing effective treatments involves analysis of several client and counselor variables, including client and counselor personal resources as well as nonspecific relationship factors.

## SUGGESTED READINGS AND RESOURCES

Numerous publications focus on training practitioners to use *DSM-IV* as a diagnostic guide and as a guide to psychological treatment. There are also many publications available on treatment planning. The following list is limited in scope but provides some ideas for further reading and study.

Frances, A., & Ross, R. (1996). *DSM-IV case studies: A clinical guide to differential diagnosis.* Washington, DC: American Psychiatric Association. Often, diagnosticians develop their skills from working through individual cases that present in a puzzling or challenging manner. This *DSM-IV* training book provides readers with numerous cases designed to enhance diagnostic skill.

Jongsma, A. E. (2001). *The adult psychotherapy progress notes planner.* New York: John Wiley & Sons. This book provides guidelines and samples for writing progress notes.

Jongsma, A. E., & Peterson, M. (2000). *The complete adolescent psychotherapy treatment planner.* New York: John Wiley & Sons. This book is one of a series of treatment planners written by Jongsma and Peterson and designed to aid clinicians in developing treatment plans for specific populations.

Jongsma, A. E., & Peterson, M. (1999). *The complete adult psychotherapy treatment planner.* New York: John Wiley & Sons. This book is the latest adult version of Jongsma and Peterson's series of psychotherapy treatment planners. Their series of publications in this area is voluminous and often used by practicing clinicians to help with treatment planning formulation.

Kutchins, H., & Kirk, S. A. (1997). *Making us crazy: DSM: The psychiatric bile and the creation of mental disorders.* New York: Free Press. In this book, the authors provide a strong critique of the development and promotion of the *DSM* system as a method of categorizing mental disorders. In particular, the chapters on homosexuality and racism are enlightening reading for budding mental health professionals.

Leahy, R. L., & Holland, S. J. (2000). *Treatment plans and interventions for depression and anxiety disorders.* New York: Guilford. This is a book and a CD-ROM with empirically supported cognitive-behavioral treatments for seven frequently encountered depressive and anxiety disorders. The educational package includes client handouts, homework sheets, diagnostic flow-charts, and facts about commonly prescribed medications.

McLean, P. D., & Woody, S. R. (2001). *Anxiety disorders in adults: An evidence-based approach to psychological treatment.* London: Oxford University Press. Consistent with the movements emphasizing empirically validated treatments, this book reviews evidence-based treatments, and practice parameters in psychiatry and psychology. It focuses exclusively on treatments for anxiety disorders.

Nathan, P. E., & Gorman, J. M. (1998). *A guide to treatments that work.* New York: Oxford University Press. This guidebook reviews treatment outcomes research and clinical lore to provide readers with an evaluation of current drug and psychotherapeutic methods that are effective. The book also identifies treatments that are, at this time, known to be ineffective.

Rapoport, J., & Ismond, D. R. (1996). *DSM-IV training guide for diagnosis of childhood disorders.* New York: Brunner/Mazel. This handbook offers guidance for practitioners who use the *DSM-IV* for diagnosing psychiatric conditions occurring usually in childhood and adolescence. Case vignettes are used to demonstrate the application of *DSM-IV* diagnostic criteria and guidelines.

Reid, W. H., & Wise, M. G. (1995). *DSM-IV training guide.* Washington, DC: American Psychiatric Association. This is the training guide designed to accompany *DSM-IV.*

Rogers, R. (2001). *Handbook of diagnostic and structured interviewing.* New York: Guilford. This text includes reviews and research perspectives on many different approaches to diagnostic and structured interviewing with mental health clients.

Roth, A., & Fonagy, P. (1996). *What works for whom? A critical review of psychotherapy research.* New York: Guilford. This is a comprehensive review of the status of psychotherapy research. It includes evaluations of various therapeutic interventions for addressing symptoms associated with various *DSM-IV* diagnostic categories.

# PART FOUR

# INTERVIEWING SPECIAL POPULATIONS

# Chapter 11

# *INTERVIEWING YOUNG CLIENTS*

> *Mr. Quimby wiped a plate and stacked it in the cupboard. "I'm taking an art course, because I want to teach art. And I'll study child development—"*
> *Ramona interrupted. "What's child development?"*
> *"How kids grow," answered her father.*
> *Why does anyone have to go to school to study a thing like that? wondered Ramona. All her life she had been told that the way to grow was to eat good food, usually food she didn't like, and get plenty of sleep, usually when she had more interesting things to do than go to bed.*
>
> —Beverly Cleary, *Ramona Quimby, Age 8* (1981, pp. 15–16)

---

## CHAPTER OBJECTIVES

As our young clients often remind us, you don't have to know much to realize that interacting with children and teens is often strikingly different from interacting with adults. In this chapter, we provide practical recommendations for interviewing young clients. After reading this chapter, you will know:

- Several special considerations for interviewing children and adolescents.
- How you can modify your interactions—and sometimes even your clothing—to make a good first impression with young clients.
- How to discuss confidentiality, informed consent, referral information, and assessment and therapy procedures with youth.
- A specific technique for talking with young clients about therapy goals.
- User-friendly assessment and information-gathering strategies.
- Methods for reassuring, supporting, and empowering youth.
- Important issues to address when ending sessions with young clients.

---

To this point, our primary focus has been on interviewing, assessment, and treatment planning with individual adult clients. However, young people present the interviewer with challenges and opportunities that are quite different than those presented by adults. In this chapter, we explore the unique considerations and interviewing procedures necessary for mental health professionals who work with young clients. We also describe difficulties associated with interviewing young clients and suggest strategies for addressing these difficulties.

## SPECIAL CONSIDERATIONS IN WORKING WITH CHILDREN

When working with children, it can be hard to stay balanced and objective. For example, there is an unfortunate tendency for adults to view each individual child as primarily a "good kid" or "bad kid." If interviewers succumb to this tendency, it often results in dreading the arrival of some (bad) child clients, while celebrating the arrival of other (good) child clients.

Similarly, interviewers, teachers, and other adults frequently either overidentify or underidentify with children. Some adults see themselves as fully capable of understanding children because of a strong belief, "I was a kid once and so I know what it's like." Adults suffering from this overidentification may fail to set appropriate boundaries when necessary, project their own childhood conflicts onto children, and/or be unable to appreciate unique aspects of children with whom they work. Other adults who underidentify with children may experience children as alien beings—not yet fully part of the human race. Adults suffering from underidentification may talk *about* a child who is sitting three feet away, as if the child were not even in the room. They also might become condescending, rigid, out of touch with issues children face, and/or unrealistic in their fears or expectations.

Children are *not* just like us, nor are they like we were when we were younger. Though different, they are not unfathomable creatures either. Instead, children are somewhere in the middle—rapidly developing, fully human, deserving of respect and age-appropriate communication and information.

To effectively interview children, there are both educational and attitudinal requirements. We encourage mental health professionals to consider their work with children as a form of cross-cultural counseling (J. Sommers-Flanagan & Sommers-Flanagan, 1997). You need to be familiar with basic cognitive and social/emotional developmental theory and have had some exposure to applied aspects of child development (i.e., you should have spent some time with children in either a caretaking or emotionally connected manner).

Additionally, effective child interviewers feel some degree of affection toward children. If children frighten, intimidate, or irritate you, it may be that you should explore these reactions by getting some counseling before you begin directly working with children. Another danger sign is a tendency to repeatedly get overly involved in children's lives. Signs of overinvolvement include continuous fantasizing about adopting or rescuing children in difficult circumstances or actually breaking traditional boundaries and doing things for children that are outside the parameters of the professional relationship. Overinvolvers need to achieve some understanding of themselves in this area and find other ways to meet their needs to rescue and provide extensive nurturing before working therapeutically with children.

A healthy professional and psychological balance is especially necessary when working with children. Children are uniquely able to push our buttons, throw us off balance, and trigger our unconscious unfinished business. Making this balance even more essential is the fact that children constitute a very vulnerable population. Adult clients most likely possess greater maturity, more education and life experience, and have a more fully developed sense of themselves. They are usually more able to defend and advocate for themselves. They have more resources and are considerably more autonomous than children. Most adults can extricate themselves from manipulative or ineffective relationships with mental health providers, but most children cannot. Most adults can express their disappointments and needs in a way that makes sense to the counselor; often, children cannot or will not communicate so directly, and when they do, they are sometimes ignored. For all these reasons, we must be especially attuned to the skills, education, and attitudes necessary to work effectively with children.

The remainder of this chapter is organized based on interviewing stages identified by Shea (1998) and discussed in Chapter 6. Because interviewing children usually requires involving the child's caretaker(s), the stage model becomes a bit complicated. Time management is important. For the initial interview, you may need to schedule an extended session so the child has adequate time for self-expression and the caretakers also feel their concerns are sufficiently addressed.

When it comes to working with young clients, this chapter merely scratches the surface. Students who want to work extensively with young clients need much more education and training. As usual, additional readings and professional resources are listed at the conclusion of this chapter.

## THE INTRODUCTION

Many, if not most, young people do *not* seek mental health services willingly (DiGiuseppe, Linscott, & Jilton, 1996; Richardson, 2001). It is unlikely they will be the ones making the initial call to request a clinical interview and/or counseling. Generally, children are referred to a mental health professional's office by their parents, guardians, caretakers, or school personnel. They may or may not have any advance ideas about whom they will meet with and/or the meeting's purpose. In some cases, they may not think there is anything wrong in their world or, even worse, they may not have been informed in advance that they have a counseling appointment. In other cases, they may be very clear regarding their distress or the distress others are experiencing because of them.

With minors, the role of the caretaker (parent, grandparent, stepparent, foster parent, older sibling, group home manager) in the interview is central and requires conscious attention. Some caretakers assume they will be present during the entire interview, and others assume they will not be present. In most cases, this determination should be made based primarily on the interviewer's assessment of what would be best given the presenting problem, child's age, and relevant clinic or agency policies. Often, experienced interviewers arrange to spend time with the caretakers and child first, allowing time for meeting with the child alone as well. Depending on theoretical orientation and the child's age, some interviewers also meet alone with the parents or caretakers.

The arrangements you make for the initial interview communicate important messages to the child. An interviewer who meets alone with caretakers may be perceived as an agent of the caretakers (or an alternative authority figure). This is especially true with adolescents. On the other hand, there are possible problems associated with not meeting with parents separately (F. Kelly, 1997). Sometimes, it is important to hear background information about the parents or the situation that is inappropriate for the child to hear. Also, it is preferable to meet with angry, hostile parents alone rather than risk subjecting the child to a barrage of negativity from the parents. However, if the child is your primary client, the child deserves, at least generally, to know what is said about him or her. Letting caretakers know that you will be summarizing and sharing any information you feel is important with the child helps set a meaningful boundary. If you are working directly with a child or adolescent, then the young person is your client to whom you are responsible for confidentiality.

# CASE EXAMPLE

*Sandy Smith, a 13-year-old child of mixed racial descent, was adopted by a mixed-race couple who later divorced. She was a gifted violinist and athlete but had begun "hanging with the wrong crowd." Her father and stepmother insisted on getting counseling for Sandy. Her mother and stepfather were less eager, but felt something must be done about her increasingly defiant behavior. All four parent figures plus Sandy's 3-year-old half brother arrived at the counseling office. Sandy's father was going to pay for the counseling and was clearly planning to talk with the counselor alone before anyone else was interviewed.*

*The counselor gave Sandy's father a warm smile, but oriented to Sandy in the waiting room, saying, "Hi. You must be Sandy. Looks like you have a pretty big fan club along with you today."*

*Sandy shrugged and mumbled, "Hi."*

*The counselor then said, "How about if everyone comes back for a few minutes so I can meet everyone?"*

*Sandy's father asked pointedly, "Can I just see you first for a couple minutes?"*

*The counselor again smiled warmly and said, "You know, it would really be better if we all come in and everyone hears a little bit about how I work with young people (significant smile is sent in Sandy's direction). Then, if at the end of our time, we haven't gotten to some of your concerns, Mr. Smith, we'll think of ways to get to them. Would that work for you?"*

*Mr. Smith nodded, a little reluctantly, and the whole group proceeded to the counselor's office.*

In this example, the interviewer was clear in advance regarding her plan, and she was capable of setting limits with a dominant (and perhaps controlling) parent. Without a clear plan and assertive behavior, interviewers dealing with children and families may end up having a dominant family member control the interview and even the therapeutic plan. Although this may be revealing, generally it's better for the mental health professional (rather than the parent) to guide the treatment plan.

The child's guardians have many legal and moral rights, but it is essential that your client—the child—realize that your primary allegiance is to him or her. This realization can be seriously hampered by too much attention to the caretakers' desires and concerns and not enough attention to the child. Therefore, early on, preferably even while appointments are being made, it is good to be clear about the role caretakers will play in the upcoming interview. For example, an early telephone conversation with a mother who wants to bring her 12-year-old son for counseling might proceed like this:

**Interviewer:** "Hello, my name is Maxine Brown. I'm returning your call to the Riverside Counseling Center."

**Mom:** "Oh yeah, I called yesterday because I want to set up an appointment for my 12-year-old son. I'm raising him by myself, and I just can't seem to get through to him. He's been so angry lately. He's impossible to deal with. When can I get him in?"

**Interviewer:** "Well, I have open times next Monday at 1:00 P.M. and 3:00 P.M."

**Mom:** "Great. I'll take 3:00 P.M."

**Interviewer:** "Sounds good. (Therapist explains fee arrangement, office forms to be completed, and directions to the counseling center.) Also, I'd like to let you know that at the beginning of the session, I need to meet with both you and your son together. During that time, I'll talk with both of you about office red tape as well as counseling goals and how I like to work with young people. Does that sound okay to you?"

**Mom:** "Yes, I guess so. So you want me to actually come in, too? I thought I could just drop him off and run back to work."

**Interviewer:** "Yes, actually it's very important for me to meet with both of you to review the goals of counseling. That should take about 20 minutes or so. Then I'll meet with your son alone so I can get to know him a bit and we can begin working together. While I meet with him, you can either run back to work or do some paperwork in the waiting room. Okay?"

**Mom:** "All right."

**Interviewer:** "Great. I'll look forward to meeting with both of you on Monday."

Whether directly on the telephone (as in the preceding example) or at the outset of the interview (as in the first example), it is essential to control caretaker involvement in therapy. Each situation is different, but establishing your own or your agency's general policies and guidelines early clears up potential confusion and allows you to develop a working alliance with the child (and parent).

## THE OPENING

*The reason that all the children in our town like Mrs. Piggle-Wiggle is because Mrs. Piggle-Wiggle likes them. Mrs. Piggle-Wiggle likes children, she enjoys talking to them and best of all they do not irritate her.*

—B. MacDonald, *Mrs. Piggle-Wiggle*

This section describes effective strategies for getting acquainted with young clients. Child interviews include two general goals. First, learn as much as possible about the child (Greenspan & Greenspan, 1991). Second, as you learn about the child, you have a simultaneous goal of establishing a warm, respectful relationship with the child. Because children and adolescents are likely to be unfamiliar with clinical interview procedures and may be shy, reluctant, or resistant, relationship-building can present a special challenge. Interviewers can carry this burden more easily if they follow Mrs. Piggle-Wiggle's lead: Young people quickly perceive whether mental health professionals like them and enjoy them. They also readily notice if professionals are threatened or irritated by child/adolescent attitudes and behaviors. If young clients do not believe they are liked or respected, there is much less chance that they will listen, open up, or, if they have any choice in the matter, choose to continue therapy (Hanna, Hanna, & Keys, 1999; M. J. Lambert, 1989; Ricks, 1974; S. Stern, 1993).

### First Impressions

First impressions are very important. Counselors need to be friendly, active, interesting, and upbeat. This usually begins with the waiting room greeting. Although it may be tempting to engage in adult talk with parents first, doing so can make rapport-building with young clients more difficult. Make efforts at connecting with young clients when initially meeting them in the waiting room. A wave or a handshake and a friendly "Hi, you must be Whitney" is a good start, followed by more quick exchanges, such as "It's very nice to meet you" or "How's it going today?" or "Great biking weather out there, huh?" You are sending the message that you have been looking forward to meeting the young person and are eager to spend time with him or her. A little adult chatter is fine, too, as long as you do not forget to connect with the child.

After you move from the waiting room into the office, maintain some focus on the young person. Children, even when cooperative and open, are best considered involuntary clients, because, for the vast majority, seeking therapy is not their idea. As with any involuntary client, the interviewer is wise to introduce a few creative choices within the interview frame. For instance, you might say something like:

1. "Hi, Bobbie. Your mom and stepdad are going to fill out some boring old paperwork while you and I talk together. I have some toys in this closet. You can pick two to bring with us to my office."
2. "Well, Sarah, I need to explain three important things to you. One is about how we will spend our time together today. One is about a word called *confidentiality*. And one is about why my office is so messy. Which one would you like me to talk about first?"

Another way to introduce choice with young people is to offer food or drink. The options, depending on your values, budget, and setting, might include milk, hot chocolate, juice, sports drinks, or sodas. Snacks might be pretzels, chips, granola bars, fresh fruit, crackers, candy, or yogurt. To feed or not to feed is a professional question we do not discuss at length in this book. Suffice it to say, feeding young people builds relationship. Hungry young people can think of little else besides their hunger, and watching the process of acceptance and consumption can provide a great deal of clinical information. Food may be an especially important therapy tool when young children are meeting with you immediately after school. Although we try to avoid beverages with caffeine and highly sugary foods, other therapists we know use such items after obtaining parental permission.

## Office Management and Personal Attire

Young clients can be turned on or off by physical surroundings. When interviewing youth, place a few "cool" items in clear view. Depending on clients' ages, items such as popular sports cards, fantasy books, playing cards, drawing pads, clay, and hats can be useful to have in your office. Trendy toys are always the mark of a cool counselor, but you have to make a commitment to being up on the trends. At the time of this writing, Gameboys, Harry Potter books, and Spider Man are in. Beanie Babies and trolls are out. By the time you buy this book, you will be left to your own devices to discover what is cool. More generically, soothing items, such as puppets and stuffed animals, can increase young clients' comfort level. Sometimes, teenagers may comment negatively about such items because they are normally associated with younger children, but the comments are probably just a cover for their comfort and dependency needs (Brems, 1993). Overall, the office should be interesting and youngster-friendly to whatever extent possible.

Rather than drawing attention to objects of interest in the office, let young clients notice particular items on their own. Their natural exploratory behavior helps them become comfortable in a new setting. In addition, their reaction to office items is valuable assessment information. For example, some children orient to the sports cards and begin estimating their resale value; others cuddle up with pillows and stuffed animals; and still others ignore everything, appear overtly sullen, and roll their eyes if someone tries to talk with them. Some clients are not able to keep their hands off certain items. In fact, materials may need to be placed in drawers or boxes if they become too distracting; others, such as clay or a doodle pad, can give the client something to "mess around with" while talking with the therapist. Having something to hold or squeeze or draw with can reduce client anxiety (Hanna et al., 1999).

Young clients in general and adolescents in particular respond better to therapists who, even in their choice of dress, indicate they can connect with the adolescent world. This does not mean you have to shop at Old Navy or Eddie Bauer. Nonetheless, we recognize that one of the most successful female therapists we know attracts and maintains relationships with difficult adolescent girl clients, at least in part, because she dresses "way cool." If you are wondering how we know this bit of information, it is because teens seen in therapy often compare notes; they talk with each other about their respective "shrinks" and often offer therapist progress reports pertaining to their friends who are seeing other therapists. Listening to these assessments can be informative.

In contrast, some clothing choices may be "uncool." For example, traditional, conservative attire (suit jacket, shirt, and tie) may be viewed by adolescents, especially those with oppositional and conduct disorder behaviors, as signs of a rigid authority figure. Delinquent adolescents have strong transference reactions to authority figures, and such reactions can impair or inhibit initial rapport (Spiegal, 1989).

Generally, more casual attire is recommended when interviewing young clients. This is not to suggest that young clients cannot overcome their reactions to a therapist's clothing choices. However, when working with youth, it is useful to eliminate even the most superficial obstacles to rapport whenever possible. Although interviewers need to present themselves and their work in a way that feels personally and professionally authentic, keeping an eye to youth-friendly accessories can be helpful.

## Discussing Confidentiality and Informed Consent

Many young people (especially teens) are sensitive to personal privacy. Therefore, you need to discuss confidentiality at the *beginning* of the first session. In addition, teenagers sometimes believe the interviewer is working as an undercover agent for their parents; they may fear that what they say in private will be reported back to caretakers or authority figures. Although written informed consent forms should be read and signed before an initial session, discuss confidentiality immediately after child and parents are comfortably seated in the office and have finished basic paperwork (K. Gustafson, McNamara, & Jensen, 1994; Handelsman & Glavin, 1988; Plotkin, 1981). When working with teens or preteens, we recommend an approach similar to the following:

> "Willy, you and your mom both may have read about confidentiality on the registration forms, or you may have heard the word before, but I want to discuss it with you for a few minutes. Confidentiality is like privacy. That means what you say in here is private and personal. Of course, I have a supervisor and I keep files, but my supervisor also will keep information private, and our files are locked and secure.

> "I will keep what you say to me private . . . I won't talk about what you say to me outside of here. Now, there are a couple of situations where I won't keep secrets. For example, if either of you is dangerous to yourself or to anyone else, I will not keep that information private. Also, if I find out about child abuse or neglect that has happened or is happening, I will not keep that information private either.

That doesn't mean I think there's anything dangerous going on with you two; I'm just required to tell you about the limits of your privacy before we get started. Do either of you have any questions about confidentiality (privacy) here?

"Now (while looking at the child/adolescent), one of the trickiest situations is whether I should tell your mom and dad about what we talk about in here. Let me tell you how I like to work and see if it's okay with you. (Look back at parents.) I believe your daughter (son) needs to trust me. So, I would like you to agree that information I give to you about my private conversations with her (him) be limited to general progress reports. In other words, aside from general progress reports, I won't tell you what your child tells me. Of course, there are some exceptions to this, such as if your child is planning or doing something that might be very dangerous or self-destructive. In those cases, I'll tell your child (turn and look to child) that he (she) is planning something I think is dangerous and then we'll have everyone (turn back to parents) come in for an appointment so we can all talk directly about whatever dangerous thing has come up. Is this arrangement okay with all of you?"

Teenagers need to hear how privacy is maintained and protected. Further, most parents appreciate their children's need to talk privately with someone outside the home and family. In the case of a diagnostic interview where results are shared with a referral source or a child study team, the child should be made aware of this. In rare cases where parents insist on being in the room continuously or constantly apprised of therapeutic details, a family therapy or family systems interview and intervention is probably most appropriate.

School and agency mental health professionals must also be very clear regarding the constraints of the position they hold and the system they work for. Young clients often assume their life is an open book. Assuring them of confidentiality and carefully explaining its limits enhance their sense of being respected participants in the relationship.

Confidentiality laws regarding working with minors vary from state to state. All mental health professionals and trainees should review their paperwork and practices with regard to regulations in each particular setting and state.

Teenagers may respond better to a modified version of the previous confidentiality disclosure. More relevant and sometimes humorous examples can be provided. For example, when turning to the teenager, the following statement may be made:

"So, if you're planning to do something dangerous or destructive, such as holding the mailman hostage, it's likely that we'll need to have a meeting with your parents to talk that over, and it's the law that I would need to warn your mailman. But day-to-day stuff that you're trying to sort out, stuff that's bugging you, even if it's stuff *about* your parents or teachers or whoever—we can keep that private."

Setting confidentiality limits may be controversial, but all interviewers must determine (preferably beforehand) if, when, and how they might inform parents if they become aware of a teenager's dangerous behavior (K. Gustafson, McNamara, & Jensen, 1994). If written confidentiality and informed consent statements are used, both parents and young clients should sign them, indicating their understanding and willingness to cooperate.

Whatever your situation, we recommend you talk about confidentiality limits with children of all ages. Confidentiality is a unique aspect of therapeutic relationship development. For example, Leve (1995) states:

> There is one last aspect of a therapeutic relationship that children find very unusual. Children are almost never told that what they say to an adult will be held in strict confidence and never be told to another adult. This indicates that the therapist respects the child in a way they have never before experienced, and it is a signal that the child's thoughts and actions are important, probably in a way they never dreamed possible. As a result, children sense that therapy is an experience very different from other adult relationships and that it will have an unusual importance in their life. (p. 245)

As an interviewer, you should develop your own way to talk with young people and their parents about counseling and confidentiality. Rehearsing different approaches to talking with clients about this important issue can help (see Individual and Cultural Highlight 11.1).

## Handling Referral and Background Information

Teachers, family members, or others who are bothered by or concerned about a particular child's behavior frequently refer difficult youth for therapy or evaluation interviews. In most cases, the interviewer should tell the child why he or she was referred. Keeping secrets about why the youth was sent to therapy can harm the working relationship. Remember, the referral source, no matter how distraught, is not your primary client.

For example, a school counselor may be contacted by a concerned teacher who, undetected, observed a student throwing up in the bathroom after lunch. At the teacher's request, the counselor may invite the student to stop by for a visit. We believe it would be a mistake to fail to mention the reason for concern. Of course, you must make your policies along these lines very clear to informants and referral sources. In some cases, the referral information source may need to remain anonymous, but the information itself, in the vast majority of situations, should be tactfully, compassionately, and honestly conveyed.

After discussing confidentiality and informed consent, it is time to begin to get an idea of the reasons the client has come for therapy. Common reasons for bringing pre-school- to latency-age children in for clinical interviews include:

- Moodiness, irritability, or aggressive behavior patterns.
- Behaviors that caretakers believe to be abnormal or especially irritating.
- Unusual fears or tendencies to avoid age-appropriate play activities.
- Unusual or precocious sexual behaviors.
- Exposure to trauma or difficult life circumstances, such as divorce, death, or abuse.
- Hyperactivity or problems with inattentiveness (predominantly boys).
- Enuresis or encopresis.
- Custody battles between parents.

This list is neither exhaustive nor comprehensive. It is intended to help you glimpse a typical young child referral. Like younger children, older children and adolescents

## Individualizing Introductory Statements with Young Clients

In this chapter, we provide sample statements for introducing yourself to young clients and introducing interviewing and counseling to young clients. These statements are a good start, but you can come up with better opening statements for yourself. Whatever you say the first few minutes should fit your personality. If you're using some standard opening with young clients, but the opening is uncomfortable for you, children will sense that there's something unauthentic or phony about you. Therefore, this activity involves formulating opening statements to use with young clients that fit with your personality. Of course, these statements should be somewhat serious and not offensive. They should focus on:

1. Introducing yourself to the child and family.
2. Describing confidentiality and its limits to the child and family.
3. Describing any other feature of interviewing and counseling (e.g., psychological assessment).

Take a few minutes to think about the words you'd like to use when discussing these issues with children. Now, shift your focus and imagine how you might change your introductory comments depending on the ethnic or cultural background of a particular child. How would your introductory comments change if you were working with an American Indian, African American, Asian American, or Hispanic child and family? What issues do you think would rise to the surface and require a comment from you? If you have an ethnically diverse background, imagine the differences that might arise if you were working with a White child versus someone from your own background. Discuss these issues with your class or classmates.

Besides the fact that youth itself can be considered a culture, many young people in the United States have the challenging task of living in one culture at home and another at school and in their social lives.

One in five children in the United States is a child of an immigrant (Wax, 2001). The stresses and strains of fitting in are sometimes magnified by having parents or caretakers who speak a different language and have customs different from people at school and in the neighborhood. Interviewers should not make assumptions about immigrant families or young people. It can be quite harmful to ignore the potential intergenerational stress created by being immigrants. It can also be harmful to assume that the immigrant family is suffering because of the bicultural demands it faces. The challenges might make family life interesting, or they may be daunting and painful. The wise interviewer finds ways to assess this particular dynamic. You might make observations and ask gentle, opening questions such as:

"I notice your mom is wearing a traditional H'mong skirt, Tu. But you've got on jeans and a T-shirt. Do you dress traditional sometimes?" or "I notice your parents have a kind of cool accent. Do you guys speak Russian or English at home usually?"

Making a few observations that are neutral or slightly positive and following that with a question about the young person's cultural involvement communicates that you are willing to ask about and listen to the struggles and points of pride involved in being a family spanning two or more cultures.

usually do not request therapy themselves. Common reasons for adolescents to be referred for therapy include:

- Depressive symptoms (usually as recognized by a caretaker or teacher).
- Oppositional or defiant behaviors (usually as experienced by authority figures).
- Anger management.
- Eating disorders or weight problems.
- Traumatic experiences (rape, sexual abuse, divorce, death in the family).
- Suicide ideation, gestures, or attempts.
- A court-order or juvenile probation mandate.
- Substance abuse problems (usually identified by having been caught using or driving under the influence).

Although it is important to have a general understanding of childhood psychopathology and typical complaints, each situation is unique and needs to be addressed with individualized concern. Every child who comes to therapy should be asked about his or her understanding of the visit's purpose. However, it is not unusual for young clients, when asked why they have come to therapy, to give vague or unusual responses:

"My mom wants to talk with you because I've been bad."

"I don't know . . . I didn't even know we were coming here today."

"Because I hate my teacher and won't do my homework."

"I'm here because my mom offered to buy me a new computer game if I came to see you."

"Because my parents are stupid and *they* think I have a problem."

Some young clients simply remain quiet when asked about reasons for counseling; it may be they are (a) unable to understand the question, (b) unable to formulate and/or articulate a response, (c) unwilling or afraid to talk about their true thoughts and feelings with their parents in the room, (d) unwilling or afraid to talk openly about their true thoughts and feelings with a stranger, or (e) unaware of or strongly resistant to admitting personal problems.

Resistant or nonresponsive children present interviewers with a very practical difficulty. How can you obtain information and begin a working alliance if the client is reluctant to speak, let alone expound on the problems in his or her life? A focus on wishes and goals, such as described next, can facilitate engagement and bypass resistance by engaging the child in a positive interaction.

## Wishes and Goals

To explore core client problems using the wishes and goals strategy, make a statement similar to the following, with the parents (or caretaker) and child present (unless the child is about 6-years-old or younger, in which case you may simply meet with the parents to focus on parenting strategies):

"I'm interested in the reasons you're here and so I want to ask you about your goals for counseling. Usually, even though parents (look at parents) may have some very clear goals in mind for counseling, I like to start by asking the youngest person in the room. So, Renee (look at the child), you're the youngest one here, so you get to go first. If you came to counseling for a while and, for whatever reason, your life got better, what would change? In other words, what would you like to have get better in your life?"

Some children/adolescents understand this question clearly and respond directly. However, several potential problems and dynamics may occur. First, the child may not understand the question. Second, the child may be resistant, or reluctant to respond to the question because of family dynamics. Third, the child may focus immediately on his or her perceptions of the parents' problems. Fourth, the parents may begin making encouraging comments to their child, some of which may even include tips on how to respond to the counselor's question. Whatever the case, two rules follow: (a) if the child/adolescent does not answer the question satisfactorily, the question should be clarified in terms of wishes (see the following), and (b) for assessment purposes, the counselor should make mental or written notes regarding family dynamics.

### Introducing the Wish

Wishing as an approach to assessing problem areas and obtaining treatment goals from young clients is useful because it involves using a language that young people are more likely to accept (J. Sommers-Flanagan & Sommers-Flanagan, 1995b). For example:

"Let me put the question another way. If you had three wishes, or if you had a magic lamp, like in the movie *Aladdin,* and you could wish to change something about yourself, your parents, or your school, what would you wish for?"

This question structures goal setting into three categories—selfchange, family change, and school change. Thus, the child/adolescent has a chance to identify personal goals (and implied problems) in any or all three of these categories. Depending on the child and on the parents' influence, there may still be resistance to identifying a goal in one or more of these areas. If there is resistance, the question may be amplified:

"You don't have any wishes to make your life better? Wow! My life isn't perfect, so maybe I should wish to change places with you. How about your parents? Isn't there one little thing you might change about them if you could? (Pause for answers.) How about yourself? Isn't there anything, even something small, that you might change about yourself? (Pause again.) Now, I know there must be something about your school or your teachers or your principle you'd like to have change . . . they can't all be perfect."

Nervous or shy children/adolescents may continue to resist this questioning process. If so, young clients should be given the chance to pass on immediately responding to the wishing question:

"Would you like to pass on this question for now? I'll ask your parents next, but if you come up with any wishes of your own, you can bring them up any time you want."

The purpose of this questioning procedure is to get young clients, in a somewhat playful, provocative, and perhaps humorous way, to share their hopes for positive change. The interaction can provide diagnostic-related information as well. Usually, clients with disruptive behavior disorders (i.e., attention-deficit/hyperactivity disorder, oppositional defiant disorder, or conduct disorder) acknowledge that the school and parents have problems but admit few, if any, personal problems. In contrast, clients who are primarily experiencing internalizing disorders (e.g., anxiety and depression) identify their own personal problems and goals (e.g., "I'd like to be happier").

*Obtaining Parental or Caretaker Goals*

After young clients identify at least one way their life is not perfect, or after they have passed on the question, the focus should shift to the parents. Direct interaction and attention to parental concerns is crucial to getting the full picture and to treatment compliance (e.g., if parents do not support therapy or provide reliable transportation to therapy, it will not continue—and to support therapy, they want their concerns addressed). In addition, it is helpful for children and adolescents to watch the therapist become serious and thoughtful when discussing important topics and problems with parents.

When addressing parents, interviewers should take detailed notes; it is important that parents know you are taking their concerns seriously. However, it is equally, if not more, important to limit the number of negative and critical comments parents make about their children, especially during the first session. Usually, three or four problem statements are enough. Setting this limit protects young clients from feeling devastated or overwhelmed by their parents' criticism. If parents indicate they have additional concerns, you can invite them to write down the concerns for you to review later. Another strategy is to shift the conversation by asking parents to name a few of their child's strengths (P. Silverman, personal communication, July 9, 1998). In some cases, after an initial rapport has been established between therapist and child, a separate meeting with parents can be conducted (with the young client's permission) to address parental concerns more completely. Similarly, you can ask young clients if it is okay for their parents to make us a list of parental concerns. If everyone has been informed of how important it is to have this information, and if an initial trusting relationship has been established, there will usually be little resistance to these information-gathering strategies.

*Assessing Parents or Caretakers*

Sometimes the parents or caretakers who bring children for an interview have more psychological problems than the children. For several reasons, this can be a tricky situation for interviewers of all ages and experience levels. However, it can be especially challenging for those with little family interviewing and counseling experience.

If parents present with extreme psychological problems or display very disturbing interaction patterns with their children, you may be professionally obligated to take actions. These actions can range from mild to extreme, depending on your perception of the severity of the parent-child problem. For example:

- You may be able to ignore the unhealthy patterns during the first session and wait until rapport has been established before providing feedback.
- You may need to provide some gentle feedback immediately.
- You may need to gather further assessment information to determine if the child is in immediate danger.
- You may need to inform the parent of your obligation to report child abuse and proceed to do so.

In most cases, it is best for you to wait for additional sessions and greater rapport to give feedback and suggestions for parental change. However, sometimes, if unhealthy behavior patterns are mild and the parent seems open to constructive feedback, you may be able to provide that feedback immediately in the first session. Alternatively, you may be able to assign some therapeutic homework for addressing the problematic behavior.

Research has shown that there are three common parenting styles: authoritarian parents, permissive parents, and authoritative parents (Baumrind, 1975; Coloroso, 1995). *Authoritarian* parents are also referred to as *brickwall* parents because they make rules that are etched in stone and govern the home with a dictatorial "my way or the highway" style (Coloroso, 1995). *Permissive* parents are often referred to as *jellyfish* parents because they have difficulty setting and enforcing family rules and values. Children of jellyfish parents tend to rule the house. In contrast, *authoritative* parents have been labeled *backbone* parents because they set reasonable rules, parent democratically, and listen to their children's ideas, but remain in a position of final authority. Unfortunately, all too often, parents find it much easier to take brickwall or jellyfish approaches to parenting, but parents who engage in backbone or authoritative parenting score higher on measures of self-actualization (Dominguez & Carton, 1997). It can be useful to assess whether a young client's parent is an authoritarian, permissive, or authoritative parent.

Divorce, remarriage, and stepfamily life are realities for many children. Assessing the family system and its unique qualities is important when working with young clients. For some children, divorce is painful, while for others, it is a significant relief. Similarly, parental remarriage and new blended families can bring both joy and terror to children's lives. To deepen your understanding of these issues in children's lives, we recommend that you read divorce information from the children's perspective (R. Sommers-Flanagan, Elander, & Sommers-Flanagan, 2000; see Individual and Cultural Highlight 11.2 and Suggested Readings and Resources at the end of this chapter).

### Managing Tension

During the wish-making procedure, tension may rise, especially if children/adolescents are asked to make wishes about how they would like to see their parents change. Despite this tension, child/adolescent wishes about their parents area crucial part of the assessment and information-gathering process. Additionally, it is reassuring to most young clients to hear the interviewer say things like "I guess your parents aren't perfect either." In addition, focusing on parental behaviors at the outset of therapy may provide a foundation for working on changing parental behaviors through counseling. Finally, as suggested previously, parent-child interactions during this goal-setting procedure sometimes reveal interesting family dynamics. For example, we have observed children who seem afraid to comment on their parents' behavior (and their parents do not reassure them), and we have seen children who are rather vicious in their wishes for parental change.

If, after help, encouragement, and humor, and after passing on their initial opportunity to wish for life change, the young client is still unable or unwilling to identify a personal therapeutic goal, the prognosis for counseling may not be promising.

### Discussing Assessment and Therapy Procedures

After initial concerns and goals have been identified, a brief review or explanation of interview procedures is appropriate. Depending on the situation, you may choose to

# Children and the Culture of Divorce

The following Divorced Children's Bill of Rights is a document written to divorced and divorcing parents from the child's perspective. It is included here to give you a deeper sense of children's views of the culture of divorce.

*The Divorced Children's Bill of Rights*

I am a child of divorce. I hold these truths to be self-evident:

I have the right to be free from your conflicts and hostilities. When you badmouth each other in front of me, it tears me apart inside. Don't put me in the middle or try to play me against my other parent. And don't burden me with your relationship problems, they're yours, not mine.

I have the right to develop a relationship with both parents. I love you both. I know you will sometimes be jealous about that, but you need to deal with it because you are the adult and I am the child.

I have a right to information about things that will affect my life. If you're planning on getting a divorce, I have a right to know, just as soon as possible. Likewise, if you're planning to move, get remarried, or any other major life change, I have a right to know about it.

Just as I have a right to basic information about my life, I also have a right to be protected from inappropriate information. This means you shouldn't tell me about sexual exploits or similar misbehavior by my other parent. You also should not apologize to me—*for my other parent*—because this implies a derogatory judgment of my other parent. If you apologize to me, apologize for yourself.

I have a right to my own personal space in each of my homes. This doesn't mean I can't share a room with my brother or sister, but it does mean that I need space and time of my own. I also need some special personal items in my own space . . . and this just might include a picture of my other parent . . . don't freak out about it.

I have a right to physical safety and adequate supervision. I know you may be very upset about your divorce, but that doesn't mean you should neglect my needs for safety and supervision. I don't want to be home alone all the time while you're out dating someone new.

I have a right to spend time with both parents, without interference. My right to spend time with each of you shouldn't be dependent upon how much money one of you has paid the other. That makes me feel cheap, like something you might buy in a store.

I have a right to financial and emotional support from both my parents, regardless of how much time I spend with either of you. This doesn't mean I expect twice as much as other kids get, it just means that you should stop worrying about what I got from my other parent and focus on what you're providing me.

I have a right to firm limits and boundaries and reasonable expectations. Just because I'm a child of divorce doesn't mean I can't handle chores, homework, or other normal childhood responsibilities. On the other hand, keep in mind that even though I may have a little sister or brother (or step-sister or step-brother), I'm not the designated babysitter.

I have a right to your patience. I didn't choose to go through a divorce; I didn't choose to have my biological parents live in two different homes, move away, date different people, and in general, turn my world upside down. Therefore, more than most children, my life has been beyond my control. This means I will need your help and support to work through my control issues.

*(continued)*

---

**INDIVIDUAL AND CULTURAL HIGHLIGHT 11.2 (continued)**

Finally, I have a right to be a child. I shouldn't have to be your spy, your special confidant, or your mother. Just because you hate to talk to each other, I shouldn't have to be your personal message courier. I exist because you created me. Therefore, I have a right to be more than a child of divorce. I have a right to be a child whose parents love me more than they've come to hate each other.

---

*Note.* From "The Divorced Children's Bill of Rights" [Guest editorial], by J. Sommers-Flanagan, 2000, *Counseling Today,* p. 9. Reprinted with permission from the American Counseling Association.

---

send parents to the waiting room with an assignment or questionnaire (e.g., a developmental history questionnaire and a problem behavior checklist). If you need a direct interview with parents, young clients can be given drawing assignments or questionnaires to complete in the waiting room. In most cases, it is useful to spend individual time with an adolescent and then to have parents return for 5 to 10 minutes at the end of the time to review therapy or follow-up procedures (e.g., appointment frequency, who will be attending appointments, or even, time permitting, a description of specific treatment approaches such as anger management or treatment of depressed mood).

## THE BODY

After obtaining child and parent versions of problem areas and possible treatment goals, it is time to shift to the body of the interview. Depending on developmental and temperamental factors, children are more or less verbal. Therefore, anyone planning to communicate fully and effectively with children must develop and be comfortable with a wide variety of methods. Textbooks, graduate classes, workshops, and even core emphases in graduate programs focus exclusively on assessment and therapy strategies with children. An effective child interviewer is familiar with principles and procedures far beyond what is included in this brief chapter (Priestley & Pipe, 1997).

### User-Friendly Assessment and Information-Gathering Strategies

The purpose of formal assessment or evaluation procedures is to obtain information about client functioning that may be used to make diagnoses and treatment recommendations and/or facilitate therapy (Peterson & Nisenholz, 1987). While many mental health professionals use traditional, formal assessment procedures (e.g., intellectual and personality testing, questionnaires) when interviewing children, many do not. Those who do not sometimes have negative attitudes toward assessment or view formal assessment as interfering with the therapy process and with understanding the "whole life of the child" rather than narrow diagnostic aspects (Gaylin, 1989; Goldman, 1972).

Young clients often express criticism and/or sarcasm when asked to participate in traditional assessment (e.g., "This test is totally lame"). They may resist completing the instruments fully and thoughtfully. Fortunately, there are alternatives to using formal assessment procedures for obtaining information. The following procedures help interviewers gather information, while at the same time, capture client interest and cooperation. Because these techniques can facilitate rapport and trust, they usually have a positive effect on cooperation with and validity of subsequent traditional, self-report assessments (J. Sommers-Flanagan & Sommers-Flanagan, 1995b; Shirk & Harter, 1996). Using these qualitative information-gathering procedures can increase youth cooperation with therapy and provide the interviewer with assessment information. They are not a replacement for formal assessment procedures, but add a great deal of information and simultaneously enhance the working relationship.

### What's Good (Bad) about You?

A relationship-building assessment procedure that provides a rich interpersonal interaction between young clients and counselors is the "What's good about you?" question and answer game (D. Dana, personal communication, September 1993; J. Sommers-Flanagan & Sommers-Flanagan, 1997). The procedure also provides useful information regarding child/adolescent self-esteem. Initially, it is introduced as a game with specific rules:

> "I want to play a game with you. Here's how it goes. I'm going to ask you the same question 10 times. The only rule is that you can't answer the question with the same answer twice. So, I'll ask you the same question 10 times, but you have to give me 10 different answers."

When playing this game, interviewers ask their young client, "What's good about you?" (while writing down a list of the client's responses). Each client answer is responded to with a "Thank you" and a smile. If the client responds with "I don't know," the response is simply written down the first time it is used; but if "I don't know" (or any response) is used a second time, the interviewer kindly reminds the client that answers can be used only one time.

The "What's good about you?" game provides insights into client self-perceptions and self-esteem. Some youth have difficulty clearly stating a talent, skill, or positive personal attribute. They sometimes identify possessions, such as "I have a nice bike" or "I have some good friends," instead of taking personal ownership of an attribute: "I am a good bike rider" or "My friendly personality helps me make friends." Similarly, they may describe a role they have (e.g., "I am a good son") rather than identify personal attributes that make them good at the particular role (e.g., "I am thoughtful with my parents and so I am a good son"). In this case, the ability to clearly state positive personal attributes is probably evidence of more adequate self-esteem.

Interpersonal assessment data also can be obtained through the "What's good about you?" procedure. For example, we have had some assertive or aggressive children request or even insist that they be allowed to switch roles and ask us the "What's good about you?" questions. We have always complied with these requests as it provides us with a modeling opportunity and the clients with an empowerment experience. Additionally, the manner in which young clients respond to this interpersonal request can be revealing. Youth who meet the diagnostic criteria for conduct disorder (or who are angry with adults) sometimes ridicule or mock the procedure; most other children and adolescents cooperate and seem to enjoy the process.

An optional follow-up to the "What's good about you?" procedure is the "What's bad about you?" query. Although asking young clients "What's bad about you?" is more negative and perhaps controversial, it can yield interesting information. Ask this negative question only five times. Young clients frequently are quicker at coming up with negative attributes than they are at coming up with positive attributes. In addition, sometimes they identify as negative some of the same traits that were included on their positive attribute list.

During both "What's good about you?" and "What's bad about you?" procedures, observe how clients describe positive and negative traits. For example, adolescents frequently use qualifiers when describing their positive traits (e.g., "I'm a good basketball player, sometimes"). When describing negative traits, adolescents may quote someone else (e.g., an adult authority figure), and they may make an excessively strong statement (e.g., "My teachers say that I'm *never* able to pay attention in school").

## Offering Rewards

With disruptive youth, impulsivity and lack of behavioral compliance is a commonly identified problem. As an assessment tool, offering rewards allows interviewers to evaluate how clients might respond to behavioral incentives. The question is whether anticipation of specific reinforcer(s) can motivate a young client to agree to reduce his or her impulsivity and increase behavioral compliance.

After the parents leave the room, ask your client what would happen if he were paid money for discontinuing a problem behavior (e.g., hitting a little brother or sister, leaving the house without seeking permission, forgetting homework at school, or refusing to complete homework). For example:

> "If I were to pay you $10 (or give a $10 gift certificate) next week for completing all homework assignments and always checking with your parents before leaving the house, do you think you could do it?"

This incentive procedure can be conducted in an "as if" mode, or as an actual reward offer.

The offering rewards assessment procedure is used for at least four reasons. First, it helps determine clients' perception of their self-control skills. While some clients are overconfident in their ability to modify their behavior, others are underconfident. Obviously, it is helpful for counselors to know if young clients are being realistic when they describe their personal potential and ambitions.

Second, offering rewards can provide diagnostic information. Specifically, children/adolescents diagnosed with attention-deficit/hyperactivity disorder (ADHD; American Psychiatric Association [APA], 2000) get excited about the money possibility, but quickly fail the homework assignment; sometimes, they fail the homework assignment even before leaving the office (Barkley, 1990). In contrast, children/adolescents diagnosed with oppositional defiant disorder (ODD; APA, 2000) often comply with the counselor's request and simply earn the money (if they feel like it). Finally, children/adolescents diagnosed with conduct disorder (CD; APA, 2000) may try to negotiate or manipulate for additional reinforcers (e.g., more money) or for payment in advance (Rutter & Rutter, 1993).

Third, this technique introduces and then models the importance of informing parents of therapeutic homework (even if the child thinks parents will not approve of the homework) and of the importance of having an objective person monitor the homework success. Although this activity is initially discussed privately with youth, toward the end of the session, the youth is told:

> "Now we need to tell your parents (or teacher) about our arrangement. We need to get their permission and have someone besides you to keep track of your success."

In school settings, where the counselor may have daily access to students, it is still wise to have parents or teachers monitor the desired behavioral change. Involving an "objective" third party, usually one affected by the behavior, can provide additional assessment information.

Fourth, parents and/or teachers can be educated as to the potential usefulness of contingency programs. Sometimes, parents are against using what they call "bribery" to obtain behavioral compliance. If parents object (or perhaps before they object), it can be explained that *bribery* is defined as "paying someone in advance, to do something illegal" (Gordon, 1991). Additionally, you can point out that positive reinforcement is a more efficient behavior modifier than punishment.(Maag, 2001); this can be emphasized by inquiring about positive reinforcers parents receive in their daily lives.

Young clients should be informed that this is only a one-time assessment. Otherwise, clients may expect payments every week. Additionally, young clients may not pay attention to the rules of the homework assignment; therefore, the rules should be clearly written out and clients should repeat the rules of the assignment back to the counselor. Finally, counselors should consider an *effort* reward for children who prove they do not have the ability to sustain attention and effort for a reward that is distant in time (i.e., one or two weeks away).

### Inferring Attachment Issues

> Some people, when they have taken too much and have been driven beyond the point of endurance, simply crumble and give up. There are others, though they are not many, who will for some reason always be unconquerable. You meet them in time of war and also in time of peace. They have an indomitable spirit and nothing, neither pain nor torture nor threat of death will cause them to give up. Little Peter Watson was one of these.
>
> —Roald Dahl, *The Swan*

Children's lives—their emotional, intellectual, and physical development, their attitudes and beliefs, their opportunities and hindrances—are directly and radically affected by their early caretakers and the quality of the attachment to these figures (Ainsworth, 1989; Bowlby, 1969; D. A. Hughes, 1998). Recently, therapists have become more oriented to attachment dynamics in children and adolescents (Bradford & Lyddon, 1994). Consequently, formal measures of attachment can now be administered to clients at the beginning of or during therapy. However, rather than relying on questionnaire administration, the approach we present here focuses on therapist ratings of client attachment behaviors based on Bartholomew's (1990) reformulation of Hazan and Shaver's (1987) and Bowlby's (1977) attachment models. Specifically, therapists can categorize their young clients' attachment behaviors into one of Bartholomew's (1990) four attachment styles:

1. *Secure prototype:* Clients appear comfortable and open interacting with the interviewer or therapist. They are capable of being emotionally close to others. There are no significant problems with separation from parents or with separation from the interviewer when the session ends.

2. *Preoccupied prototype:* Clients seem to want to be exceptionally close to the interviewer or therapist. There is an apparent desire (spoken or unspoken) for more and more time with the interviewer. Sometimes it seems as if these children/adolescents would gladly go home and live with a therapist after only a few minutes of counseling.

3. *Fearful prototype:* Clients seem to want to be emotionally close, but are fearful of being hurt. This often occurs with children in foster care because they've had numerous experiences of being close to adults and then being emotionally hurt because of a placement change. These clients are likely to put the interviewer through tests of trust (Fong & Cox, 1983).

4. *Dismissing prototype:* Clients appear disinterested in emotional closeness. They like to feel self-sufficient. It is important to distinguish this prototype from the fearful prototype because the fearful prototype may act disinterested to protect himself or herself from emotional hurt. These clients may be more prone to violence and other emotionally distancing behaviors.

Be sure to remember that although attachment styles may have implications for psychopathology, they are not diagnostic entities representative of particular forms of pathology. Instead, these categories help interviewers understand early childhood dynamics that now influence the ways that an individual child/adolescent interacts with others.

The role of protective factors versus risk factors can also be addressed in the context of assessing attachment (Rutter & Rutter, 1993). Although the preceding attachment styles are described in a categorical manner, individual clients display attachment behaviors falling along a continuum within the secure, preoccupied, fearful, and dismissing prototypes. In addition, as the Roald Dahl quote at the beginning of this section suggests, there are rare children who display amazing resilience, even in the face of extreme adverse childhood experiences.

## Traditional Assessment and Feedback

In many situations, using traditional assessment procedures with children and adolescents is recommended. Traditional assessment procedures include questionnaires, parent/teacher rating scales, projective tests, intellectual testing, and more. When interviewers use such procedures, children and adolescents are curious about assessment procedures and should be informed of the purpose of particular assessment devices and offered feedback regarding their test scores. Young clients in general and adolescents in particular are likely to feel anxious and distrustful of adults who are evaluating them. Your explanations and feedback need to be carefully geared to both age and level of understanding present in the child. For example, when administering the Minnesota Multiphasic Personality Inventory–Adolescent version (MMPI-A; Archer, 1992) to an adolescent (of at least average intelligence), we might make a statement similar to the following:

> "As a part of our work together, I'd like you to fill out a questionnaire called the MMPI-A. The MMPI-A has been given to thousands of teenagers. It's really long and probably boring to most young people who take it. I'm having you take it because it can give us useful information about certain personality traits you have. You know how sometimes people can have too much of a certain trait or quality, or a healthy amount, or even too little of a particular quality. After you have taken the test, I'll have it scored and we'll look at the results together and I'll explain what the different scores mean. If you want, at the end of counseling, you can take the test again and we can see if there have been any changes."

Obviously, we would not use MMPI-A unless there was a specific purpose for its administration. The reason we have explained its use in the preceding example is that evaluators can be reluctant not only to explain this test, but also to give clients feedback regarding MMPI-A scores. Because the MMPI-A is a test designed to measure pathology, it can be difficult to give constructive feedback to clients who obtain elevated scale scores. On the other hand, just as therapists should avoid writing notes that they would not want their clients to read, therapists should also avoid administering tests to their clients if they are nervous about providing oral or written feedback regarding the client's test results. In almost every case, we recommend showing clients their test profiles and explaining the meaning and interpretation of each clinical scale of the MMPI-A. For example, sample verbal or written descriptions of clinical elevations on MMPI-A scales 1 (hypochondriasis) and 6 (paranoia) are provided next:

> "Scale 1 of the MMPI is called the *hypochondriasis scale.* That's a pretty long and weird word. The scale includes test items primarily related to physical health and physical discomfort. As you probably know, some people are healthier than others are, and some people worry about their health more than others do. People who score high, such as yourself, usually either have some physical health problems or they're worried about having physical health problems in the future. Also, people with scores like yours are more likely than the average person to feel physically sick or physically uncomfortable when under stress. Do these descriptions sound at all like you?"

Notice from the preceding paragraph that the evaluator is giving straightforward and nonpathologizing feedback. Also, whenever giving feedback, we recommend asking clients if the descriptions or interpretations seem to fit for them. Here is another example:

> "Scale 6 of the MMPI is called the *paranoia scale.* Now, just because the scale is called paranoia doesn't mean that people who have high scores are paranoid. In fact, really, the scale is a measure of sensitivity. People with high scores are more likely than the average person to be sensitive to how other people act and what they might be up to. Sensitive people notice little things that an average person might not even notice. As you can see, your scale 6 is a little higher than average. Therefore, I'd guess that you are a keen observer and you notice how other people's actions relate to you. An example might include noticing that other people are laughing and then wondering if maybe they are laughing at you. Also, higher scores on scale 6 are associated with intelligence. So your high score here might mean that on your good days, you are intelligent and sensitive, but on your bad days, days when you're experiencing lots of stress, you can become touchy and suspicious of others. Does any of this seem to fit how you see yourself?"

Perhaps more important than the specific scores obtained by young clients who complete such questionnaires is the manner in which the tests are administered and feedback is provided. Openness with young clients regarding the purpose of formal assessment procedures and results can facilitate the development of trust. Because assessment procedures, depending on *how* they are used, can either interfere with or facilitate trust development, select specific procedures carefully and present them to clients in an open and honest manner.

Considerations of when, why, and how to administer formal assessments should be informed by graduate training in appraisal, test construction, and diagnosis. With regard to young people, it is especially important to note that formal assessment can have a strong impact on the therapeutic relationship and often does not yield as much information as you might have hoped.

## General Considerations for the Body of the Interview

When using play or physically interactive strategies with children, think through stated and/or unstated ground rules and be prepared to set limits that fit within your theoretical framework. In an assessment situation, the fewer rules, the better, as this allows the child more free expression. However, children often test limits. They try leaving the room, tinkering with items on your desk, opening windows, or even placing a call on your phone. More infrequently, they try mild aggression toward you: poking with a tack, spitting a spitball, swearing, and blowing smoke (literally). Rather than having stated rules covering all such potentials, it is better to be prepared to set firm limits as needed. Some theoretical orientations prefer to leave all rules unstated; others suggest the statement of one or two basic rules (Landreth & Lobaugh, 1998; Priestley & Pipe, 1997). The most common rule is usually stated something like this:

> "Billy, you're welcome to play with things in my office (or things from the toy closet). We don't have too many rules about playing here, but it's important that you know my one basic rule: It is not okay to break things or hurt yourself or anyone else with the toys or the art supplies."

Cleaning up and putting things away is also an assessment activity. It is challenging to keep time boundaries that include cleanup time before moving into the closing few minutes of the interview. Doing so provides information about how the child interacts when play is ending. An abrupt shift in attitude toward the toys or game may occur. The emotions directed at the toys may be an important signal about how the child feels about endings. In addition, note behaviors directed toward you. Does the child refuse to cooperate? Does he or she scurry around, cleaning frantically to impress you? Those few cleanup minutes at the session's end can be very revealing.

The following section describes tools and supplies helpful in working with children; Putting It in Practice 11.1 lists these supplies and suggests a group art assignment.

### Arts and Crafts

Drawing is a favorite activity of many children and even a few adults (especially in the form of doodling through long boring meetings). All that is necessary are a few sharp pencils with good erasers, paper, and a nice flat solid surface. When interviewers invite children to draw, they often suggest a subject for the drawing. Kinetic family drawings, draw-a-person, and house-tree-person drawings are old favorites, but there is much to be gained from all sorts of drawings (Machover, 1949; Oster & Gould, 1987). More abstract and sometimes spontaneous assignments, such as "Draw me a quick sketch of how you feel about math" are sometimes quite informative.

When the child is busy drawing, the interviewer might wonder what to do. There is the option of drawing too, but it should be carefully considered. Children can get distracted and begin watching you, even comparing your work with theirs. This can provide meaningful information about the child, but can also become uncomfortable at times. Choice of subject, shape, size, and style of drawing by the interviewer can subsequently influence the child as well. Simply watching the child draw, or making a few supportive, nondirective comments or observations can often enrich the material gen-

==================== **Putting It in Practice 11.1** ====================

## Art Therapy: Supplies and Practice

Art therapy is a specialized professional endeavor in which practitioners generally obtain master's level training. However, the use of art in working with young people does not require a degree in art therapy and can be rewarding for both you and your client. Most materials are neither complicated nor expensive. However, you should be familiar and comfortable with their use. Therefore, convince your graduate faculty or fellow graduate students to pool your resources and obtain the following:

Colored chalk

Watercolor paint sets

A few basic color tubes of acrylic paint

Some bottles of tempera paint

Drawing pencils (or charcoal pencils)

Colored pencils

Fat markers and crayons

Skinny markers and crayons

Oil pastels

Colored plasticine clay

A big stack of nice white paper

A roll of newsprint paper

A big box of old magazines

A few aprons

Egg cartons for paint mixing

Paintbrushes

Good-quality paper towels

Rags

Chocolate (optional)

Right before finals is an excellent time for an experiential art party. Get a group together and do some expressive art. Pair up and reflect on the process with each other. Remember to be open, nondirective, and nonjudgmental—with yourself as well as with your partners. Ask indirect or open questions like "Tell me about your work" or "How did it feel to do this work?" or "What do you notice about your work?"

Treat each art piece respectfully. Notice the medium you chose. Clay is the "loosest"; colored pencils might be considered one of the more controlled choices (I. Rafferty, personal communication, June 8, 1998). In suggesting art as a modality to your client, you will be much more effective, insightful, relaxed, and convincing if you have recently used and played with art yourself.

erated by the drawing. Children often spontaneously explain core aspects of what stimulated their drawing choices.

Play-Doh is a familiar commodity in child therapists' offices. It provides a tactile, expressive modality and is considered fun by most children. Having a cleanable surface is essential. If your office is carpeted, a plastic tablecloth can solve some management problems. Play-Doh accoutrements include all sorts of molds and machines, but we prefer the more projective quality of letting the child create things free-form.

Clay (plasticine) is similar to Play-Doh but will not dry out and requires more working before becoming malleable. Clays that require firing are generally more difficult to use in controlled, meaningful ways unless the professional is quite familiar with this medium.

Painting is one of the more expressive modalities used in art therapies (Simonds, 1994; Thomson, 1989/1997). Although messier and harder to control than drawing, painting often elicits more emotion. Given the opportunity to work with tempera or watercolor paints, some children go from nonresponsive and uninvolved to happy, verbal, and very connected to the process.

Collage-building (using pictures or words) has become a favorite therapeutic use for old or unwanted magazines. Glue (or tape), scissors, magazines or picture calendars, and posterboard are the essential ingredients. You can ask clients to select pictures or phrases that help illustrate any number of things: life events, internal states, family troubles, school worries, and so on. They can attach their selections in any way they wish, sometimes creating an intense representation that would have been impossible to achieve with words.

## CASE EXAMPLE

*Kerry was a 12-year-old intellectually gifted boy struggling with an overcontrolling father and clinically depressed mother. He was born late in his parents' marriage; his mother was now 55 and his father was 61. His elderly grandparents on his mother's side lived in the family home. Both grandparents were frail and needed constant care, which was provided by Kerry's mother. Kerry was referred for individual counseling by his school counselor because his grades had slipped significantly, he was refusing to engage in his usual social activities, and he was making self-destructive comments in class. The interviewer invited Kerry to build a collage that illustrated his family life. Until that point, Kerry had, with his large, impressive vocabulary, indicated acceptance of his grandparents' needs and pride in his mother for caring for them. However, the collage was filled with pictures of young parents with little children and peppered with happy, upbeat words from advertisements. As the interviewer observed the contents, Kerry burst into tears and shared his longing for a "normal" family with young parents and happy, healthy grandparents. Although the therapist obviously couldn't change Kerry's family situation, the collage project provided a starting point for identifying and working through Kerry's grief and particular family needs.*

### Nondirective, Interactive, and Directive Play Options

"Children's play is both a result of their emerging ability to distinguish between appearance and reality and a causative factor in their further development of this important cognitive achievement" (J. Hughes & Baker, 1990, p. 46). For children, play is the stuff of life. It is the means by which they work out pain, achieve mastery, explore new terrain, and take new risks. It is also a means by which they can distance themselves from things too difficult to deal with directly (Bateson, 1972).

Clinicians vary greatly in their use of play in working with children. Some prefer to model themselves after Virginia Axline, who advocated a nondirective, minimally interactive play therapy format, beautifully described in the book *Dibs* (Axline, 1964). Others use play and storytelling to enhance the therapeutic relationship and explore themes in the child's life (J. Sommers-Flanagan & Sommers-Flanagan, 1997). Still others find ways to use play and playful interactions to teach greater interpersonal empathy or more adaptive ways to behave (Brems, 1993; R. Gardner, 1971).

Not all interviewers have the luxury of a full set of potential play items. However, the following list of possibilities commonly used in child interviewing and therapy can be used to facilitate playful child-interviewer interactions.

**Action figures** is a category that includes such known and loved cultural icons as G.I. Joe, Ninja Turtles (which, according to our sources, are no longer considered cool *at all*), X-Men (and women), Pokemon, and Ken and Barbie. It also includes generic soldiers or Wild West figures. You do not need an elaborate or expensive collection; even a few "gray guys and green guys" are enough for children to create a sizable war or city or extended family if given the chance.

**Sand trays** come in all sizes and shapes. Working with a sand tray is a specialized skill that can become a central treatment modality (Thomson, 1989/1997). However, it can also be used simply for play or "fiddling around" while talking. Sand is a tantalizingly movable medium that many children can't resist. A good, sturdy lid and adequate floor covering is essential. You can collect items to play with, such as tractors, trucks, action figures, stones, and so on.

**Stuffed animals** are a comforting presence in a clinical office (Brems, 1993). Sometimes, child-oriented mental health professionals collect quite a set of stuffed animals. If more than one is present, children often create relationships among the animals. Varying the size and even collecting a whole family of stuffed bears enhance this likelihood.

**Dress-up clothes** are not as common as some of the categories in this list, but are easy to obtain for potential spontaneous use. A small suitcase of dress-up clothes can facilitate a breakthrough with an otherwise unresponsive child. Outfits such as cowpoke, firefighter, artist, plumber, and ballerina can easily be assembled. The suitcase itself can also elicit interesting play themes. It is amazing how young children can be powerfully drawn toward dress-up activities.

**Construction sets** vary in size, numbers of parts, and age-appropriateness. Lego, Lincoln Logs, and Tinker Toys are all helpful in engaging young clients in therapeutic activities. They should not be used with small children who might swallow them, and you should be wary of using them with children who have impulse control problems or violent histories. They can very easily become weapons.

**Aggression items** are a matter for consideration, but certainly provide vivid enactments with certain children. Your own values, professional training, and general background dictate your comfort level with toy guns, knives, swords, and other play weapons. They certainly allow for expression of aggressive urges. Some worry that they are too provocative and promote violent expression; others worry that having them in an office suggests a sort of approval of violence on the part of the counselor. These are issues for research and discussion in classes and with supervisors and colleagues as you determine what play items you are comfortable having in your office.

**Dollhouses** or other environments are classic props for allowing the child to reenact life dramas and traumas. The dollhouse is a time-honored play therapy tool. Many toy companies now produce schoolhouses, gas stations, playgrounds, whole city blocks, and other plastic-molded environments complete with figures, vehicles, pets, furnishings, miniature toys, and so on. Children love the props these settings provide and often build entire communities of friends, enemies, and families. Themes emerging in the play are usually central for the child and provide many insights for an astute observer.

**Anatomically accurate** figures or dolls are common for particular kinds of interviews, but are not without controversy. For a short time, therapists who evaluated potential sexual abuse in small children were urged to use anatomically accurate dolls. If children then had the dolls interact sexually, this was interpreted quite concretely to indicate sexual exposure. Controversy quickly arose regarding the appropriateness of such interpretations (Koocher, Goodman, White, & Fredrick, 1996). Although anatomically accurate dolls still serve many useful functions, it is *essential* that the interviewer using them seek adequate training and supervision before doing so.

A final comment regarding collecting your toys: Be aware that you can inadvertently collect toys that reflect a certain cultural or socio-economic class exclusively. Find toys and dolls that are not overly expensive, that have different racial features, and are sturdy, inviting, and not easily broken.

*Fantasy and Games*

This category includes activities that require verbal interactions. They are described here because they do not involve direct interviewing procedures (e.g., questions and answers).

Storytelling procedures have captivated and/or influenced children for many centuries. Inviting the child to listen to a story, to make one up, or even to share the process back and forth can be entertaining and revealing (R. Gardner, 1971). There are many ways to use stories and storytelling activities (J. Sommers-Flanagan & Sommers-Flanagan, 1997). Very few materials are needed, but sometimes an active imagination is required. Lacking that, it may be helpful to have some favorite stories firmly memorized (see Putting It in Practice 11.2).

Acting or miming is a highly projective activity with children. Often, children love to make up a play and assign the acting parts. This activity can uncover themes of great importance in the child's life. Having the child write a script and then act it out can reveal things to both interviewer and child—especially as the child assumes the roles of the various characters in the play.

Familiar child games such as checkers and Candy Land, or card games such as Crazy Eights and Uno, can help break the ice and establish relationships with children. Assessment information can be obtained by observing the child's handling of setup, turn-taking, rule obedience, disappointing events, strategy, and eventual winning or losing.

Therapeutic games are available through a number of companies that serve mental health professionals' needs. They vary in their format, themes covered, appeal, and sophistication. It is worth obtaining a catalogue and checking out a few options, depending on the type of interviewing work you intend to do (see Suggested Readings and Resources).

Sometimes, children spontaneously generate an idea for a game. The level at which you choose to participate (if you participate at all) is a decision worth forethought. For example, one 7-year-old girl, referred because of social skill problems, decided it would be fun to play a form of hide and seek with a stuffed animal, a very fuzzy raccoon. Her inexperienced interviewer agreed and closed his eyes. The child climbed up the back of

---

**Putting It in Practice 11.2**

## Storytelling

Some people believe that good storytellers are born, not made. We beg to differ. For this activity, you will need a partner and access to the creative side of your personality. If you're worried, try to reassure yourself by remembering that everyone has a creative side to their personality—even you.

Sit with a fellow student and start telling a story. You can tell any story you want. The only rules are that the story should have a beginning, a middle, and an ending. It also helps if the story includes some characters (e.g., people, Martians, ants) that have thoughts and feelings. The story can be about you, about animals, about spaceships, about anything. Simply start telling the story. Then stop telling it, while it is still incomplete, after about 30 to 60 seconds. At that point, the other person takes over telling the same story, using his or her unique storytelling style. Then, after about 30 to 60 seconds, switch storytelling authors again. The goal is to generate a story together with your partner or partners. The purpose is to loosen up your storytelling inhibitions, thereby allowing yourself to further develop your storytelling skills and talents. At the end of the story, you may provide one another with gentle interpretive statements (e.g., "I noticed Howard always brought conflict or tension back into the story, but Joyce seemed to always get everything resolved so that all the characters were feeling good again."). However, be sure to request permission before interpreting the meaning of anyone else's storyline. This activity will help prepare you for creative storytelling activities with young clients. You may also want to look at various storytelling resources (i.e., R. Gardner's *Mutual Storytelling Technique;* 1971; Chapter 5 of our *Tough Kids, Cool Counseling* book; see Suggested Readings and Resources).

---

the couch and placed the animal directly on the filament of a halogen lamp. The odor of burning polyester provided an excellent clue for helping the student interviewer locate the singed raccoon.

Creative ways and means to work effectively with children are abundant in the treatment literature (Brems, 1993; Priestly & Pipe, 1997). It is important to assess the needs, skills, and development level of the given child, the ramifications of the identified problem areas, your setting and its limitations, and your own exposure and comfort levels with the various tools listed.

## THE CLOSING

Children experience time differently than adults. In fact, even the linear, nonreversible quality of time is not fully grasped by young children (Kovacs & Paulaukas, 1984). Therefore, telling a child there are 10 minutes left during a session may be less helpful than saying something more concrete, such as:

> "We just have a little bit of time left together. Probably enough time to read one more page (color one more picture, tell one more short story), and then I'll sum-

marize what we've talked about and see if I remember everything. Then we'll make a plan for next week, okay?"

As with adult interviews, you will probably always wish you could gather more information than you were able to get in 50 minutes. Unfortunately, you need to stop playing or gathering information and begin to wind down activities to ensure a smooth, unhurried closing with your child client.

## Reassuring and Supporting Young Clients

Young people need support in their efforts to relate to you, so be sure to offer support throughout the interview. Especially during the closing, provide reassuring, supportive feedback. Make comments such as:

"You did some neat things with that Lego set."
"I know you told me this is your first time in counseling, but know what? You're pretty good at it."
"I appreciate all that you told me about your family and your teachers and you."
"Thanks for being so open and sharing so much about yourself with me."

Because most child clients do not come to therapy on their own, it is all the more important to let them know you appreciate them and the risks they have taken. Some young clients, especially challenging adolescents, may have behaved rudely or engaged in defensive, resistive actions. You might experience countertransference impulses such as urges to withdraw, reprimand, or even punish the child (Willock, 1986, 1987; J. Sommers-Flanagan, Sommers-Flanagan, & Palmer, 2001). It is certainly permissible to note the difficulty of being "dragged off to counseling" in an empathic comment and notice that the client seemed to have some reluctance about being open with you. However, as with adults, expressing anger or disappointment toward young clients who are resistant, defensive, or nondisclosing is inappropriate; such reactions make it less likely they will seek professional help again in the future. Instead, if your client is defensive, try to remain optimistic:

"I know it wasn't your idea to come in and talk with me today, and I don't blame you for being a little upset about it. We might be able to find some ways, together, to make this less of a pain. In fact, I might even know some ways that would make this whole thing go by pretty fast and then you'd be all done with counseling."

(For more information on termination strategies with difficult young clients, see "Termination as Motivation," in J. Sommers-Flanagan & Sommers-Flanagan, 1997.)

## Summarizing, Clarifying, and Seeking Involvement

The most important closing tasks with young people are: (a) clearly summarizing your understanding of the problem areas; (b) making connections between the problems and possible counseling interventions (assuming you see such connections); (c) reminding the client about ways caretakers will or will not be involved; and (d) if possible, seeking some kind of positive involvement by the child. Two case examples follow. The first is an example of a 7-year-old struggling with nightmares. The second is an adolescent who repeatedly has been caught stealing from classmates.

## CASE EXAMPLE 1: CLOSING

*"So, Beth, our time is almost up. You've sure helped me understand what it's like for you trying to go to sleep at night. You get pretty frightened. Then everybody gets mad at you for not staying in bed. I think there are some things we can do to help you, but it'll mean coming back to talk some more . . . I hope that's okay with you. It also might mean having your mom and dad and big brother come in so I can talk with them about ways to help you. But you'll be here with me when I do that, and you and I will make a plan first. I'm thinking it would be good for us to see each other again in three days. Would that be okay with you? We might draw some more pictures, and I have a story I want to read to you. Do you have any questions before you go?"*

## CASE EXAMPLE 2: CLOSING

*"Tommy, we've got a few minutes left together. I know this hasn't exactly been fun, but hey, you got out of English and a little bit of study hall, right? People are pretty upset with you for taking stuff—and even though you think you're borrowing stuff, it seems to be getting you in more trouble than it might be worth. I really appreciate the time you've taken to tell me what you think about all this and to answer all my questions about your family and stuff. I think we could work together to get things to chill out a little in your life. It wouldn't take too long because you're pretty smart about things, but at least a few more sessions to work together. I doubt if we need to involve your mom much, unless you get in more trouble. It can be just some planning and thinking between the two of us. You're pretty good at thinking about stuff. I bet we could come up with some ideas that would help. But I'd have to understand more about your life. It'll mean talking. Think you can stand coming back and talking with me a few more times?"*

### Empowering Young Clients

Because young people do not have final authority over many aspects of their lives, they usually respond well to being given choices and opportunities to ask questions. Leave time in your closing to shift the focus and allow the child time to ask questions and reflect on the process of being together with you:

"You know, I've done all the questioning here. I wonder if you have any questions of me?"

"Has our time together been like you thought it would be?"

"Is there anything about this meeting we've had that's bothering you?"

"Is there any last thing you want to say that I should have asked about?"

"I wonder if you felt there was anything I could have done in this interview that would have helped you feel more comfortable (or helped you talk more freely)?"

These queries help give the young client a sense of power and control. Although, as Foley and Sharf (1981) point out, it is important to maintain control toward the end of an interview, it is also important to share that control (carefully) with the child.

## Tying Up Loose Ends

With young people, reconnecting with their parent or guardian is an essential piece of closure. Children are not able to arrange the details necessary to get themselves back to another session or follow through on recommendations resulting from the interview. Therefore, the interviewer must clear these things with the caretaker, preferably with the child present. Other related matters, such as fee payment and scheduling, can be addressed as well.

## TERMINATION

The same general principles are true for children as for adults regarding conscious and unconscious termination concerns. It may be helpful for you to review the termination section in Chapter 6 as you prepare for a child interview. The main differences to anticipate are a matter of degree rather than substance. Children are often more overt and more extreme. An adult may *wish* to hug you but refrains, whereas a child may snuggle right up for a hug. An adult may fantasize telling you to "F___ off" toward the end of your time together, but an adolescent might just do it. Adults may feel a bit sad; children may burst into tears. Adults may register some disappointment; children may give you an ugly look, complain vociferously that their time is up, or even deliver a swift kick in the shin. They may even try refusing to leave or just announce they are tired of this and leave early. The interviewer needs to assume the role of observer, empathizer, and gentle limit-setter. Sometimes, children feel things, reflect things, and enact things quite acutely and dramatically. It is all part of the goodbye process.

## SUMMARY

In many ways, interviewing children is qualitatively different from interviewing adults. This chapter identified basic differences between children and adults and discussed ways to professionally address these differences. In the introduction phase of the interview, the role of the child's caretaker must be considered and clarified. However, it is imperative for the interviewer to pay attention to the child, address him or her directly, and help him or her to understand the upcoming interview.

During the opening phase, if young clients are unable or unwilling to identify personal goals for therapy, we advocate using a procedure called *wishes and goals* to establish a positive tone, allow the child to engage in the process, and give parents a sense of being heard as well. With young clients, there are special issues in confidentiality that must be addressed. The child is a legal minor, and therefore, parents and guardians have certain rights to therapy information.

Obtaining assessment information during the body of a child interview is enhanced by the use of many nonverbal play tools and strategies. In addition, specific user-friendly assessment and information-gathering strategies should be used to assist the interviewer in obtaining information at the same time as developing rapport. When formal assessment instruments are used with young clients, their use should be explained to the client and assessment feedback should be provided.

Closing and termination procedures with children are similar to processes with adults, but they become more complicated for several reasons: There are more players to consider, more time demands to balance, and children may express their reactions to their interview experiences more overtly or bluntly than adults.

# SUGGESTED READINGS AND RESOURCES

Brems, C. (1993). *A Comprehensive Guide to Child Psychotherapy.* Needham Heights, MA: Allyn & Bacon. This book includes important areas relevant to working with children: Legal and ethical issues, interview strategies, culture, environment, issues in assessment, various treatment modalities, and termination are all addressed.

Gardner, R. A. (1971). *Therapeutic storytelling with children: The mutual storytelling technique.* New York: Aronson. Gardner's book provides a good foundation for practitioners who like to use storytelling with their young clients.

Hibbs, E. D., & Jensen, P. S. (1996). *Psychosocial treatments for child and adolescent disorders.* Washington, DC: American Psychological Association. This edited volume strives to bring research and application together, considering both theory and environment in addressing common childhood disorders. Chapter foci include anxiety disorders, affective disorders, attention-deficit/hyperactive disorders, socially disruptive disorders, autistic disorders, and general treatment guidelines.

House, A. E. (2002). *The first session with children and adolescents.* New York: Guilford Press. This book will help you prepare for conducting initial interviews with young clients.

Hughes, J. N., & Baker, D. B. (1990) *The clinical child interview.* New York: Guilford Press. This text offers both theoretical and practical information for professionals engaged in assessing and treating children. It is applicable for school and agency settings.

Jongsma, A. E., Peterson, L. M., & McInnis, W. P. (2000). *The adolescent psychotherapy treatment planner.* New York: John Wiley & Sons. This treatment planning guide is set up in step-by-step fashion. It includes comprehensive coverage of most adolescent disorders and presenting problems and includes treatment goals and objectives as well as specific therapeutic interventions for each disorder.

Jongsma, A. E., Peterson, L. M., & McInnis, W. P. (2000). *The child psychotherapy treatment planner.* New York: John Wiley & Sons. This is another treatment planning guide designed for developing treatment plans for child clients. Similar to the preceding resource, it includes childhood disorders, presenting problems, treatment goals and objectives, and therapeutic interventions for each disorder.

Kelly, F. (1997). *The clinical interview of the adolescent: From assessment and formulation to treatment planning.* Springfield, IL: Charles C. Thomas. The process and procedures for interviewing difficult adolescents is described in this short book (216 pp.). It is a handy resource for students or professionals who work primarily with adolescent clients.

Richardson, B. (2001). *Working with challenging youth: Lessons learned along the way.* Philadelphia: Brunner-Routledge. Richardson offers over 50 "lessons" he has learned about providing counseling to difficult or challenging youth. Not only does it offer numerous practical ideas about counseling youth, but also this book is well-organized and written in a style that makes for pleasant reading.

Sommers-Flanagan, J., & Sommers-Flanagan, R. (1997). *Tough kids, cool counseling: User-friendly approaches with challenging youth.* Alexandria, VA: American Counseling Association. What can we say? This is just a magnificent book. Seriously, the book has a distinctly applied focus. The many suggested techniques and strategies have in common a goal of establishing and deepening the therapy relationship with young people who may not be relationship-oriented. The chapters on suicide and medication issues are especially practical and relevant.

Sommers-Flanagan, R., Elander, C. D., & Sommers-Flanagan, J. (2000). *Don't divorce us!: Kids' advice to divorcing parents.* Alexandria, VA: American Counseling Association. This book is based on interviews and surveys of individuals, both children and adults, who have experienced divorce firsthand. The book emphasizes the children's perspective and covers issues ranging from predivorce, parent-parent conflict during and after divorce, and new families.

# Chapter 12

# *INTERVIEWING COUPLES AND FAMILIES*

*All happy families resemble one another; every unhappy family is unhappy in its own way.*

— Leo Tolstoy, *Anna Karenina*

*The fact that something is difficult must be one more reason to do it. To love is also good, for love is difficult. For one human being to love another is perhaps the most difficult task of all, the epitome, the ultimate test. It is that striving for which all other striving is merely preparation.*

— Rainer Maria Rilke, *Letters to a Young Poet*

---

**CHAPTER OBJECTIVES**

Not all interviewers are up to the task of interviewing couples and families. From our perspective, working with couples and families in a therapeutic setting can be one of the most exciting and intimidating situations a mental health professional can face. Although reading this brief chapter does not provide you with adequate information and training for working competently with couples and families, it provides an important overview. After reading this chapter, you will know:

- Some classic ironies of working with couples and families, including the fact that clinicians often have less time to work with more clients.
- How interviewers commonly define couples and families.
- How to apply the interviewing stages and tasks reviewed previously in this text to interviewing couples and families.
- Different formal couple and family assessment instruments.
- Practical and philosophical issues in identifying, managing, and modifying conflict (and setting limits) in couple and family interviews.
- Several family therapy concepts, such as identification, projection, joining, and avoiding.
- When (and if) shifting from individual to couple or family therapy is appropriate (or ethical).

---

Clinical interviewing with an individual is a challenging endeavor. Not surprisingly, when simultaneously interviewing more than one individual, the task becomes even more complex. Instead of assessing and addressing one client's problem areas and motivations and expectations, when interviewing couples, you have two people *and* their relationship in the room with you. All the diverse problems, motivations, and expectations of two different individuals attempting to maintain a relationship and to love each other must be assessed and addressed. In addition, when working with families, interviewers must assess and address motivations, expectations, and relationships in an entire family system. As the number of individuals increases, so does the complexity and difficulty associated with therapeutic assessment and treatment.

Although this chapter reviews basic strategies for interviewing couples and families, our coverage of this complex topic merely scratches the surface and necessarily reflects our own biases and orientations. This chapter exposes you to general principles for interviewing couples and families, but you will not obtain all the knowledge, skills, or training necessary to competently interview couples and families. Throughout, we refer to experiences, readings, and activities to help prepare you to interview and work with couples and families.

## SOME IRONIES OF INTERVIEWING COUPLES AND FAMILIES

Working with couples and families involves several rather ironic truths, discussed next.

### More Clients, Less Time

Despite the fact that interviewing couples and families is more complex than interviewing individuals, most therapists must work faster with couples and families than they do with individuals. This is because, on the average, couples and families do not stay in counseling as long as individuals (Hampson & Beavers, 1996; Lowry & Ross, 1997; Luquet, 1996). There are several possible reasons for this shorter period.

Couples and families usually come to counseling with different motivation levels, expectations, and agendas among the members. Some of the family or one of the couple may be openly reluctant to even try counseling. This imbalance may lead to premature termination. Additionally, most insurance companies and many managed care organizations do not provide insurance reimbursement for couple or family therapy. This reduces the length of time the family or couple can afford therapy, thus further increasing the pressure to provide efficient interviewing and counseling services. Finally, logistically, it is hard for busy couples or families to find a time when everyone can consistently attend therapy sessions. Difficulty scheduling may reduce the time couples and families spend in counseling.

### Defining Couple

Another ironic fact about working with couples or families is that before you begin, you must define the terms you use to describe your client.

There is disagreement and discomfort in the professional and general population regarding how to define a *couple* (e.g., Hawkins, 1992; B. Murphy, 1992). Some professionals advertise marriage or marital therapy; others use the term *couples counseling* or *couples therapy.* Our position on the couple versus marital therapy issues is based on inclusion. Throughout this chapter, we refer to interviewing and counseling techniques that include two people who are pursuing a romantic relationship together primarily as *couple work.* Couple counseling may involve therapy with unmarried gay and lesbian couples, unmarried heterosexual couples (who never plan to marry), unmarried couples (who are pursuing premarital counseling), couples who have made a life commitment they regard as marriage, even though not legally recognized, and traditional, legally married couples. It also includes couples who are divorced and reconciling. In contrast, *marital therapy* refers specifically to therapeutic efforts occurring between two people committed to each other through the bonds of matrimony, as defined by the laws of the state.

Couple counseling has also been referred to as *relationship therapy* or, more specifically, *relationship enhancement.* However, unless you are using the specific approach entitled *relationship enhancement therapy* (Guerney, 1977), we recommend avoiding this term because it does not distinguish between couple therapy and family therapy or even more specific interventions such as mediation. Frequently, two family members (e.g., mother and daughter, father and son) pursue therapy together in an effort to improve their relationship. This is most aptly referred to as *family therapy* because it includes two members of one family who are not romantically involved.

## Defining Families

Like the definition of a couple, the definition of a family has, unfortunately, become a politically loaded topic. It is difficult to make statements about families without encountering opposition. We believe families come in all shapes and sizes. Family theorists and therapists differ with regard to whether they will treat subsets of family members when conducting family therapy (Goldenberg & Goldenberg, 2000). However, in our transient, mobile society, at any given time, the family may be defined and configured differently than it was a week ago or than it will be next week.

Children in coparenting situations often see themselves as actually having two or more families. Children raised in extended kinship systems, as reflected in many American Indian and other cultures, may live for periods with grandparents, aunts, uncles, or older siblings. Families may contain foster children, elderly relatives, and part-time members. They may be headed by one parent, two parents, a grandparent or two, a parent and stepparent, and so on. Sometimes, people who consider themselves family do not reside together, either by choice or by law. For instance, it is not uncommon to do family therapy with a family in which one member is living in a juvenile detention facility or group home.

The family-oriented mental health professional must find both a comfortable working definition of family and a theoretical basis for determining appropriate treatment modalities. Learning to effectively interview a family and then proceed with family therapy requires serious study and close supervision. At this point, theoretical approaches to interviewing families and conducting family therapy are diverse and sometimes contentious. This theoretical and practical diversity, along with the complexities noted previously, requires that beginning interviewers *not* conduct family interviews or family therapy unless they have close supervision. Our preference is for beginning interviewers to obtain training experiences by conducting family interviews in conjunction with their immediate supervisors or with a team of fellow therapists (i.e., reflecting team; Andersen, 1991; Bertolino & O'Hanlon, 2002). This *apprenticeship* model is especially important when learning family interview, assessment, and therapy techniques.

## The Generic Interview

In this chapter, important aspects of interviewing couples and families are described. We also identify problems and possible solutions associated with these interview populations. However, when it comes to interviewing either couples or families, practitioners from various theoretical approaches strongly disagree with each other regarding appropriate and effective interviewing strategies. In fact, some practitioners might argue that there is no such thing as a generic or atheoretical approach to interviewing families or couples because the initial interview is based on the professional's theoretical and treatment orientation. We believe, however, that there are basic elements in family interviews common to most accepted family treatment theories. These elements, therefore, are important considerations for beginning interviewers who work with couples and families.

## INTERVIEWING STAGES AND TASKS

Similar to work with individuals and children or adolescents, clinical interviewing with couples and families can be divided into Shea's (1998) five stages. We briefly describe these stages and their associated tasks with regard to interviewing couples and families next.

### The Introduction

The introduction stage of interviewing with couples and families includes telephone contact or scheduling, initial meeting and greeting, and client education.

*Telephone Contact or Scheduling with Couples*

When couples refer themselves for professional assistance, one partner is often more eager than the other to engage in counseling. Ordinarily, the person who makes the initial telephone call is more motivated for treatment than the other party. However, this is not always the case. On occasion, one party calls at the insistence of the other. For example:

Client: "Hello, my name is Bert Smith. I'm calling to schedule an appointment for marriage counseling."

Interviewer: "Okay, before we go ahead and schedule the appointment, let me give you some information about our services and ask you a few questions." (The interviewer proceeds to inform the client about the agency's fee structure, ask about insurance, ask about best appointment times, etc.)

Client: "Yeah, well, we can come in on Friday afternoons. You know, my wife told me to make this call or I could just forget about our marriage. She thinks we need counseling. So I'd like to get this appointment scheduled right away."

As you can see from this example, the caller informs the person scheduling the appointment that although he is not personally motivated to pursue counseling, he is quite motivated by his wife's ultimatum. In cases where one party has made an ultimatum, the less motivated party sometimes makes the call. The less motivated party also usually makes his or her attitude known early in the telephone conversation. This can also be true when the more motivated person makes the call. For example:

"I'm calling to make an appointment for marriage counseling. Our marriage is falling apart. I've been trying to get my husband to come for counseling for years.

Now, I'm just making an appointment. Either he'll come with me or I'll come by myself."

Couples are notorious for engaging in what therapists refer to as *triangulation*. Triangulation occurs when one member of a couple relationship establishes an allegiance with a third party, usually to gain sympathy or power. Often, the person calling for couples counseling begins, even during the initial telephone contact, to actively seek sympathy from the interviewer. Triangulation frequently occurs in couples and families; it is generally viewed as a less-than-optimal (and sometimes pathological) strategy for increasing a person's power in the couple or family system (Horsley, 1997; Scarf, 1995).

Often, the sex of the therapist is an important variable when couples call for an appointment. In training clinics, it can be possible for an opposite-sex cotherapy team to work with couples and families. Although doing cotherapy can add therapist communication problems to the already complicated mix, it is usually seen as advantageous, especially in training clinics. Inexperienced therapists gladly look to each other for support and direction when they are unclear regarding how to proceed. In contrast, more advanced therapists sometimes regard cotherapy as a burden. Already confident regarding how to proceed, they find comments from a cotherapist detracts from an efficient therapy process. However, assuming the cotherapists are theoretically compatible and capable of communicating well with each other, having two perspectives usually offers couples and families a more comprehensive service.

Unfortunately for clients, rarely do counselors work together in mental health clinic or private practice settings. There are exceptions, and even some theoretical orientations in which having two therapists involved is foundational to the work (Young-Eisendrath, 1993). Generally, however, it is too costly for two professionals to work jointly with a couple or family. In some training clinics, the option for either a male or female therapist is presented when couples counseling has been requested:

**Interviewer:** "Sometimes, people who are coming for couples counseling prefer to see a male or a female therapist. Do you have any preference?"

**Client:** "Hmm. Actually, she never said whether she wants to work with a lady or a man. I guess she'd probably rather work with a lady counselor, but I'd rather talk to another man about this. Yeah, you better schedule us with a man."

In this example, the husband briefly struggles with whether to go with his or his spouse's preference for a male or female counselor, then opts to go with his preference over his wife's. This choice may represent an initial hope for triangulation. That is, the husband is hoping that a male therapist might see things more from his perspective than his wife's perspective. Hoping for or attempting to enact triangulation, although a possible sign of couple pathology, is fairly natural for couples seeking therapeutic assistance. As usual, we recommend that interviewers make mental notes of first impressions from the outset of their telephone contact, including whether the client who telephoned was trying too hard to gain sympathy or support from the interviewer.

## Meeting and Greeting Couples

Interviewers should be careful to greet couples with relatively equal warmth and mild enthusiasm. Couples may be watching for subtle signs that the interviewer favors one client over the other. Whenever possible, avoid even the appearance of being triangulated by one member of the couple; equal treatment is the order of the day.

Not surprisingly, potential triangulation makes chitchatting with couples in the waiting room a task requiring thought and observation. If you talk about the weather, the woman may take offense because she is already angry with her husband, who she believes talks about the weather too often (instead of "more important" issues). If you talk about how it was to locate the office, they may plunge quickly into a conflict regarding who "took the wrong turn" or who really "knew the best way" to navigate to your office. When meeting and greeting seriously conflicted couples, virtually anything you say can and will be used against you.

Despite prospective dangers, try to make a few comments and engage in small talk when greeting couples in the waiting room. Stick with relatively neutral trivia, shake hands with both people, and generally avoid comments that might be interpreted as too personal or as evidence that you like or identify more with one client than the other.

## Telephone Contact or Scheduling with Families

Much of the previous advice can be applied to initial family therapy telephone contacts. The primary difference is that it is unusual for a family member to call with a clear request for family counseling. The request for help usually centers on a description of certain troubling patterns of behavior in the family, or (more commonly) in one or more members of the family. Both theoretical orientation and clinical judgment must be involved in determining whether family therapy or individual therapy with or without family member consultation is the treatment of choice.

When someone calls to request help with a situation that might best be handled by family therapy, it is advisable to arrange a time when all family members can be present for an initial interview. You may not continue to have all members attend, but meeting everyone who lives in the family home is standard when initiating family therapy. Many family therapists or clinicians with a family systems orientation are insistent about having every family member living in the home come to the first session (Goldenberg & Goldenberg, 2000). Further, some family therapists welcome or even encourage initial participation by extended family members. An example of a telephone conversation follows:

**Interviewer:** "Ms. Wilber? This is Tina Jones. I'm a counseling trainee at the University Counseling Center, returning your call."

**Ms. W:** "Yes, I'd like to make an appointment to talk with someone about my husband and my daughter. Well, actually, Bill said he might be willing to come too, but I just wasn't sure what would be best. Do you have any openings? Dr. Green said your center would be good because we don't have insurance right now and you do a sliding fee."

**Interviewer:** "Yes, we have openings. I have several late afternoon openings right now. It sounds like you want some help with relationships in your family. Is that right?"

**Ms. W:** "Well, I don't know. My husband, Bill, is just so upset these days with our daughter, Kim. She's 15, and she's got a mouth on her, if you know what I mean. And she's been pushing him. He's a quiet guy most of the time. Our son, Wally, is just kind of lost in the fighting. And maybe I should just bring Kim in, but she says it isn't her fault. She says she won't come if her dad doesn't come too."

**Interviewer:** "Kids growing up can be hard on everyone. One of the ways I've been trained to help people is through family therapy. It's best if all of you could come in for at least the first few times. Do you have others living at home besides your husband, son, and daughter?"

**Ms. W:** "No. That's it. Sometimes, that feels like a few too many."

**Interviewer:** "So, do you think everyone could come in for an hour and a half next Thursday at 4?"

There are an infinite number of variations on the themes in this phone call. Parents who call for counseling may not be aware that family therapy is available and are often confused as to what might help with some of the struggles they face. Initial phone calls require at least minimal amounts of clinical judgment and education to set up for a family therapy intake interview.

## Meeting and Greeting Families

As with couples, small talk with families is also fraught with important considerations. Generally, it is better to find global comments that pertain to the whole family than to single out a few individuals. Some theorists have emphasized orienting to the youngest family members first, even in the waiting room (Whitaker & Burnberry, 1988). If the physical surroundings allow it, greet each family member by name before going to the counseling room.

## Couple and Family Education

As in interviewing individuals, couples and families must be educated regarding counseling procedures and the general plan for the interview. It is important to cover confidentiality very carefully and go over the legally mandated reasons you might break confidentiality. You should have your own professional ethics and your agency's policies firmly in mind. For instance, it is important to explain your policy with regard to meeting separately with each member of the couple or family, whether you will take phone calls from one member of the couple or family that might involve discussing couple or family issues, and whether you will agree to keep any secrets, temporarily or on an ongoing basis. A common scenario follows:

> Jill, a psychology intern, meets with Betty and Barney for the first time. The session starts out with Betty bursting into tears and saying she is sure Barney doesn't love her anymore. Barney gets angry and defensive, and verbally dominates the meeting. Betty cries throughout the session. Jill does her best to get both involved in helping her understand their background and needs as a couple, but it is tough going. The session ends with Jill feeling she needs two or three more hours with them before she can establish good treatment goals. She sends them home with a marital satisfaction inventory to complete and return to the office. The next day, Barney calls and explains to Jill that he is having an affair, but he feels it is better that Betty not know. He would like to stay with Betty until their youngest graduates next year, which is why he agreed to come to counseling. He has assumed Jill will not tell Betty anything unless he gives her permission to do so.

Clarity about your willingness to keep secrets is essential in couple and family therapy. Specifically, as the International Association of Marriage and Family Counselors (IAMFC; 1993) ethical code states, if Jill has not stated otherwise, Barney's assumption is correct:

> Unless alternate arrangements have been agreed upon by all participants, statements by a family member to the counselor during an individual counseling or consultation contact are not disclosed to other family members without the individual's permission. (p. 75)

Other areas of confidentiality also require special attention in couple and family work. Concerns about child physical or sexual abuse might arise, as well as concerns about custodial rights, should the relationship end in divorce. It is important to explain these possible eventualities carefully and be very clear about both the law and your office policies.

It is also important to educate the couple and/or the family about what will be expected of them during the interview and what behaviors are unacceptable. Mental health professionals who work with couples or families range in their willingness to tolerate open conflict, destructive interactions, profanity, raised voices, and so on. Novices are well-advised to maintain control through guidelines that disallow potentially destructive conflict. We cover this area more extensively later in the chapter.

An example of setting up rules to limit conflict for a couple follows:

"Betty, Barney, I want to let you know a little bit about how we'll work together. We'll probably be talking about some pretty difficult, emotional things and I am going to reserve the right to interrupt if either of you gets too far off track or too wound up. Sometimes, counselors like to let couples actually get into a big argument to see how that goes, but that doesn't fit with how I work. I know it's hard sometimes, but we're going to work together on constructive ways to solve the problems you face."

One student who was working with a family that included a very vocal, controlling, middle-aged man simply made the following statement:

"Mr. Smith, I should tell you this room is only partially soundproofed. So, when you raise your voice that much, the secretary and the people upstairs can hear you."

From that point on, Mr. Smith did a much better job of keeping his voice within reasonable limits.

Besides dealing with shouting and other forms of destructive conflict, it is important to address your activity level and style. Most couple and family counselors are active and directive, as compared to those doing individual work. They redirect client statements, rephrase, check in, have people move about the room into different seating arrangements, and even stand in for one person during role plays. They give assignments, homework, and mini-lectures on the nature of communication, the nature of coupling, the needs of families, their theoretical beliefs, and so on. Clients deserve fair warning about these activities and interventions.

Couples and families also learn about interview process and ground rules by observing interviewer behavior. From the beginning, the interviewer should make sure everyone is aware of general information obtained in the process of setting up the interview. This involves the interviewer clearly restating the basic information he or she obtained over the telephone. By restating this information, a no-secrets approach to counseling is modeled:

**Interviewer:** "It's nice to meet both of you. Sandy, you made the call and set up the appointment, so I just want to let Rick know what we talked about. Rick, when Sandy called, she said you had both agreed to try counseling, but that it was a little bit more her idea. If I remember right, she said you'd had one trial separation last year, but it upset the kids so much you moved back together. Did I get all of our conversation, Sandy?"

**Sandy:** "Yeah, that's about it. But there's a lot more to why we're here. Rick has been pretty mean."

**Interviewer:** (interrupting) "Thanks, Sandy. At this point, I just want to make sure Rick knows the basics of what we've talked about so we're all on equal footing. We'll get into the issues that brought you here in just a couple of minutes. Rick, does that fit with what you knew?"

**Rick:** "I knew she called and that's right . . . I'm not too jacked about being here. But I guess we have to do something."

**Interviewer:** "Thanks, Rick. It's important that both of you know what I know. There are always at least two sides to relationship problems. It's my policy when working with couples not to keep secrets about what either person says to me separately. After I talk a bit about how I work and give you some information, I'll ask each of you about the problem areas, okay?"

This quick but important check-in provides a natural link to the topic of secret-keeping and individual contacts between one member of the couple and the therapist. Policies and orientations vary, so try to establish your own stance (based on theory, supervision, and agency policy; see Putting It In Practice 12.1 for a discussion of secret-keeping with couple clients).

## The Opening

The opening in a family or couple interview varies depending on theoretical orientation. One very important component of the opening for couples, no matter what comes next, is to obtain fairly complete information from each person about why they have come for counseling. A simple, balanced statement can help begin this portion of the interview. It may be unrealistic to expect everyone to participate equally, but it is important to hear from each member during the opening phase.

### The Interviewer's Opening Statement in Couple Counseling

After asking for any final procedural questions they might have, the interview opening begins with a statement such as:

"I want to hear about what each of you believes brought you here and what you want to work on as a couple. It doesn't matter who starts, but I will want to hear from each of you. I know you might disagree on some things, so you can check in with each other along the way, and I will too."

It is informative to monitor how the decision is made as to who goes first. Couples express their feelings toward each other and about counseling via voice tone. In many cases, these feeling expressions are less than subtle.

Bornstein and Bornstein (1986) provide an alternative example of an opening statement:

My plan for today's session is as follows. First, I'd like to get to know you folks a little. Second, I'll need some information about what brings you in. Third, while I want to hear from you, I will be asking a considerable number of questions today. Finally, by the time we are

---

**Putting It in Practice 12.1**

## To Keep Secrets or to Not Keep Secrets?

Think about the case of Rick and Sandy presented in the text. Imagine the following scenarios:

When she calls for the appointment, Sandy tells you that Rick has been very depressed and lethargic. She tells you about the fact that he shows no sexual interest in her anymore, and she thinks it is related to the biology of depression. She also mentions that Rick's father committed suicide last year. How much of this information do you repeat to Rick during the initial session?

When she calls for the appointment, Sandy tells you that she had been having an affair for the past year, but that she has stopped seeing the other man. She also tells you that she hasn't informed Rick about the affair and that she's not sure she needs to. What do you tell her about your policy on secret-keeping in couple therapy?

Rick calls you for the appointment and tells you that he's lost sexual interest in Sandy because she's gained 20 pounds over the past two years. He also tells you that he's developed a pornography addiction and he's spending lots of time on the Internet, rather than interacting with Sandy. When they both come in for their first session, do you share this information with Sandy? What if Sandy had called for the appointment and had described the same situation (that she had gained 20 pounds and that she suspected Rick was addicted to pornography)? Would you be more or less inclined to share the information with Rick during the first session?

As you can see from the preceding scenarios, deciding what to share with a couple during the initial meeting is challenging. Should you have a policy where you always tell everything the caller tells you? (If so, you must make this policy clear *before* the caller starts telling you all about their relationship problems.) Alternatively, do you *selectively remember* what the first caller has said . . . do you bring it all up later . . . and if you don't bring it up, what message does that send to the first caller about secret-keeping and a possible coalition?

Before you begin taking couple therapy referral calls, get clear on your policy. We know some therapists in our community who not only refuse to keep secrets, but who also directly ask possible couples therapy clients if there is an affair happening. If the caller indicates there is an affair (or a suspected one), these therapists refuse to initiate therapy until the "love triangle" has been discussed and terminated by the couple.

Consider your position. Will you keep secrets between romantic partners? Will you work with partners who are having an active affair? How will you decide your position on these issues?

---

finished, I'd like to be able to give you some initial feedback and let you know if I think I can be of service to you. (p. 54)

Note that in this sample opening statement, the interviewer is providing the couple with greater structure and direction. The Bornsteins' opening statement is dictated, to some degree, by their behavioral orientation. They want to control the direction and course of couple interviews.

## Maintaining Balance

Simultaneously attending to whoever is currently speaking as well as the other party is important. If you observe nonverbal signs of anger, pain, or disagreement, you can model a balanced approach by saying:

> "Just a minute, Betty. Barney looks like he might need to say something. I know you aren't done, but let's check in with him for just a minute."

> (Turning to Barney) "Barney, I noticed you winced and looked away when Betty spoke about the television issues. Betty isn't quite done explaining her perceptions. Would it be all right with you to have her finish and then come back to this area, or do you need to check in with her?"

Even though you have just begun to get the reasons for their visit, by actively structuring their initial communications, you model your style and orientation. It is poor modeling to allow one member of the couple to ignore distress displayed by the other, but also balance and fairness is essential to good couples work. Therefore, if Barney indicates he needs to correct Betty's rendition of the television issue, allow him a bit of time, summarize his concerns, and get back to Betty, saying:

> "Thanks, Barney. It's helpful to know you have some differences. I bet we'll discover quite a few areas where you two don't see eye to eye, but we'll work on that. Let's let Betty continue now."

Although it is important for interviewers to orient toward nonverbal signs of client distress, it is equally important to recognize that some clients continually interrupt their partners through intrusive nonverbal messages. If nonverbal interruptions become a pattern or otherwise problematic, interviewers should begin acknowledging, but minimizing, nonverbal reactions:

> "Hang on a moment. I can see that Barney is having some pretty strong reactions to what you're saying, Betty. Barney, I can see you're getting upset, but I want to hold back your reactions and keep focusing on just trying to listen and understand Betty's version of what brings you both here for counseling. You will get your chance to give your perspective in just a minute."

## Evaluating Couple Interactions and Behavior

As couples discuss their main reasons for counseling, it is useful to observe their interaction and behavioral tendencies along several dimensions.

Couples often differ in their needs for intimacy and autonomy. For example, one partner may consistently push for more time together, while the other expresses (either directly or indirectly) a strong interest in being alone or away from the relationship. It is not unusual for these intimacy and autonomy differences to manifest themselves during an initial interview. Sometimes, this has the feel of a chase scene or drama occurring in the relationship: One partner is chasing and the other is running for cover.

Intimacy and autonomy issues are sometimes attributed to general sex differences. In this framework, men are viewed as cooler, more distant, and more autonomous; and women are viewed as warmer, closer, and more intimate. Although viewing couple conflicts as stemming primarily from male-female differences may be helpful and even desirable at times, sex-typed behavior models tend to be overused and abused (Gray, 1992;

Tannen, 1990). Indeed, you may find that men are more often seeking autonomy and women are more often seeking intimacy in the work you do with couples; however, such an observation should not lead you to assume that an autonomous style in males and an intimate style in females is either normal or desirable. Instead, watch for partner preferences and tendencies to more deeply understand couple dynamics and thereby assist the couple in attaining more adaptive or healthy dynamics.

Recently, John Gottman, a marriage and family researcher from the University of Washington, has focused on the importance of "emotional bids" in working with couples (Gottman & DeClaire, 2001). He emphasizes that loving partners offer up emotional bids to each other and, if the relationship is healthy, they receive and respond empathically to each other's emotional needs. For example, continuing with the scenario, Betty might claim:

> "I spent all day Saturday cleaning the garage while he was watching his football game. And then, when I came in and told him I was all finished, instead of supporting me, he just said, 'Boy, you sure took a long time cleaning up our tiny garage.'"

As you can see, Betty is offering a bid for emotional support and connection, a bid that Barney completely misses. Watching for these missed opportunities can help interviewers gain insight into negative communication patterns.

Psychoanalytic therapists view interpersonal attraction as based on complementarity. *Complementarity* refers to the tendency for couples to be complementary rather than similar in their personality and behavioral traits. Complementarity theory suggests that relationship partners are attracted to each other in part because of opposite qualities. It seems that just as two opposite puzzle pieces fit together well, so do intimate partners with opposite qualities.

Complementarity is not without its strong critics. Nevertheless, observations by clinicians suggest that complementarity, to some extent, is frequently present in clinically referred couples (I. Myers & McCaulley, 1985). Therefore, it behooves the interviewer to observe ways that couples are different and ways they are similar. Of course, the classic complementary couple system is characterized by the compulsive husband and the hysterical wife. Once again, although we think that observing for complementary traits or styles during the interview may be useful, we recommend against systematic stereotyping of men, women, or any other subgroup.

### The Family Interviewer's Opening Statement

Referral needs and theoretical orientation dictate both tone and content of your opening statements as a family interviewer. Sometimes, when tension is high, it can be reduced by mild humor, reflected in comments such as:

> "I suppose you're all wondering why I called you together."
>
> "What's a nice family like you doing in a place like this?"

We hasten to add that such humor is often a very bad idea. It requires clinical judgment and at least a minimal comfort level on the interviewer's part. After getting everyone settled, it is important to thank people for coming and state something such as:

> "We're going to spend the next hour together, getting acquainted. I'll be doing some of the talking, and I hope each of you will get a chance to do some too. It is

important that I get an idea of what's been going on and what brought you here. I hope we can also talk about how family therapy might help."

Family therapy openings are wide-ranging, depending on the interviewer's theoretical orientation. Another guide is from Virginia Satir (1967):

> In the first interview, the therapist starts out by asking questions to establish what the family wants and expects from treatment.
>
> a. He asks each person present, though not necessarily in these words:
>    "How did you happen to come here?"
>    "What do you expect will happen?"
>    "What do you hope to accomplish here?" (p. 109)

### Maintaining Balance with Families

A classic situation in family work is the "identified patient" phenomenon (Goldenberg & Goldenberg, 2000; J. Patterson, Williams, Grauf-Grounds, & Charmow, 1998), wherein the entire family system claims that one member is the cause of all family problems. Satir (1967) was among practitioners who have pointed out that, in a family, the disturbed person may be reacting to a family imbalance and, through his or her symptoms, is trying to absorb the family pain. Such situations illustrate why maintaining balance in family work goes beyond simply making sure everyone gets a chance to speak. Even in the opening minutes of an initial interview, your job is to make sure one person is not attacked or scapegoated by the rest of the family. It is also your task to determine how and when you begin to alter the system. Again, theory, supervision, and experience are essential components of developing this important skill.

## CASE EXAMPLE

*The Ragsdale-Hagan family came in for therapy because their 14-year-old, Theo, was extremely aggressive toward his 9-year-old sister, Sira. The parents, Thomas and LaChelle, disagreed on how to handle it, but agreed that Theo was way out of line. After hearing the basic confidentiality information and the counselor's opening statement, Thomas took the floor and complained bitterly that his son seemed bent on killing his sister. "I ought to pound that boy once a day. Maybe more. But his mother won't hear of it." LaChelle put her hand on Thomas's arm and said, "Now, Baby. You know he'll be bigger than you before you know it. He's not going to change 'cause you pound him, are you, Theo?" Theo said to the counselor, "He's not my real dad. He's been with my momma a long time, but he's not my dad. He's her dad, though."*

*The parents started into why the biology didn't matter. Theo was clearly directing the interactions. Sira was completely silent. In this case, to achieve balance, the interviewer would need to intervene and redirect the conversation in a way to involve Sira.*

### Evaluating Family Interactions and Behavior

From the opening to termination, the family therapist's powers of observation must be on high alert. The family is your client. It is a complex organism, always communicating simultaneously with you and among its members. The potential number of communiqués at any given moment are staggering to consider and daunting to observe, let alone manage. However, such observation and management is the heart of most family therapy approaches. It is important to note *both* verbal and nonverbal communication patterns.

## CASE EXAMPLE

*A family of four had brought their youngest daughter (age 14) for counseling, claiming she had a lot of "bizarre" ideas that made them wonder if she was "crazy." The daughter was expressing fears of crowds, she heard voices as she fell asleep at night, she seemed overly attached to her boyfriend, and she was skipping school and underachieving. The older daughter no longer lived in the home. The counselor asked both parents to attend the initial interview with their daughter to determine whether family or individual therapy would be a better fit. The parents talked openly about their professional lives, their religious convictions, and their pride in their daughters. The daughter was also verbally active and had a quick sense of humor, which she interjected frequently. The parents were not overly blaming of their daughter and expressed concern for her well-being. The student interviewer was impressed with the sophisticated vocabulary and open communications and had begun to think this was a very nice, normal family. Then, out of the corner of her eye, she noticed the daughter had slipped off her shoe and was stroking the top of her father's shoe, under his chair, with her bare foot. The father was completely ignoring this action, and the daughter did nothing to call attention to it either.*

Needless to say, this behavior is not ordinary father-daughter behavior in an initial counseling session. It alerted the student counselor that there was more going on here than was apparent on the surface. Although it would have been a mistake to draw attention to the foot-stroking until she had built more of a relationship with the family and knew more about the dynamics, her observations led her to investigate a number of potential problem areas more thoroughly. Consistent with her supervisor's theoretical orientation, she also determined that she would need to meet with members individually and perhaps in dyads to fully understand the coalitions in the family and the reasons for these coalitions.

### The Body

The body of the family or couple interview, like the opening, is strongly influenced by the interviewer's theoretical orientation. After hearing about the chief complaint(s), inquiry is directed toward central feelings, behaviors, and thoughts (or beliefs) related to the problem areas. However, before going more deeply into these areas, it is appropriate to explain the theoretical orientation that guides your work, including the use of certain techniques, such as having everyone speak, assigning homework, listening skill practice, questionnaires, and so on. It is important, on an ongoing basis, to assess each person's willingness to participate and/or cooperate with your strategies and plans.

### Theoretical Orientations with Couples

There are many ways to approach working with couples. Some are based in the traditional theories of psychotherapy and some are more skill- or value-based, such as therapy specifically oriented toward improved sexual functioning or, in contrast, toward compliance with religious beliefs about how couples should relate to each other. Some examples follow.

Therapists with behavioral orientations systematically inquire about desirable and undesirable behaviors that occur within the couple context. They emphasize that couples who rate their relationships as positive and satisfactory usually report a higher frequency of mutually pleasing or mutually enjoyable interactions (Jacobson, 1996). However, when evaluating what each partner desires from the other, behaviorists proceed carefully because if couples are simply asked what they would like to get more often from their relationship partner, listing these desires may be viewed as only a new and improved list of partner demands. Instead, when eliciting desirable behaviors from each partner, behaviorists often inquire first about what each partner is willing or able to do that he or she *believes* his or her partner would find desirable. Focusing on specific behaviors that each partner is willing to initiate or increase can take the demanding quality out of mutually pleasing or mutually enjoyable behavior lists.

Cognitive therapists have extended their treatment philosophy into the arena of couples counseling (Baucom & Epstein, 1990; A. Ellis, Sichel, Yeager, DiMattia, & DiGiuseppe, 1989). Their perspective emphasizes the importance of some or all of the following cognitive variables in shaping couple interactions:

1. Perceptions about *what* events occur.
2. Attributions about *why* events occur.
3. Expectancies or predictions of what events *will* occur.
4. Assumptions about the nature of the world and correlations among events.
5. Beliefs or standards about how things *should* be. (Adapted from Baucom & Epstein, 1990, pp. 47–90)

Consequently, from a cognitive therapist's perspective, much of what occurs in the body of a couple interview involves active assessment of and education about the role of cognitions in causing and shaping couple conflict.

Relationship enhancement couple work draws heavily from Carl Rogers's person-centered theory (Guerney, 1977), focusing on teaching a couple skills for listening to each other that are very similar to the skills person-centered therapists use professionally. Jungian theory and concepts are evidenced in a number of couples therapy modalities, including imago relationship therapy (Hendrix, 1988) and dialogue therapy (Young-Eisendrath, 1993). These and a number of other couples therapies include, at least to some degree, a couple communication orientation. Early on, an interviewer with a communication orientation might begin, during the body of the interview, to instruct couples in basic listening skills and have each member of the couple try one or two simple paraphrases to demonstrate the power and effectiveness of these skills (Bornstein & Bornstein, 1986). They might assign homework requiring each partner to spend time listening and sharing with each other.

One common issue often discussed when educating couples about communication skills is to whom the clients should direct their oral communication in the session. Couples frequently begin discussing their problems and conflicts directly with the interviewer, sometimes in a manner that suggests the other person is not even present. Although this might be natural, therapists who emphasize communication skills training often tell the clients something similar to the following:

"I know this may seem strange, but most of the time in here I want the two of you to talk with each other. In other words, instead of directing your comments and questions toward me, I want you to direct your comments toward each other. When speaking about anything that has to do with the two of you, I want you to look at and talk to each other. It's my job to interrupt and help you change your communication patterns, but I can do that best if I watch you communicate with each other."

Even after this instruction, couples often keep turning to the interviewer to make statements such as:

"I just don't know how to tell if he is interested in talking with me. I come home and he says hello, but he doesn't initiate conversation and I just feel so alone."

In a communications model, the interviewer intervention often consists of:

"I'd like you to turn to Barney and restate what you said, only this time, talk to him."

An underlying assumption of this model is that it is more important for Betty and Barney to learn to communicate effectively with each other than it is for them to learn to communicate effectively with the interviewer (Bornstein & Bornstein, 1986).

In contrast, psychoanalytic or object relations couple therapists formulate relationship problems in terms of individual psychopathology. Consequently, they may not even view conjoint couples therapy as an appropriate treatment modality for addressing conflict. For example, Strean (1985) states, "In most instances, but far from all, the psychodynamically oriented therapist has favored individual long-term therapy for the treatment of marital conflict" (p. 69). Therefore, strange as it may sound, some psychoanalytically oriented clinicians view couple therapy as of little use. Instead, they believe that psychologically healthy relationships are based on psychologically healthy individuals. Therefore, the treatment of choice is individual therapy.

The preceding descriptions are by no means an exhaustive list of couples counseling modalities. Many other approaches exist (see Gurman & Jacobson, 2002). To give these diverse approaches appropriate consideration, you would need to read the original texts and obtain specific training and supervision. The Suggested Readings and Resources section includes introductory and/or advanced readings from various theoretical perspectives.

## Theoretical Orientations with Families

The following quote from Lewis Thomas's *Lives of a Cell,* included in Minuchin and Fishman's (1981) book, *Family Therapy Techniques,* captures the flavor of the orientation foundational to much of family therapy: "There is a tendency for living things to join up, establish linkages, live inside each other, return to earlier arrangements, get along whenever possible. This is the way of the world" (p. 147).

Most family therapy theorists and modalities come from a systems (Goldenberg & Goldenberg, 2000) or ecological (Brofenbrenner, 1979, 1986) perspective. Such perspectives, though quite similar to each other, are a radical departure from seeing counseling as a process that cures or eliminates the pathologies of an individual or even of a family. The context for the manifestation of the dysfunction is as important, and in some cases, more important, than the actual dysfunction itself. From Whitaker's symbolic-experiential family therapy to Bowenian theory and therapy with its concepts of differentiation and multigenerational transmission, writers and therapists with a family orientation attend to a much broader domain than those focusing on individuals or even nuclear families (see Goldenberg & Goldenberg, 2000).

A family therapist working in the structural family theory model approaches the family as a living organism, which leads to an open definition of both family and normality (J. Patterson et al., 1998). During an initial interview, the therapist absorbs all aspects of family functioning to begin to draw a family map. This map, or schema, allows for an analysis of structural strengths and weaknesses in the family.

Orienting to a family and to the family's distress *systemically* will substantially change interviewer-client interactions and interviewer inquiry. For instance, in the body of a family interview, coming from an ecosystemic approach, Amatea and Brown (1993) recommend seeking answers to the following:

1. What is the nature of the problem and what solutions have been tried to solve this problem?
2. Who else has been involved in helping with this problem?
3. If you were to bring in anyone to help with this problem, whom would you invite?
4. Who would be the last person(s) to bring in to help with this problem?
5. If this problem were solved, how would things be different?

The authors also advocate assessing the entire ecosystem that surrounds the problem and intervening at whatever junctions in the system seem most likely to positively effect change. Amatea and Brown draw heavily from the MRI (Mental Research Institute) approach, which stems from the early work of Gregory Bateson, Paul Watzlawick, Don Jackson, Jay Haley, Virginia Satir, and others (see Goldenberg & Goldenberg, 2000, for review; Bertolino & O'Hanlon, 2002; Fisch, Weakland, & Segal, 1982).

Using a systems or ecological perspective to some extent, behavioral family therapy shares similarities with behavioral couples therapy. Behavioral family therapists believe that families develop behavioral patterns that may be counterproductive or maladaptive, but these behaviors represent the family's best efforts to respond to their situation (I. Falloon, 1988). Behavioral therapists' intentions are to conduct a functional analysis of the problem(s) and begin altering behaviors through traditional behavioral change strategies. Education and communication training are also important features of behavioral family therapy.

To summarize, the body of an initial family interview most likely involves seeing the family from a systems or ecological perspective. Problems, tensions, and distress are discussed in relation to the context in which they occur, rather than to the pathology of one or more family members. Many, if not most, family counselors send the family home with homework or experiments, or at least new ways to think about their situation. The bulk of the interview body provides the foundation for designing and implementing these interventions.

### Common Areas to Address

Regardless of theoretical orientation in working with couples or families, there are certain assessment domains that should be considered and, in most cases, explored during the body of an initial interview. These domains are described in the following section. The first three assessment domains—sex, money, and level of commitment—are specific to couples.

## Sex

When working with romantic partners, satisfaction with sexual intimacy is a central area to assess. However, it can be difficult for interviewers to ask questions about sexual functioning. Therefore, you should practice asking unusual or difficult questions. One of our favorite homework assignments for interviewers consists of the following: "During the next week, spend several hours loudly discussing the details of your sex life with your class partner while out at a crowded local restaurant."

Of course, after giving this assignment, we follow it with: "Okay, if you'd rather not complete the original assignment, then simply discuss sex with each other quietly, in a very private and confidential setting." The point is that interviewers, as well as couples, need to become comfortable talking about sex.

For the most part, you may find relief in the fact that couples probably have a more difficult time answering your questions about their sex life than you have asking, which makes your comfort with this aspect of couple functioning all the more important. In the first interview, you may or may not get a chance to ask about sex, and in addition, when you do ask, you may get a quick "Oh, fine. We're fine in that area." Later, after more trust has been established, very different answers to questions about sexual functioning may surface. What matters is that you ask about sexual functioning, compatibility, and satisfaction in a natural, caring way.

## Money

Although easier to ask about than sex, money is often a difficult issue for couples. Questions about money practices include who pays the bills, whether checking accounts are joint or separate, if there is agreement with regard to saving and spending, and so on. By evaluating how couples manage money in their relationship, interviewers may also glimpse how power is managed (or abused) in the relationship.

## Level of Relationship Commitment

Only a minority of couples enter counseling because they simply want to improve their relationship. They arrive excited and interested to explore ways to increase their relationship satisfaction, and are fully committed to continuing the relationship. Other couples come to counseling to repair or work on certain troublesome areas in their relationship but have not seriously considered ending the relationship. They are committed, but are experiencing significant distress. Still other couples come to counseling with a marked imbalance in their commitment, with one deeply questioning whether to stay in the relationship and the other desperately committed to keeping things together. Finally, there are couples who come to counseling as a last resort; they are not very committed to each other anymore and hold little hope for continuing their relationship.

Either directly or indirectly, you need to obtain a clear idea of where the couple you are interviewing fits along this continuum. The Stuart Couples' Precounseling Inventory provides each client with questions that interviewers can use to assess commitment without asking about it directly in front of the other partner during an interview (Stuart & Stuart, 1975). Additional couple relationship measures range from the 280-item Marital Satisfaction Scale (D. K. Snyder, 1979) to the 32-item Dyadic Adjustment Scale (Spanier, 1976; see Sporakowski, Prouty, & Habben, 2001, for a brief review).

## Family of Origin

It is certainly not feasible to devote a great deal of time to each person's upbringing and family of origin relationship patterns, but it helps to at least get an overview of this important area, both in couple and family work. You can gain a great deal of information by designing your intake paperwork to include the family history of each member of the couple with regard to relationships, deaths, divorces, and so on. It is also helpful to know about siblings' marriages. However, beginning interviewers may have the following question when working with couples: Should I interpret the couple's unresolved family of origin issues early on?

Despite our belief that unresolved family of origin issues can strongly influence couple or marital interaction, we strongly advise against family of origin–based couple conflict interpretations during initial interviews. Premature interpretation in the couple context is generally inappropriate and certainly can turn couples off to counseling. Instead, make a mental note or written progress note indicating that family of origin issues may be fueling couple conflict. Additionally, it may be appropriate to acknowledge this likelihood, but not describe the dynamics in an initial session. For example:

> "As you both probably know, your childhood experiences, your relationships with your mother and father or brothers and sisters can shape the way you relate to each other. I'm not sure if this is the case with the two of you, but as we work together, it may be useful for us to occasionally discuss how your family of origin experiences may be contributing to your current conflicts and the ways you go about trying to resolve these conflicts. But, because this is our first session, I won't even venture any guesses about how your childhood experiences might be influencing your relationship."

As some theoretical perspectives suggest, family of origin issues may be deeply influential, but they may also be outside client awareness (Gurman & Jacobson, 2002; Odell & Campbell, 1998). Consequently, as in the case of psychoanalytic interpretations (discussed in Chapter 5), family of origin interpretations must wait for sufficient rapport and supporting information (or data) before they can be used effectively. As a family therapy technique, interpreting intergenerational family themes is probably less threatening, but should still be approached carefully.

### Genograms

Most modes of family therapy and some modes of couple therapy use a schematic drawing of the family tree of both parents, including stepparents and half siblings. There are slight variations in the construction guidelines, but knowing how to do a basic genogram is essential in working with families (Hartman, 1995; McGoldrick & Gerson, 1985). The counselor may not actually do a genogram with the family present but may accumulate the data necessary to complete one. However, it is a common activity to do with families early in treatment. Numerous books are available for teaching interviewers how to complete genograms (Hood & Johnson, 1997; McGoldrick & Gerson, 1985).

### Gathering Family Therapy Goals

Many family therapists, when gathering information during the body of an interview, maintain balance by systematically orienting toward each family member. For example, Lankton, Lankton, and Matthews (1991) state: "We always ask each member what he or she would like to have changed in the family and how, and even if members contradict each other, each input becomes the basis of a goal" (p. 241).

A key to gathering goals in family therapy is to emphasize inclusion and minimize scapegoating or constant references to the identified patient. It is crucial to explore the range and quality of strengths and deficits of all family members and to begin determining how they are influencing the identified patient (I. Falloon, 1988).

## Willingness to Make Changes

A close corollary to the level of commitment in couple interviewing is each person's willingness to do homework, try new things, experiment with change, and try out new perspectives. Besides asking directly, a good way to assess this area is to have each member try a new behavior or listening skill during the interview. This can be as simple as saying:

> "Barney, I wonder if you could take Betty's hand for a minute and just let her cry."

> "Mom, it seems like you and Karen are sitting closer together than anyone else. I wonder if you could have Karen sit by her brother for a few minutes while Dad moves over here and we talk a bit further."

If the couple or family agrees to homework or to setting aside talking time, interviewers should inquire as to exactly when such a new behavior might fit into their schedules.

## Kids, Parents, Neighbors, Friends

Often, couples and/or families are the core of a circle of wider relationships, all of which contribute to one another's well-being or struggles. Getting an idea of these interpersonal and role demands operating on the couple or family system is important. Grandparents, children and their friends, stepchildren, in-laws, close friends, and other associates can play influential roles in the happiness or unhappiness of a couple or family and can contribute to, or use up, many relationship resources. Considering the rich and interactive ways in which many outside factors influence couples and families is a core concept of the ecological approach to therapy (Brofenbrenner, 1979, 1986).

## Drugs, Alcohol, and Physical Violence

Intake forms may help with gathering information about concerns in these areas. Sometimes, this opens the door to further sharing regarding fears of alcohol abuse or instances of past violence. This, like sex, may be an area wherein you get a simple "Everything's fine" answer until much later, when trust has been established. However, simply asking, either in writing or verbally, begins the process of letting everyone know that you are open to hearing about trouble in these areas. When questionnaires or intake forms are used to inquire about sensitive issues, interviewers should review the forms thoroughly and discuss significant issues with the couple or family. Depending on your perspective, it should be made clear to couples and families that any issues mentioned on questionnaires or intake forms are *not confidential* in the family or couple system and, therefore, may be discussed during the interview.

## The Closing

Watching the clock closely is essential, but very difficult, in an initial interview with families and couples. There are more clients to manage and profound issues may be raised with just moments left in a session. We believe that when new issues are raised at the session's end, it is appropriate, unless the issue represents a true crisis, to close the session by stating something such as:

"Rosa, I'm glad you brought up the fact that you want to change your curfew. Unfortunately, we're out of time for today. So, next time, I want you to remind us about the curfew issue and we can discuss it earlier in the session, when we have enough time to deal with how everyone feels about it."

When working with families, it is often best to meet for an hour and a half or even two hours, but interviewers should be careful to stay within whatever time boundaries are originally agreed on. Make sure you allow plenty of time to "put things back together" because the session may involve some intensely emotional material. You cannot be responsible for making each person feel better about the situation, nor is it ethical to minimize the problems so everyone leaves feeling artificially hopeful. On the other hand, it is in your power to support and compliment everyone's efforts in coming for help. It is in your power to provide structure that enables each person to regain composure. In addition, it is usually in your power to offer a sense of direction for the family counseling work.

As with all closings, summarization is an important tool. Couples or families who come and share their problems and fears need to be reassured that they have been heard. They also need help finding closure and preparing to leave. A thorough, sensitive summary helps facilitate these goals:

"Well, today we certainly covered a lot of important material. Your family has been through a lot and you have ideas about things that you would like to work on. Grandma's death seemed like it would be much easier than it has been, given she had been ill for so long. Her death, along with Peter's recent legal trouble and Ginny's decision to move in with her boyfriend next month, has just seemed like too much, and your old comfortable ways of talking with each other seem to have disappeared. Dad, you're often angry. Mom, you feel torn 50 different ways. Ginny, you feel nobody pays much attention to you, and Peter, everyone pays *too* much attention to you. Now, I may not have repeated everything, but I think that catches some of the main areas. Did I miss any big ones?"

Another common closing tool for many theoretical orientations is the homework assignment. This might involve communication time, journaling, charting behaviors, going on dates, reading, listening to instructional tapes, or any number of activities. The important thing to remember is that your opening explanation of how you work should alert the couple or family to the notion that you would be asking them to do something between sessions.

Finally, in closing with multiple people, try to acknowledge that their lives will continue to intersect after the session. You may want to devise a short statement, the essence of which communicates "This will be different at home." An example is:

"Being in counseling together, with me here to guide, ask questions, and even boss people around, is obviously different from when you are together at home. We've talked about some areas that are really troubling and hard. I'm sure you'll continue talking about them at home, but I hope you will remember to try some of the guidelines we've used today. If it gets too damaging, or too hard, we'll have more time to work on things next week. It's okay if everything doesn't get solved at once."

## Termination

As noted earlier, working with couples and families is complex simply because of the number of people involved. In some situations, it can be complicated to schedule the next meeting, so a few minutes for this need should be allocated at the session's end. It is awkward and unprofessional to run out of time and leave people unsure of when the next meeting time is.

Concluding comments should be brief, reassuring, and upbeat. Again expressing your respect for their choice to come in, your appreciation for their work, or noting events upcoming in the week (birthdays, travel plans) can be good transitional termination talk.

## FORMAL COUPLE AND FAMILY ASSESSMENT PROCEDURES

Numerous couple and family assessment devices exist. It is beyond the purpose of this book to provide detailed descriptions of these devices. Therefore, instead of providing an exhaustive review of couple and family assessment procedures, we have listed some of the most popular instruments and procedures, along with their original references, in Table 12.1.

Table 12.1.   Couples and Family Assessment Instruments

| Instrument and Citation | General Description |
|---|---|
| Family Environment Scale (FES), Moos and Moos, 1986 | The assumption underlying this measure is that environments, such as families, have unique personalities that can be measured in much the same way as individual personality. Thus, the 90-item family environment scale seeks to measure the unique social climate within the family. |
| The Family Genogram, McGoldrick and Gerson, 1985 | The family genogram is a procedure that enables therapists to graphically represent family structure. It is very popular among family therapists. The genogram is essentially a visual map of family relationships. It contains factual information such as names, ages, deaths, divorces, etc., as well as relationships. |
| Marital Satisfaction Inventory (MSI), D. Snyder, 1981 | This instrument is a self-report designed to assess marital interaction and marital distress. It includes 11 subscales (e.g., problem-solving communication, disagreement about finances, sexual dissatisfaction). The inventory should be completed by both partners and results are graphed on a single profile so that partner differences can be identified, discussed, and addressed in counseling. |
| Myers-Briggs Type Indicator (MBTI), I. Myers and McCaulley, 1985 | Widely known as the MBTI, this instrument is often used to help couples understand their differences and similarities. The MBTI emphasizes normality rather than pathology, and therefore couples are given feedback about their normal differences and how to live together more efficiently. |
| Stuart Couples' Precounseling Inventory (SCPI), Stuart and Stuart, 1975 | This questionnaire assesses couple relationship areas such as communication, conflict management, relationship change goals, and others. It emphasizes a social learning approach to relationship change. Consequently, the instrument focuses on descriptions of current interaction patterns, rather than personality characteristics. |

## SPECIAL CONSIDERATIONS

The following discussion focuses on situations and issues that interviewers who plan to work with couples and families should consider. These situations and issues are unique to working with couples and families.

### Identifying, Managing, and Modifying Conflict

Couples or families who come for help are frequently there because they have encountered serious conflicts in their relationship and lack the skills to resolve them. Therefore, interviewers must identify, manage, and sometimes modify the ways couples and families express their conflict. Some couples and families seem to fight more readily and naturally than they do anything else. There are a number of issues related to conflict that manifest when interviewing couples or families.

### Conflict Process versus Conflict Content

Couples come to counseling with numerous conflicts. For example, three of the top areas of ongoing conflict reported by couples are money, sex, and in-laws. Of course, there are many other potential couple conflict areas, including division of labor, child rearing, and recreational and religious pursuits/preferences (D. K. Snyder, 1979). Similarly, families arrive in counseling with a variety of common conflict areas. Shared duties, chores, children's individuation needs, and fairness in family resource allocation are some of the most common family issues presented in counseling.

*Conflict content* refers to *what* is argued about. In contrast, *conflict process* refers to *how* everyone argues. This is an important distinction, and clinical interviewers must, during the first session, help couples and families identify both *what* they are arguing about as well as *how* they are arguing with one another.

Most couples and families who come to therapy are engaging in destructive or inefficient conflict process. This is an assumption, albeit a relatively safe one. Specifically, we are assuming that couples and families who come to counseling have, at least to some extent, conflict resolution skill deficits. They are having problems with the *how* of conflict. Most human beings are not completely equipped with healthy and effective conflict management skills (Wilmot & Hocker, 1997). Of course, there are occasions when couples and families have significant conflict in numerous content areas and have tried various adaptive strategies to resolve their differences.

Both conflict content and conflict process are manifest during an initial family or couple counseling interview. Both are important. Further, it is likely that the interviewer may have personal reactions to both *what* families and couples argue about and *how* they argue.

### How Do You Feel about Conflict?

Not everyone enjoys open conflict. Some people are conflict avoiders and others are conflict seekers (Wilmot & Hocker, 1997). This is true about counselors as well as clients. If, as an interviewer, you find yourself having strong conflict avoidance qualities, you may not be well-suited to becoming a couple or family counselor. Generally, before entering the marriage and family counseling field, it is advisable to explore how you respond to interpersonal conflict and what conflict issues push your buttons (see Putting It in Practice 12.2).

---

**Putting It in Practice 12.2**

## Exploring Your Conflict Buttons

To explore, in advance, how you might respond to various couple and family conflict scenarios, reflect on some of the following questions:

1. Do you have any conflict topics that push your personal or emotional buttons? For example, some interviewers with extensive problems with their in-laws bring so much personal baggage into the session that they cannot help but reveal their biases when couples begin discussing in-law issues.
2. Do you have any strong biases about the ways that couples have to behave to continue in a marriage or partnership, or ways parents, children, and other family members must behave to be a "healthy" family? For example, some counselors may have idealistic visions of couple or family relationships. Having an overly idealistic attitude toward relationships may cause you to become rigid regarding how families or couples should relate to one another to maintain their relationship.
3. Do you carry conflict home with you? Working with families and couples is usually quite emotionally charged work. The conflicts you witness, help manage, and sometimes become a part of can be very draining.
4. When you were growing up, what conflict content issues and process styles were characteristic of your family? Did your mother and father avoid conflict with each other, or did they engage in scary and threatening conflicts? Or, did they handle conflict gracefully?

---

### How Much Should You Let People Argue and Fight during the Session?

As you might guess from material covered thus far in this chapter, our answer to this question is: Not much. As noted, usually families and couples come to counseling partly because their joint conflict resolution skills are poor or dysfunctional. Therefore, if you allow them to engage in open conflict without intervening and changing the process, they simply recapitulate their dysfunctional conflict patterns. It is the interviewer's responsibility, among other things, to disrupt these patterns and help people establish new, different, and more adaptive conflict and conflict resolution patterns.

The only reasonable rationale for allowing couples or families to engage in their usual dysfunctional conflict patterns is to gather assessment information. It can be useful for an interviewer to have a glimpse of how people usually argue and fight with one another. However, this observation period should be relatively brief, followed by a more analytic discussion of what happens when the couple or family system experiences conflict. To help couples or families transition from deeply emotional conflict to a more intellectual analysis of their conflict patterns, make a statement similar to the following:

> "Okay, I'd like you two (or in the case of families, everyone) to stop your argument now."

Depending on the intensity of the conflict, this statement may need to be repeated or stated in a strong, authoritative manner. Continue your statement:

"You've given me a glimpse into how you sometimes handle your conflicts. Let me tell you what I saw. First, Judy, I saw you express criticism toward Bill about his lack of involvement in housecleaning. Then, Bill, I saw you defend yourself by complaining that Judy's housecleaning standards are too high. Then, Judy countered Bill's statement by suggesting that his housecleaning standards are abysmally low. And then, Bill, you started talking about how usually, men and women have different cleanliness standards and that Judy needs to loosen up. And finally, the reason I interrupted your argument is that you both seemed to be getting more and more frustrated because little progress was happening. Is that right?"

As you can see from this relatively tame example, conflict interactions accumulate a great deal of material very rapidly. Many things happen simultaneously. It can be daunting for an interviewer to perform the "simple" task of tracking and then accurately summarizing conflict process. This simple task is not so simple. It requires exceptional listening skills and concise communication. It requires sensitivity. Couples are especially wary about whether the interviewer is siding more with one partner than the other. Aligning with a certain family member in family work is a potent intervention and should never be done inadvertently (Odell & Campbell, 1998; J. Patterson et al., 1998). Managing conflict also requires tact because interviewers must determine when and how to interrupt couple conflict.

Interestingly, some theoretical orientations emphasize that the couple conflict process is guided and sometimes determined by unresolved family of origin issues (Luquet, 1996; Strean, 1985). While managing interpersonal conflict, it is also wise to note both content and process with this intergenerational view in mind. Putting It in Practice 12.3 provides a sample couple conflict scenario.

Conflict interactions can escalate quickly. This is especially true in cases of physically or emotionally abusive couples or families. Abusive or highly conflicted couples

---

**Putting It in Practice 12.3**

## Couple Conflict Intervention

Imagine you are the interviewer for the following scenario. As you read the example, evaluate how comfortable you believe you would feel during the session. Write, word-for-word, an intervention you might try after the couple had returned to your office. Compare and contrast your answers with those of others.

Darren is a 58-year-old American Indian. He is married to Anita, a 45-year-old Caucasian. It is Darren's third marriage and Anita's second marriage. During the first few minutes of their initial session, Anita erupts in anger toward Darren. She accuses him of physical abuse, tells him she now understands why he's been divorced twice before, and marches out of your office. Darren jumps up and runs after her. They both return about one minute later. Anita continues to look angry and Darren is pleading with her to stay in the session and try to work things out. Anita turns to you and says that she refuses to speak to Darren for the remainder of the session, but she will stay if you will try to "talk some sense into his head."

Reflect, either on your own or with a partner, how you might handle this couple's counseling situation.

and families often have so much emotional energy and baggage that their conflicts erupt in powerful outbursts. We have had clients refuse to speak for the remainder of a session, try to hit or kick each other in the counseling office, and abruptly leave sessions amidst a flurry of profanity. The potential emotional explosiveness of couple and family interviews requires that interviewers maintain control throughout the session (Bornstein & Bornstein, 1986). Generally, with more disturbed couple or family systems, you must use greater structure and control to moderate the session. In extreme cases, you may act as an intermediary, paraphrasing almost everything that is said and sometimes not allowing the conflicting parties to speak directly to each other.

In summary, allowing families or couples to act out their emotionally based, destructive conflict processes during counseling is almost always ill-advised. Clients should not be allowed to yell at one another, raise accusations in an abusive manner, or repeatedly use ineffective communication skills. Instead, interviewers must structure the session and become more active, especially when working with high-conflict families and couples (Gurman & Jacobson, 2002; J. Patterson et al., 1998).

## Limit-Setting in the Service of Therapy

Besides the bad modeling and potential damage done by allowing too much conflict in the couple or family work, the conflict itself can become a distraction. It is the interviewer's job to control and minimize distractions so that the necessary work can get done. However, minimizing distractions often involves limit-setting that is uncomfortable for the beginning interviewer to enact. Putting It in Practice 12.4 helps you explore your ability to set limits when interviewing couples and families.

## Diversity Issues

Working with gay and lesbian couples or couples and families from different cultural backgrounds can present interviewers with unique problems (Green, 1996; Igartua, 1998). As discussed in Chapter 13, when an interviewer and client have clear and unmistakable differences, the client may initially scrutinize the interviewer more closely than if the client and interviewer are culturally similar or of the same sexual orientation. These circumstances call for sensitivity, tact, and a discussion of the obvious. The following case example illustrates one scenario requiring multicultural counseling skills.

## CASE EXAMPLE

*Jim and Ollie had been together for three years when they began encountering difficulties in their relationship. Both were students and had limited budgets, so they decided to seek couple counseling at a counseling clinic on campus, staffed by counseling interns. When Jim called for the appointment, he simply indicated he wanted to see someone for couple counseling. The receptionist asked a few basic questions and set up a time for Jim and his partner to come in and see Mary, a fourth-year counseling graduate student. The receptionist had mistakenly assumed Ollie was female, so naturally, Mary was somewhat surprised to meet Jim and Ollie.*

*Mary decided to use the receptionist's error to start a discussion regarding the fact that Jim and Ollie were a gay couple and she was a heterosexual female therapist with very little background in working with gay or lesbian couples. With a warm*

=== **Putting It in Practice 12.4** ===

## Limit-Setting with Couples and Families

Imagine the following scenarios:

*Scenario 1:* Antonio and Lucy have been married four years and are struggling as a couple. They have an 8-month-old baby girl. Unfortunately, they were unable to obtain a babysitter and therefore arrive at their intake interview session, much to your surprise, with their little girl. Although she is very quiet during the session's initial 10 minutes, she progressively becomes more and more distressed and begins wailing and screeching in such a manner that it is impossible to continue the interview. Discuss the following questions with your class, discussion group, or supervisor:

1. Would you be able to end the session politely and then reschedule another appointment?
2. Would you be able to gently ask the parents to leave their child with a babysitter during the next appointment time?
3. How would you respond if, despite your gentle reminder, the parents showed up at the next appointment with their daughter and stated, "We really tried to get a babysitter, but we really couldn't come up with one."
4. If the parents insist on meeting with you while their daughter is present, can you imagine any circumstances under which you would agree to meet with the parents even though they have brought their fussy 8-month-old child?

*Scenario 2:* The Johnsons have been referred by youth court for family therapy. The family includes Margie Johnson, mother of twins Rick and Roy Johnson, and Calvin, Margie's live-in boyfriend. Margie is 37 and the twins are 15. Calvin has lived with Margie and the twins for the past three years. His daughter, Mollie, visits on weekends. The boys' father is currently in prison for forgery and has not seen the boys since they were infants. During the initial visit, Margie, Roy, Rick, and Calvin are all present. The twins begin having a burping contest and Margie gets the giggles. Calvin does nothing. The counselor waits until things settle down and then asks another question. Roy and Rick both burp in response. Margie begins laughing again. No one responds to the question. Discuss the following questions.

1. What is your initial response to the scene? Do you imagine wishing you could call youth court and send back the referral? Do you imagine laughing along with Margie or sitting stone silent, like Calvin? Do you imagine feeling intimidated or disgusted or hopeless?
2. Can you think of ways to get some cooperative interactions going?
3. What are your reactions to the thought of simply burping for a while with the boys?
4. For whom do you have the deepest empathy? How could you use this empathy in the service of therapy?

*smile, Mary said, "Ollie, it is very clear to me you are a guy. Apparently Jane, our receptionist here at the clinic, assumed 'Ollie' could be a woman's name. Funny how our stereotypes fool us sometimes, huh?" Jim and Ollie smiled but didn't say much. They were clearly nervous. Mary continued, "Well, I bet you guys encounter a number of stereotypes and even some bad attitudes. I'm sorry for any misunderstandings. Let me tell you a little bit about how I work with couples and then let's talk about whether it seems like my way of working could be helpful for you."*

*Mary then proceeded to briefly explain her relationship enhancement orientation. Jim and Ollie relaxed a little and were able to say they felt learning some new ways of understanding and handling conflict would be helpful to them. Mary then said, "Yeah, I think this model is excellent for many couples. But I know you face some unique situations and have unique needs as a gay couple. I've read a couple of books that address gay and lesbian couples' needs, but I may miss some things. I hope you will be honest with me if you feel I've made a wrong assumption."*

In her work with Jim and Ollie, it is Mary's responsibility to occasionally check in regarding her possible blind spots. As a heterosexual, she may need specialized supervision to enhance her work with Jim and Ollie (Bailey, Kim, Hills, & Linsenmeier, 1997). Finally, it is up to Mary and her supervisor to refer Jim and Ollie to a different counselor if she finds herself, for whatever reason, unable to nonjudgmentally proceed with couple counseling.

Cultural, religious, and racial differences are expressed in families and couples more fully than in individual therapy. Therefore, these differences and how they are handled can play a pivotal role in the therapy success. This area is covered more thoroughly in Chapter 13, but its importance cannot be underestimated.

### Shifting from Individual to Couple or Family Therapy

As noted throughout this chapter, interviewers should treat all couple and family members equally. We also have emphasized the tendency of relationship partners and family members to triangulate interviewers in an effort to have greater power or control in the therapy and family settings. For these reasons, we usually avoid the ubiquitous temptation to shift from individual to couple or family therapy with people from the same family system. We also advise against simultaneous individual and couple or family work by the same counselor. Our rules for handling this issue are:

- Once an individual client, always an individual client. Generally, we will not do individual counseling with someone and then initiate couple or family work that involves that person. Instead, we refer those involved to a competent colleague.
- Following completion of couple or family counseling, on rare occasions, we might consider working in individual therapy with one of the family members. However, when doing so, we always make it clear: Once we start individual therapy, we will not return to couple or family therapy.

For a number of reasons, many therapists do not abide by these suggestions; consider the following scenarios:

An individual client says something to the therapist such as, "Because we've already been working together, I trust you. I don't want to start all over and go see someone else for marriage therapy. And my husband says he doesn't mind."

A teenage boy and his therapist mutually conclude that family therapy is needed. The boy states, "I absolutely refuse to go to therapy with anyone else but you! There is no way I'm going to see a different shrink!"

Therapists may want to prolong therapy with a person because they enjoy working with that client or because they need to maintain their caseload for financial reasons.

Clients may believe that a particular therapist is the best choice because he or she is already well-versed in the couple's or family's therapy issues. It feels safe to stay with the same professional.

You may have noticed that previously we referred to the potential shift from individual to couple or family therapy as the "ubiquitous temptation." From a therapist's perspective, it is almost always tempting to continue counseling when there has been some success with a client, or when a client expresses a strong preference to continue counseling with you, or when there is potential financial gain from continuing counseling. We also refer to this as a temptation because close inspection of the reasons for shifting from individual to couple or family therapy reveals many potential problems or counterarguments. As you read about and reflect on our views regarding this issue in individual/family therapy, keep in mind that we are expressing our professional opinion and bias—there are many therapists and counselors who disagree with this position.

## Conflicts of Loyalty

Perhaps the greatest reason to avoid shifting from individual to couple or family therapy is that conflicts of loyalty inevitably ensue. Specifically, unless the therapist makes great efforts to build trust and rapport with the original client's romantic partner or family, the new parties are likely to believe the therapist holds a deeper loyalty to his or her original client. Additionally, if the therapist, for whatever reason, sides with the new therapy client against the original client, the original client may feel betrayed and abandoned. Consequently, the therapist can become stuck in a no-win therapy bind; both or all clients may quickly suspect the therapist has already "sided" with the original client, or has switched allegiances. Such dynamics can add unnecessarily to an already difficult therapy task.

## You Are (Almost Always) Not the Only (Competent) Therapist in Town

An excuse often offered for doing individual, couples, and family work interchangeably with the same people is that the people involved insist on it. Underlying their preference is their belief that you have done excellent work. This is flattering, but not a convincing argument. Choosing to cross the boundaries and do the additional work can, in fact, undo some of the good work you did in the first place. Avoiding dual roles, an ethical guideline present in all mental health professional ethics codes, includes avoiding being someone's family therapist and individual therapist if being in both roles may cause you to lose objectivity (ACA, 1995; American Psychological Association, 1992).

Catering to the clients' ideas that you are the best or only option is, in fact, not even necessarily healthy. Helping clients attain a more flexible manner of functioning in the world and increasing their capacities for relationships are goals that undergird most forms of therapy. Encouraging an individual to try a different therapist because you were his or her couple counselor can be an important vote of confidence in the client. It communicates that you believe the client can connect with another professional and can use that therapeutic relationship to grow and change. It is rarely, if ever, justified to allow or encourage client dependence on you as the counselor. Obviously, in some rural settings, managing (or juggling) multiple therapy relationships in one family may be unavoidable. In fact, you may not be the *only competent* therapist in town, you may be the *only* therapist in town (Welfel, 2002).

## Identification, Projection, Joining, and Avoiding

Working with couples and/or families comes as close to proving the existence of the unconscious as any professional activity we can think of. You will find it challenging to keep your *own* early learning, beliefs, attachment issues, and the resulting current (conscious and unconscious) struggles from affecting your professional work with couples and families. The common term for this reaction is *countertransference,* mentioned in Chapter 5. Couples and families elicit significant countertransference reactions worthy of consideration.

Adding to the complexity is the fact that effective assessment and assistance is enhanced by interviewers' life experiences. Even if it were possible to exclude your own personal family and relationship issues from your work (including the unconscious processes and conflicts these entail), it would be inadvisable. Common experiences form part of the foundation of any relationship and assist us in understanding other peoples' experiences. Individual and Cultural Highlight 12.1 describes a technique to help you explore your own relationship and family issues.

Working with couples and families usually involves a joining that is more pronounced than in individual work. It is analogous to empathy but perhaps more inclu-

---

**INDIVIDUAL AND CULTURAL HIGHLIGHT 12.1**

### Family Choreography

*Family choreography* is a technique developed by Peggy Papp (1976) and used in many treatment programs. To explore some of your own family of origin material, choose members of the class to represent all the salient members of your family of origin and position them physically according to the roles they played in your family. Then position yourself in your own role. You can hold a particular arrangement for a minute or two and feel the power of the rigid positions, or direct movement and interactions that represent your family dynamics. Then have someone stand in for you and walk around the creation you have fashioned, observing the stand-in family members. Finally, change the action or structure in some way that would have been positive for you. Move positions, change interrelationships, remove members. Do whatever you like and, again, view what you've done.

After everyone sits down, share your feelings about the experience. Also, invite those who were involved to share whatever reactions they had.

As you explore your unique, personal family dynamics within a group setting, it is especially revealing to examine issues associated with culture and ethnicity. Specifically, in the context of your class, you may have individuals who are male, female, disabled, gay, lesbian, straight, Asian, African American, American Indian, Hispanic, older, younger, liberal, conservative, and so on. If your class is up to the task, take time to discuss the major differences in family style between these different unique individuals.

sive. This joining involves coming not only into the worldview of each individual, but also into the worldview of the relationship(s). In the process, you bring your own points of view. Your presence in the system, of course, alters the system. In addition, your views are altered by having joined the system. Keeping a professional perspective in the midst of all this exposure is not easy. Sometimes, counselors "overjoin" and lose perspective completely. Other times, they avoid joining at all, staying aloof and clinically removed. This is safer, but far less informative and probably less therapeutic.

Minuchin and Fishman (1981), among others, have discussed the concept of *joining:*

> Joining is more an attitude than a technique, and it is the umbrella under which all therapeutic transactions occur. Joining is letting the family know that the therapist understands them and is working with and for them. Only under this protection can the family have the security to explore alternatives, try the unusual, and change. Joining is the glue that holds the therapeutic system together. (pp. 31–32)

In addition, the exposure caused by joining a relationship or set of relationships increases the likelihood of tripping our own unresolved family or relationship issues. A big problem with unconscious unresolved issues that might affect our work is that, of course, they are unconscious. The following list is intended to help you glimpse areas that may be active conflicts for you. Consistent patterns of reactions provide clues to areas that might be ripe for personal exploration and growth.

- Do you have any topics that you would rather not talk about? For example, as we discussed earlier, it can be difficult for couples and interviewers to bring up sexual matters in counseling. Mothers-in-law, stillborn babies, the use of belts for punishment, the denial of pets, forced consumption of food—we all carry wounds, sore spots, and fears that can be triggered by common family or couple issues.
- Do you have any biases about clients from diverse cultural or ethnic backgrounds? For example, some counselors have difficulty accepting patriarchal or macho styles associated with some Hispanic couples, religious couples, and others.
- Do you have biases against gay or lesbian people? Further, do you have beliefs about the appropriateness of lifetime exclusive romantic commitments between people of the same sex (i.e., gay and lesbian marriages)?
- Do you find you cannot get certain conflicts or client problems out of your mind? This may manifest by finding yourself thinking about a family or couple excessively, or dreaming about them, or barely resisting talking about them with family or friends.
- Are certain areas of conflict or trouble guaranteed to cause you to condemn one person or be overly sympathetic to the other?

This is, of necessity, not an exhaustive list. It is important to register your reactions and ways of being on an ongoing basis and to seek professional supervision and collegial support when you suspect your own background, values, beliefs, or conflicts are getting in the way of your work with couples or families.

## SUMMARY

In this chapter, we provided an overview of issues relevant to interviewing couples or families. To begin professional development in this area, you must define the terms *fam-*

*ily* and *couple.* Both meanings have values and political issues embedded in them. The complexities of working with families and couples are compounded by the fact that, usually, they do not stay in counseling as long as individuals.

The introduction phase of the clinical interview with couples and families must involve clarity regarding confidentiality, who will attend sessions, and some basic education regarding therapist style and orientation. The opening statement helps further orient clients and establishes norms regarding the inclusion of everyone's voice. The body of the interview is most influenced by theoretical orientation and presenting problem. The chapter cited examples of such orientations and included content areas that are important to cover regardless of therapeutic orientation. The closing is important to manage, both informationally and emotionally; it usually requires significantly more time than closing with an individual. Termination, too, has complications because of the number of people involved in this type of interview.

A number of formal assessments are used effectively with couples and families. Special considerations for couple and family interviewers include: (a) managing interpersonal conflict, (b) setting limits, (c) seeing an individual in the family system for individual therapy, and (d) working with gay or lesbian couples and families.

Finally, ways that countertransference plays an unavoidable role in couple and family work were described and discussed. Suggestions for recognition and management of interviewer countertransference were offered.

## SUGGESTED READINGS AND RESOURCES

American Association for Marriage and Family Therapy. (2001). *AAMFT code of ethics.* Washington, DC: Author. This is the code of ethics for members of the American Association of Marriage and Family Therapy. It is a must-read for AAMFT members and for individuals who plan to frequently conduct couple or family therapy.

Brofenbrenner, U. (1979). *The ecology of human development.* Cambridge, MA: Harvard University Press. This is Urie Brofenbrenner's classic text on ecological formulations of human development.

Gottman, J. M., & DeClaire, J. (2001). *The relationship cure: A five-step guide for building better connections with family, friends, and lovers.* New York: Crown Publishers. Gottman is currently the premier marriage researcher and writer in the United States. His books are based on his vast research and knowledge of marriage and family functioning.

Gray, J. (1992). *Men are from mars, women are from Venus.* New York: HarperCollins. We should be clear that by listing this book, we are not necessarily endorsing its underlying philosophy. It emphasizes male-female differences (rather than similarities) and an "accept me as I am" philosophy more than we prefer. However, it has become so popular that all couples counselors should be familiar with it and its implications.

Gurman, A. S., & Jacobson, N. S. (2002). *Clinical handbook of couple therapy* (3rd ed.). New York: Guilford. This 716-page text offers broad coverage of many couple therapy interventions and theoretical perspectives. It also includes material on divorce, multicultural couple therapy, and how to work with couples who struggle with various medical or psychiatric problems.

Hendrix, H. (1988). *Getting the love you want: A guide for couples.* New York: Holt and Company. Hendrix's book is a popular homework reading assignment for couples who are in counseling. It emphasizes how unconscious and biological factors influence human attraction and coupling. It also provides numerous couple exercises for breaking out of relationship struggles.

International Association of Marriage and Family Counselors. (1993). Ethical code for the International Association for Marriage and Family Counselors. *Family Journal: Counseling and Therapy for Couples and Families, 1,* 73–77. This is another ethics code for another marriage and family counseling group. Again, although it is similar to the AAMFT guidelines, marriage and family practitioners benefit from reading and committing many of its principles to memory.

Jacobson, N. (1996). *Integrative couples therapy: Promoting acceptance and change.* New York: Norton. The late Neil Jacobson of the University of Washington was one of the United States' foremost leaders in couples therapy research and practice. This book is based on two decades of clinical research and practice.

McGoldrick, M., & Gerson, R. (1985). *Genograms in family assessment.* New York: Norton. This book provides thorough background and instruction in constructing the classic family genogram. Using famous families for illustration, it is also enjoyable reading and provides comprehensive coverage of not only construction but also interpretation and suggestions for ways to use the genogram in work with families. We highly recommended it because nearly all family therapy approaches acknowledge the family genogram's utility.

Odell, M., & Campbell, C. E. (1998). *The practical practice of marriage and family therapy: Things my training supervisor never told me.* New York: Haworth. In contrast to more theoretical and sterile approaches to writing about and teaching marriage and family therapy, this book has a strong practical and clinical focus. For example, it includes such chapters as "It Ain't Like the University Clinic" and "So What Do I Do after the Intake?" This practical approach is usually appreciated by beginning students who have had enough of reading and discussing theory.

Scarf, M. (1995). *Intimate worlds.* New York: Random House. In this book, popular mental health and relationship writer Maggie Scarf explores family dynamics. Her approach to studying families involves numerous in-depth interviews, and her orientation is generally family systems with a psychodynamic flavor. She emphasizes use of the Beavers Scale of Family Health and Competence for determining levels of family functioning. Scarf is an excellent writer, and this book provides readers with good background information about family functioning from a systems-psychodynamic perspective.

Skerrett, K. (1996). From isolation to mutuality: A feminist collaborative model of couples therapy. In M. Hill & E. D. Rothblum (Eds.), *Feminist perspectives* (pp. 93–105). New York: Harrington Park Press. This chapter briefly describes a feminist approach to couples counseling.

Tannen, D. (1990). *You just don't understand: Women and men in conversation.* New York: William Morrow, Ballantine. This book explores sex differences in human communication.

Chapter 13

# *MULTICULTURAL AND DIVERSITY ISSUES*

*with Darrell Stolle*

*Let me be quite succinct: the greatest sin of the European-Russian-American complex which we call the West (and this sin has spread its own way to China) is not only greed and cruelty, not only moral dishonesty and infidelity to the truth, but above all its unmitigated arrogance toward the rest of the human race.*

—Thomas Merton, *A Thomas Merton Reader*

*Many counselors may be continuing to suffer from cultural encapsulation and the self-reference criterion in their counseling practice.*

—Paul Pedersen, *Counseling across Cultures*

*Counseling has been used as an instrument of oppression as it has been designed to transmit a certain set of individualistic cultural values. Traditional counseling has harmed minorities and women. Counseling and therapy have been the handmaiden of the status quo.*

—Derald Wing Sue

---

### CHAPTER OBJECTIVES

We live in a multicultural society and, consequently, no matter what our own ethnocultural background may be, we occasionally (or often) work professionally with people who are much different from ourselves. This fact makes it crucial for us to broaden our perspectives and increase our cultural sensitivity. After reading this chapter, you will know:

- About the imperative of cultural competence and the importance of understanding your cultural biases and cultural self.
- Basic issues in interviewing clients with American Indian, African American, Hispanic American, and Asian American ethnocultural backgrounds.
- Basic issues to address when interviewing gay, lesbian, transgendered, disabled, or religiously committed clients.
- The importance of context to understanding client ethnocultural orientation, family environment, community environment, communication style, and language usage.
- Different culture-bound syndromes and matters of etiquette to consider when interviewing minority clients.

## RELATIONSHIP IN THE CONTEXT OF DIVERSITY

Throughout this text, we emphasize the importance of the therapeutic relationship. We believe that relationship is foundational to everything mental health professionals do—including clinical interviewing. Many mental health professionals emphasize the centrality of a therapeutic relationship in doing effective multicultural counseling (Ho, 1992; Paniagua, 1998, 2001; D. W. Sue & Sue, 1999). But what are essential components of such a relationship? What are helpful but optional components? Toward what should we be striving, as we become more multiculturally sensitive interviewers? How can we avoid cultural arrogance, the self-referencing syndrome, and counseling as oppression when working with diverse clients? This chapter provides food for thought and pieces of the puzzle, but obtaining the answers to these profound questions is a life-long endeavor.

### The Imperative of Cultural Competence

The 2000 U.S. census indicates steady population growth of cultural and ethnic minorities over the past several decades (U.S. Bureau of the Census, 2001). Of the 281 million people living in the United States, approximately 80 million identify themselves as other than White, or of Hispanic origin (U.S. Bureau of the Census, 2001). The census shows that diversity is increasing in nearly every state, making it more likely that mental health professionals in every setting will work with clients of different ethnocultural backgrounds than themselves. This is an exciting and daunting possibility; exciting for the richness that a diverse population extends to our communities, and for the professional and personal growth that accompanies cross-cultural interactions; daunting because of the increased responsibility of having to employ culturally relevant approaches in our work. Hall (1997) makes a case for the idea of "cultural malpractice" for those who practice with inadequate knowledge of cultural dynamics and warns that without significant changes in the way cultural issues are addressed, psychology will become obsolescent. The imperative is clear, especially in the context of the clinical interview. To remain a viable helping resource for our whole population, we must have the necessary knowledge and understanding of culture as it impacts mental health.

### Interviewer, Know Thyself

> *You say you're White, that you're American. Don't you know that MEANS something? Where I come from, being Black MEANS something!"*
>
> —Victor; from the movie *The Color of Fear*

Culture can be generally understood as the medium in which all human development takes place. Everything we value, know to be real, and assume to be "normal" is influenced by our past and present cultures. From a counseling perspective, answers to overarching questions such as, "What constitutes a healthy personality?" or "What should a person be or become" are largely influenced by the counselor's culture of origin (Christopher, 1996). For these reasons, the best place to begin in our quest to be culturally competent interviewers is with a thorough examination of ourselves as cultural beings. What does it mean to be from the culture we are from?

According to D. W. Sue, Arredondo, and McDavis (1992), increasing awareness of your own culture is a precondition for moving from an ethnocentric, culturally encapsulated perspective to a truly multicultural perspective. When we have the ability to un-

---

**Putting It in Practice 13.1**

## Counselor as a Cultural Being

Being aware of yourself as a cultural being has been described as a prerequisite for competent multicultural counseling. In fact, the first multicultural competency discussed by D. W. Sue, Arredondo, and McDavis (1992) states, "Culturally skilled examiners have moved from being culturally unaware to being aware and sensitive to their own cultural heritage and to valuing and respecting differences" (p. 482).

For this activity, you should work with a partner.

A. Describe yourself as a cultural being to your partner. What is your ethnic/cultural heritage? How did you come to know your heritage? How is your heritage manifested in your life today? What parts of your heritage are you especially proud of? Is there anything about your heritage that you are not proud of? Why?

B. What do you think constitutes a "mentally healthy" individual? Can you think of times when there are exceptions to your understanding of this?

C. Has there ever been a time in your life when you experienced racism or discrimination? (If not, was there ever a time when you were harassed or prevented from doing something because of some unique characteristic that you possess?) Describe this experience to your partner. What were your thoughts and feelings related to this experience?

D. Can you relate a time when your own thoughts about people who are different from you affected how you treated them? Would you do anything differently now?

E. How would you describe the "American culture"? What parts of this culture do you embrace? What parts do you reject? How does your internalization of American culture impact what you think constitutes a "mentally healthy individual"?

At the conclusion of the activity, take time to reflect and possibly make a few journal entries about anything you may have learned about your cultural identity.

---

derstand how our thinking, feeling, and knowing are influenced by our culture, we begin to obtain the capacity to understand another's perspective without imposing our own. D. W. Sue et al. defines specific parameters for practicing in a culturally competent manner (see Putting It in Practice 13.1).

### Cultural Competence

Self-awareness is only the beginning of multicultural awareness and competence. Many variables are included in cultural competence. Specifically, three critical characteristics have been identified as essential for cultural competence: (a) scientific mindedness, (b) skills in dynamic sizing, and (c) proficiency with a particular cultural group (S. Sue, 1998).

*Scientific mindedness* requires forming and testing hypotheses, rather than making faulty assumptions and/or conclusions about the status of ethnoculturally different clients. While there may be universal human experiences, you cannot assume every client's needs are the same. It is important for interviewers to move beyond the *myth of sameness* when working with clients of diverse culture and ethnicity (Wilson, Phillip, Kohn, & Curry-El, 1995).

## CASE EXAMPLE

*A 14 year-old Hopi Indian student was referred for counseling at his school because his teachers reported increasing social withdrawal and failing grades. The school counselor, on reviewing the past year's records, discovered that the boy's academic and social behavior had declined after a younger brother had died in a drowning accident approximately nine months before. During their first session, the boy reluctantly admitted to witnessing his brother's death and indicated that he had not spoken about the incident to anyone.*

*In this particular case, it would be quite natural for a school counselor to attribute the boy's school and social troubles to unresolved grief and to design a treatment plan to help the student express his feelings associated with his loss and trauma. Although this is a plausible explanation, there might be others to consider, and, regardless, the treatment plan would be a serious mistake.*

*Scientific mindedness requires the interviewer to search for alternative explanations for the boy's silence, his withdrawal, and his failure in school. Without exploring less commonly known and understood explanations, the school counselor might never know that the boy's silence was because of traditional Hopi belief about death. Without engaging in scientific mindedness, the counselor might inappropriately push the boy to talk about his brother's death.*

*For the traditional Hopi, when a person in a family, or close to a family, dies, it is best not to talk about him or her because it increases the likelihood that the person's spirit will visit them in the night. Imagine the trauma that might be induced if, according to standard operating procedure, the counselor encouraged this boy to talk openly and freely about his brother. Not only does scientific mindedness require counselors to explore all reasonable explanations for behavior, but also it requires treatment techniques that are compatible with cultural practices and beliefs.*

*Dynamic sizing* is the second cultural competency characteristic described by S. Sue (1998). This concept requires the interviewer to know when generalizations based on group membership are appropriate and when they are not. You need to know the general characteristics of the client's culture of origin, yet at the same time, allow for differential internalization and/or expression of those characteristics.

For example, the concept of *machismo* is often discussed in relation to Hispanic men. However, it is naïve to assume that all Hispanic men express *machismo;* doing so can influence your expectations of client behavior. On the other hand, you would be remiss if you were ignorant of *machismo* and the possibility that it influences Hispanic male behaviors. When dynamic sizing is used appropriately, the pitfalls of stereotyping clients are avoided, while at the same time, the interviewer remains open to significant cultural influences.

Another facet of dynamic sizing involves therapists' knowing when to generalize their own experiences. S. Sue (1998) states, "A person who has experienced discrimination and prejudice as a member of one group may be able to understand the plight of those in another group who encounter the same experiences" (p. 446). However, having similar experiences does not guarantee accurate empathy. Dynamic sizing requires the interviewer to both *know* and understand and *not know* and not understand at the same time. This elegant combination of deep understanding and openness is a crucial component of culturally competent interviewing.

The third characteristic of cultural competency is *culture-specific expertise.* Culture-specific expertise involves the continuous acquisition of information about cultural groups, including sociopolitical dynamics, as well as effective interventions and techniques geared toward specific cultural groups. It has been argued that mental health professionals cannot know every nuance of every culture on the face of the earth. Of course, this is true. However, this fact does not excuse cultural ignorance. Learning about the life experiences and belief systems of other humans never ends. Competent mental health professionals seize every opportunity to increase their understanding of the diversity of life around them. Therefore, in some ways, multiculturalism is an attitude or philosophy as much as it is an applied field.

The next section of this chapter contains basic, noncomprehensive coverage of concerns specific to groups of people identified by race and/or cultural background. In addition, brief sections addressing persons with different sexual orientations, persons with handicapping conditions, and persons with deep religious convictions are included. An argument could be made for including women, the elderly, and other groups who have experienced oppression or do not fit the mold of young, White, and male (Atkinson & Hackett, 1998; Wilkinson & Kitzinger, 1996). There are many ways people find themselves grouped together and many ways these groupings affect identity formation, functioning in the world, and quality of life in the dominant culture. As D. W. Sue et al. (1996) state:

> Each client (individual, family, group, organization) has multiple cultural identities which most likely do not progress or expand at the same rate. For example, a man may be quite aware of his identity as a Navaho but less aware of himself as a heterosexual or Vietnam veteran. As such, comprehensive multicultural therapy may focus on helping him and others like him become ever more aware of the impact of cultural issues on their being. (p. 17)

Being a multiculturally oriented clinical interviewer involves an orientation toward diversity that is open, affirming, and appropriately curious. The following information on cultural groups provides barely enough information to whet the appetite and acknowledge basic potential cultural differences among clients. The old adage "The map is not the territory" is especially pertinent here, as these descriptions are meant to simply orient the interviewer. The actual cultural landscape will be unique to the individual and will most likely look quite different from the following map.

## THE BIG FOUR

In the introduction to *Growing up Latino* (Augenbraum & Stavans, 1993), Ilan Stavans writes:

> Today, at the center of the conflict is the Hispanic, the man, woman, or child who speaks Castilian Spanish as his or her mother tongue, or whose ancestors did so. We in the United States often perceive Hispanics as a monolithic or amorphous group. They have divided loyalties, we say, and live between two cultures and two languages. But this is a narrow definition, a figment that Americans have created to fill our need to make these diverse peoples into a single one that we can then understand. (p. xvi)

Stavans was writing about Hispanics, but he could have inserted any of the larger or smaller minority groups in the United States and been equally accurate. Our groupings are huge, with an astonishing amount of diversity within each one. The same can be said for what is often referred to as White culture, or the dominant culture. We would be hard pressed to define *White* (D. Scherer, personal communication, October 13, 1998). Would we include Italian Americans? Would we include Jewish Americans? Does the word *Anglo* communicate more accurately than *White*? Even if we said "persons of Western European descent," it would not be clear as to who would be in and who would be out. In what century must the descendence begin to fit this category? With apologies for these obvious gross generalizations, we make divisions to compare and contrast very broad differences between cultures. For example, we use the word *White* to refer to the dominant Caucasian culture in the United States. However, we readily acknowledge that our generalities are so broad as to be of limited usefulness. We hope this section stimulates your desire to develop your cultural competency.

## American Indian Cultures

*Oona was only five years old but she was already trained in many of the ways of a good Ojibway. She knew almost all that she could not do and all that she must learn to do. She went to her grandparents and stood before them with eyes cast down, knowing she could not speak the many questions she wished to ask, for they who are wise must speak first. Always, the first words spoken should be from the older people.*

—Ignatia Broker, Ojibway elder and storyteller, *Growing up Native American,* ed. by Pat Riley

According to the 2000 census, there are approximately 500 tribes represented in the United States; not surprisingly, each tribe has distinct values, customs, and histories. Historically, Berkhoffer (1978) points out, more than 2,000 cultures were represented on the North American continent when Europeans first arrived in the late fifteenth century. These cultures had diverse languages, practices, and friendly or warlike interrelationships. They did not think of themselves as a single people. It is a mistake to assume more commonality among American Indians than exists. On the other hand, there are aspects of past and current Indian life that allow American Indians from different tribes to find much common ground.

One such area of common ground is that American Indians experienced genocidal practices at the hands of European settlers for more than two centuries (personal communication, G. Swaney, September 15, 2001). The trauma and intergenerational grief and despair associated with these experiences are still readily in evidence in most tribal cultures and still take a toll in many tragic ways. Although American Indians come to counseling for all the reasons anyone in the dominant culture might come to counseling, we must remember that, as a people, their cultures were systematically decimated. Consider Chief Sitting Bull's response to the American policy of assimilation in the late nineteenth and early twentieth centuries:

I am a red man. If the Great Spirit had desired me to be a white man, he would have made me so in the first place. He put in your heart certain wishes and plans, in my heart he put other and different desires. Each man is good in His sight. It is not necessary for eagles to be crows. (as cited in Deloria, 1994, p. 198)

Cultural decimation and assimilation still have direct counseling ramifications, especially if the counselor represents White European culture. While genocidal policies in the

United States are now mainly historical, contemporary struggles regarding land use and impingement on tribal sovereignty are relics of the same policies. White European counselors bear little responsibility for past events. However, they can still be *perceived* as representative of a dominant culture encroaching on the rights of Indian people. From a relationship-building perspective, establishing trust may require extra sensitivity.

The danger of overgeneralization notwithstanding, here are a few specific cultural variables that can be used to help orient an interviewer working with Indian clients.

### Tribal Identity

Asking an Indian client about his or her tribe is an important component of an initial interview. The client may choose not to tell you very much, but nearly all Indian people identify themselves as belonging to a tribe, band, or clan (Sutton & Broken Nose, 1996). Although it may reveal your unfamiliarity with the tribe named, interviewers should not be shy about asking for the correct pronunciation and spelling. Even Indian counselors do not know the names and practices of every existing tribe (although most would be far ahead of the average non-Indian counselor). No matter how much or how little tribal identity exists in a given individual, it is an important component of Indian culture (D. Wetsit, personal communication, July 11, 1998). Asking about tribal affiliation and identity begins an important process between the counselor and the Indian client. After clients identify their tribes, an easy follow-up question is: "Tell me the things you value most about being Assiniboine." When non-Indian interviewers pretend to know too much about Indian life or tribal issues, they risk damaging rapport with Indian clients. Respectful questioning about tribal affiliation is more appropriate and much less presumptive.

### The Role of Family

Across most or all tribes, extended family is deeply important to Indian people. Kinship systems vary, but the roles of adopted and biological grandparents, aunts, uncles, cousins, and siblings are central and important. Funerals, weddings, births, and community and family celebrations are occasions of great import and often supersede other obligations. Sometimes, the family considers tribal elders and medicine people as family members; under some circumstances, these members may be appropriate to include in family-based interventions or interviews.

Tribal customs for family roles vary, as do parenting practices. Given the importance of these areas, asking about differences can provide helpful information if your clients come from families with mixed tribal backgrounds (Ho, 1992).

### The Role of Spirituality

It would be a gross overgeneralization to say that every Indian person is spiritually oriented. However, for many Indians, there are a number of spiritual, sacred connections: among tribal members—living, dead, and those yet to be born; between nature and humans; between Creator and created. These connections affect the way life is lived in the present and the way family and tribal society is viewed. In gatherings of American Indians, a prayer (or song) is usually offered. Respect toward spirituality is basic to establishing a strong therapeutic relationship.

### Sharing and Material Goods

Traditionally, Indians accord great respect to those who give the most to other individuals and families, and then to the band, tribe, or community. (Sutton & Broken Nose, 1996, p. 40)

Sharing among Indians is in stark contrast to our capitalistic culture in which giving takes a backseat to acquisition. This clash of values can be a source of confusion and distress for Indian young people who are trying to maintain cultural identity and lead successful lives as measured by dominant cultural standards.

## Time

Many cultures view the passage of time in a much more relaxed, circular fashion than do dominant European and U.S. cultures. Arriving at the agreed-on time for an appointment is a given for most persons of European descent. However, arriving on time is not always related to the clock for Indian people (and people of many cultures). "On time" can mean arriving at the time that things worked out to arrive. A corollary to this, often experienced by our interns who work at tribal college counseling services, is a reluctance on the part of some Indian people to schedule weekly meetings. Although no-showing for scheduled appointments is quite common, the walk-in center receives brisk business. Indian people are more oriented to the here-and-now and less oriented to the future than Whites of European descent (Herring, 1990). When there is a felt need for counseling experienced in the present, it is sought. However, agreeing to an arrangement in the future may or may not work out, depending on what is happening when the future becomes the present.

## Communication Styles

Many American Indians believe silence is a sign of respect. Listening carefully to another is a great compliment, and not listening is seen as very disrespectful. However, there are culturally appropriate ways to demonstrate attentive listening that are quite different from common White listening habits. The liberal use of questions is not a common sign of listening; in fact, asking too many questions can be seen as rude. Therefore, the interviewer should keep questions brief and limited in number. In addition, you should not expect many questions from the Indian client. Strive for clarity and pause liberally when you ask if the Indian client has any questions. The client may want time to formulate one well-worded question rather than ask many.

Eye contact in many Indian cultures is different from the dominant American culture. Respect is communicated to others by listening quietly and avoiding direct eye contact. This is especially true when the Indian person is wishing to communicate respect to an elder or someone of perceived higher status.

For some Indian clients, note-taking during the initial interview may not be experienced as a listening behavior (Ho, 1993). It is wise to watch for nonverbal signals that taking notes is seen as rude (Paniagua, 1998), and stop taking notes if possible. If you must take a few notes, simply explain the function of your notes and try to compensate for the distraction they represent.

A case example of an initial interview and case formulation with an American Indian is provided in Putting It in Practice 13.2.

## African American Cultures

*I am Kikuyu. My people believe if you are close to the Earth, you are close to people. What an African woman nurtures in the soil will eventually feed her family. Likewise, what she nurtures in her relations will ultimately nurture her community. It is a matter of living the circle.*

—Wangari Waigwa-Stone in *Refuge: An Unnatural History of Family and Place*, by Terry Tempest Williams

Similar to the experience of American Indians, the relationship between African Americans and European settlers did not begin as a mutual, voluntary relationship. Both American Indian and African American cultures experienced the decimation of family structure, severe illness, loss of property and custom, and loss of liberty because of their involuntary contact with Whites. Between the years 1518 and 1870, approximately 15 million Africans were captured and brought by force to serve as slaves in the New World (Black, 1996). The resulting intergenerational trauma, role confusion, grief, and loss reverberate in the African American culture as it rebuilds itself. There are spectacular success stories and examples of healing, depth, and wisdom throughout African American culture, but the costs of these traumas are still evident.

### The Role of the Family

People of African descent place great importance on nuclear family and extended kinship systems. This pattern of family relationship was true in Africa before they were brought to North America and was reinforced by the extreme conditions families faced as slaves. Every family member, no matter how remotely related biologically, is highly valued.

---

**Putting It in Practice 13.2**

## An Initial Interview with an American Indian Client

Willard is a 26-year-old, single Navajo male who grew up on the Navajo reservation in rural New Mexico. He served four years in the Navy immediately after high school and is now a junior in college majoring in mathematics and education. College administration required Willard to seek counseling after he was arrested for assault during a fight in the dorm, and his status in school was contingent on completion of five sessions. The incident report noted that he and two other students became involved in an altercation after one of the other students made inappropriate gestures toward Willard's girlfriend.

During his first session, it was noted that he was a large, well-muscled young man with long hair freely falling around his shoulders. He did not smile upon introduction. However, he did make direct eye contact. He indicated that he was aware of the conditions placed on his continued enrollment, but he was not enthusiastic about participating in counseling.

Working in small groups or dyads, consider how you might proceed with the initial interview with Willard. Begin by creating a list of items that need to be considered given the circumstances of his referral. (For example, what is the impact of being force-referred to counseling?) Which of the items on your list have cultural implications? Next, consider the issues that are relevant to establishing a therapeutic relationship with Willard. How would you begin the interview? (Practice this with your small group or dyad.) Finally, what information would you want to know about Willard that would influence your work with him in the future? Do stereotypes or assumptions that you might have about Native Americans influence anything on your list? (For example, one might be curious if any of the participants in the fight were under the influence of alcohol.) Discuss these with your group.

Interviewing individuals, couples, or families of African descent should involve sensitivity to family roles. The family head may be the father, the mother, or older siblings. In addition, unrelated community members (godparents, pastors, and close friends) may serve important familial roles. Although a genogram can help with assessment or treatment, African American kinship systems may contain information not openly acknowledged. Hines and Boyd-Franklin (1996) state, "Illegitimate births, parents' marital status, incarcerated family members, or deaths due to AIDS, violence, or substance abuse may be 'secrets' unknown to all family members or information that members are hesitant to discuss with an outsider" (p. 71). Obviously, trust should be established before you can expect open sharing of such information.

### Religion and Spirituality

The role of the church, religion, and/or spiritual pursuits is central to many African Americans. Meaningful and emotionally charged religious services that began during slavery continue today. Deep involvement with a faith community might be as influential and central as family. Church members or church leaders may sometimes be effectively invited into the counseling process.

### Couple and Gender Roles

The African American male has been said to suffer from marginalization in many ways. Franklin (1993) coined the term *invisibility syndrome,* referring to White culture's fear-based tendencies to treat African males as if they were invisible. African American males have a lower life expectancy than White males or than females of either race because of murder, incarceration, mental and physical disabilities, drug and alcohol abuse, and dangerous employment situations (Hines & Boyd-Franklin, 1996). This invisibility can creep into the clinical interview, either in the form of stereotyped assumptions about the male who is present in the family system, or about the absence of the male in a family system.

Dating back to African practices, African American family roles tend to be more egalitarian than those in the White patriarchy, where women's roles were limited to childbearing and homemaking (Willie, 1981). African American women are likely to work for the family's sustenance as well as function in an equal or dominant parenting role.

Couples counseling often occurs because of child-focused concerns (Hines & Boyd-Franklin, 1996). Also, African American women have been noted to stay in a dysfunctional relationship because of a reluctance to add further distress to the burdened lives of African American men (McGoldrick, Garcia-Preto, Hines, & Lee, 1989). This reluctance to take care of themselves out of deference to "their men" can be very frustrating for counselors working with African American women.

### Language

For an interviewer unaccustomed to street talk, or Black English, a client using such can be a challenge to understand. However, we do not see this issue as qualitatively different from any other bilingual challenge. Some African Americans speak perfect Standard American English and can switch to nearly indecipherable (for the interviewer) Black English at will. Some White Americans can do the same. However, it is unlikely that most White counselors easily understand street talk or Black English. You simply need to acknowledge your inability to understand and ask for help. The important thing to remember is that it is the interviewer's language deficit, not the language-speaker's problem. A polite attitude with a bit of a sense of humor goes a long way toward bridging language barriers that might exist.

## Issues of Assumptions

There are approximately 30.8 million Americans of African descent (U.S. Bureau of the Census, 1992). They make up the largest non-White cultural group in the United States. Statistically, African Americans are poorer, have less education, suffer from more unemployment, and have more teen pregnancies as compared to White Americans. Our country has been torn by racial strife, with much of the violence and loss suffered between Whites and African Americans. We mention this because it is good to remember that a little knowledge is a dangerous thing. It is tempting to believe that because we once had an African American friend, roommate, girlfriend, or boss, we somehow know how to work with people of African descent. Such assumptions are hazardous with regard to any person from another culture, but seem especially likely between Whites and African Americans.

An example of an initial interview with an African American client is included in Putting It in Practice 13.3.

---

**Putting It in Practice 13.3**

### Working with an African American Client

Marvin was a 36-year-old African American male who had been married for 12 years and had two children, ages six and eight. He referred himself for counseling a short time after receiving a substantial promotion at the accounting firm where he had worked for the last five years. He indicated a preference for working with an African American counselor; however, he didn't feel he could wait for the next opening (estimated to be six months). He, therefore, reluctantly agreed to meet with a white male counselor who was about his age.

Marvin appeared uneasy on meeting his counselor. He shook hands, made brief eye contact, and offered a pensive smile. He reported feeling an enormous amount of stress a few months before his promotion. Fulfilling his role as a husband and father was nearly impossible while meeting the demands of his work. Then he said, "but you being White probably don't understand." He continued angrily, "There's NO WAY you can know what it's like to be a Black man in a White man's business!—Hell, in a White man's WORLD!"

Take a few minutes to contemplate this scenario. What stereotypes of Black men might emerge in your mind after this interaction? How would you deal with them? What would you feel?

How would you respond to Marvin? One option would be to say something like this, "You're right, there's no way I can truly understand what it's like for you, but I'd like to try. Can you tell me more about being Black in your place of work?"

What would a question like this accomplish? What other responses might you try?

## Hispanic American Cultures

> . . . it was the American phenomenon of ethnic turnover that was changing the urban
> core of Paterson, and the human flood could not be held back with an accusing finger.
>   "You Cuban?" the man asked my father, pointing a finger at his name tag on the
> navy uniform—even though my father had the fair skin and light brown hair of his
> northern Spanish family background and our name is as common in Puerto Rico as
> Johnson is in the United States.
>   "No," my father had answered, looking past the finger into his adversary's angry
> eyes. "I'm Puerto Rican."
>   "Same shit." And the door closed.
>
> —Judith Ortiz-Cofer, *Silent Dancing*

For the purposes of this chapter, we take our meaning for the term *Hispanic* from Marin and Marin (1991), who indicate that Hispanic people are "individuals who reside in the United States and who were born in or trace the background of their families to one of the Spanish-speaking Latin American nations or Spain" (p. 1). This term is not perfect, in that some Mexican Americans prefer the term *Latino* because it does not harken back to the conqueror, Spain (Dana, 1993). However, *Hispanic* is the term most commonly used at present, so it is our choice for this section.

The people thus grouped together represent many different countries, cultures, sociopolitical histories, and reasons for being in the United States. Therefore, an important place to begin a clinical interview is to ask about the client's country of origin.

> Proclaiming their nationality is very important to Latinos: it provides a sense of pride and
> identity that is reflected in the stories they tell, their music, and their poetry. Longing for
> their homeland is more pronounced when they are unable to return to their home either
> because they are here as political exiles, or as illegal aliens, or because they are unable to
> afford the cost of travel. In therapy, asking the question, "What is your country of origin?"
> and listening to the client's stories of immigration helps to engage the therapist and gives
> the therapist an opportunity to learn about the country the client left behind, the culture,
> and the reasons for leaving. (Garcia-Preto, 1996, p. 142)

### Religion and Related Belief Systems

The Catholic Church is very influential in many Hispanic cultures. The priest, therefore, is often central in helping solve individual and family problems. Mental health problems are sometimes seen as being caused by evil spirits, and, therefore, the church is the logical place to seek assistance (Paniagua, 1998). As a result, mental health professionals may be contacted only after all other avenues in the church and community have been accessed.

Sometimes in the Hispanic culture, it is believed that individuals bring on their own mental and/or physical problems by engaging in certain forms of behavior, and that others can be inflicted with such problems by *mal de ojo* (the evil eye) directed at them (Paniagua, 1998). Such beliefs are related to a fatalism that some have identified as common to many Hispanic cultures (Neff & Hoppe, 1993). *Fatalism* is a belief that a person cannot do much about his or her fate—adversity and good fortune are out of the control of the individual. In counseling, this belief can be counterproductive when the therapist is trying to encourage clients to take control and begin making changes. On the other hand, it can absolve individuals of blame for traumatic life circumstances that are indeed out of their control. It is ill-advised to strongly confront Hispanics regarding their fatalistic or external locus of control orientation. In some cases, encouragement to become or stay involved with the church may help.

## Personalism

Hispanic cultures are known for placing great emphasis on interpersonal relationships and valuing warmth, closeness, and honest self-disclosure (Axelson, 1999). These values may dictate the choice of counselor more than credentials per se. As an interviewer, you might be surprised by the level of inquiry and interest in your personal life and tastes, but the intention is not invasiveness, it is simply connection. However, it is advisable to remain more formal initially, to signal the boundaries of the relationship. Using last names and acting with deliberate respect during the first interview can help this process.

In addition, this personal orientation finds expression in the giving of gifts to the counselor during therapy. Paniagua (1998) points out:

> Therapists working with Hispanic clients need to recognize and acknowledge the conditions under which it is culturally appropriate to accept such gifts (e.g., during Christmas, the therapist may receive from a Mexican American client a wooden cup made in Mexico) and those conditions under which it may be clinically appropriate to reject the gift (e.g., receiving the cup as a form of payment for therapy). (pp. 42–43)

## The Role of the Family

Similar to other cultures discussed in this chapter, family is extremely important to Hispanic people and is more broadly defined than traditional White American nuclear families. Family members have most likely been consulted before an individual comes for counseling; and in many cases, involving the family directly is helpful. There is a strong emphasis on the family's needs and the needs of the group over the needs of the individual.

However, in contrast to other nondominant cultures in the United States and in contrast to White culture, role flexibility in the family is not condoned in the Hispanic community. The father is the head of the household and is to be respected as such. The mother is the homemaker and cares for the children. The sense of family obligation, honor, and responsibility runs deep for most traditional Hispanic families (Garcia-Preto, 1996).

## Gender Roles

*Machismo* and *marianismo* are central notions that tend to dictate interpersonal relationships, especially between the sexes. *Machismo* denotes masculinity as evidenced in physical prowess, aggression, attractiveness to women, and consumption of large quantities of alcohol, thereby commanding respect from others. This respect has many important dimensions in Hispanic culture. The term *respeto* (Comas-Díaz & Duncan, 1995) refers to respect accorded persons in the culture based on age, social position, sex, and status. A person who shows appropriate *respeto* is seen as someone who has been well educated or well reared.

*Marianismo,* or traditional Hispanic womanhood, is based on the Catholic worship of the Virgin Mary. It connotes obedience, timidity, sexual abstinence until marriage, emotionality, and gentleness. According to Comas-Díaz (1989), the concept of *marianismo* includes a belief in the spiritual superiority of women, who endure all the suffering produced by men.

Needless to say, machismo and marianismo are not generally socially acceptable gender-role guidelines in the dominant culture in the United States. Families who immigrated experience conflicts as younger generations acculturate and refuse to conform to these traditional roles and expectations.

A case example of working with a Hispanic client is provided in Putting It in Practice 13.4.

## Asian American Cultures

*We were sitting in a makeshift kitchen where the staff crowded in for lunch. The speaker was Laotian. A H'Mong coworker placed a straw basket packed with "sticky rice" in the center of the table; a Japanese counselor added short-grained rice from a rice cooker; a Chinese American clinician added a bowl of long-grained rice. The different varieties of rice silently spoke to the different philosophical, ethnic, cultural, historical, and religious traditions represented around that table. And yet we were all considered to be "Asian." Both viewpoints contain aspects of the truth.*

—Christina Chao, "We Do Not Even Eat Rice the Same"

---

### Putting It in Practice 13.4

### Working with a Hispanic Client

Rosa is a 19-year-old single female whose family (mother, father, and five siblings) moved from Mexico to Michigan 15 years ago. She has two sisters, ages 16 and 21, and three brothers, ages 14, 17, and 22. She and her family live in a community that is primarily Mexican American and where Catholicism is a significant part of people's lives. Rosa is living at home while she studies journalism at a local college, where she has consistently been named to the Dean's list for academic excellence.

She came to counseling because she had been feeling depressed over the last two months. She noted that she is not sleeping or eating well, and is "having a hard time just getting through each day." She stated that it was difficult to come to counseling because her family would not approve of her discussing personal things with an outsider, but she came anyway because friends at her college strongly encouraged her.

When asked about her life, she burst into tears. She was thoroughly enjoying college until she noticed that her family was treating her differently. Looking back, she thought it started as soon as she began college, but the novelty of the experience helped her overlook the differences. Rosa said her brothers, especially, were keeping their distance from her and when they spoke to her, they treated her like she wasn't like them anymore. One time she overheard her older brother accuse her of trying to be better than them. She also noticed that she couldn't relate as well to her old friends. When they met, they often ran out of things to say after a few awkward minutes. She finally said, "It's just not worth it to me—I'm going to quit college. I just don't know who I am anymore!"

How would you explore the importance of family with Rosa?

What else would you need to know about her? Her friends?

How would you ask?

Would you consider incorporating other helping sources in your work with Rosa?

Discuss these with a partner.

Asian Americans are only the third largest multicultural group represented in mental health services in the United States (Paniagua, 1998), yet they hail from the world's largest continent both in land mass and in population. Asia is diverse in terms of geographic features; it is even more diverse in terms of religion, custom, lifestyle, and ancestry. The major countries comprising South Asia are India, Bangladesh, and Pakistan; those making up Southeast Asia are Burma, Cambodia, Laos, Vietnam, Malaysia, Indonesia, and the Philippines. East Asia's major countries are China, Japan, North and South Korea, and Taiwan (Axelson, 1999).

## The Role of the Family

Again, among Asian peoples, we find stronger, more inclusive family roles than is true in most White cultures. Similar to Hispanic family structure, the father is considered the head of the household and holds the dominant role. In fact, each family member's role, based on sex, birth order, and marital status, is fixed and cannot be changed (Paniagua, 1998).

Individual acts, therefore, reflect quite directly on the family. Individualism is not viewed positively. Decisions that affect the family (which include most or all decisions) should be decided by the family rather than the individual. The family should be strong enough, wise enough, and have enough resources to handle problems encountered by the individual. Failing this task and seeking outside help in the form of counseling brings a shameful loss of face (Chao, 1992). Therefore, an interviewer conducting a first session with an Asian American client or family must consider the fact that it took a great deal of stress to cause the client(s) to seek help. Consequently, the situation is probably quite serious and must be approached as such.

Further complicating the first visit is the fact that such a visit and the problems that made the visit necessary might be experienced as shameful. The client may not be forthcoming but may, instead, minimize problem areas or attempt to describe them in vague, impersonal ways.

Asian families living in the United States are almost all in some phase of acculturation. The children often become bilingual, therefore assuming a power in the family that upsets traditional roles. Further, some families have members living in the home country and some members living here, which adds more relational and role strain (E. Lee, 1996).

## Orientation toward Authority

Many Asian cultures are rigid and hierarchical in structure (E. Lee, 1996; Reischauer, 1988). This is directly related to a concept called *filial piety,* which refers to the honor, reverence, obedience, and loyalty owed to those who are hierarchically above you (Kitano, 1969). The deference toward authority manifests in a number of ways. Asian American clients expect a counselor to be an expert and to act with authority.

In the same vein, verbal communication with a mental health professional may not be direct and certainly is not confrontive. It is likely that an Asian American client, when faced with uncertainty, simply offers the most polite, affirmative response available. Among Asians, as among many American Indian tribes, silence is a sign of respect. Also similar is the pattern of eye contact. Direct eye contact is invasive and disrespectful, especially when interacting with persons of higher status or authority (Paniagua, 1998).

Even during a first interview, many Asian American people expect concrete and tangible advice. This runs contrary to most training models for beginning interviewers; therefore, you need to practice how to give quick advice. This practice is necessary, too, because the advice being offered will likely be coming from a non–Asian American; the chances of giving culturally appropriate advice are improved by extensive reading and serious advance consideration.

It is important to be respectful to all clients, but Asian American clients may respond especially well to being treated with formal respect. Using Mr., Mrs., and Ms. and a last name is a signal of respect and should not be discontinued until the client directly invites a first-name address. However, be aware that traditionally, in most Asian countries, women keep their own family surnames and may wish to be called by that surname even if, because of customs in the United States, she has begun to use her husband's surname. A simple inquiry along these lines indicates respect.

### Spiritual and Religious Matters

A common practice among many Asian cultures has been the keeping of an ancestor altar. A reverence toward ancestors and various beliefs regarding ancestral spirits, wishes, or presence in family matters can be central to individual and family function-

---

**Putting It in Practice 13.5**

## Working with an Asian American Client

In a recent issue of *Psychotherapy,* John Chambers Christopher, a colleague of ours, reports on the following case:

Simon, an East Asian international student, referred himself to the university counseling center after about one year of studying in the United States. Simon reported low self-esteem, difficulty concentrating, and problems with socializing. His stated goal for therapy was to become "more assertive in his interactions with others" (Christopher, 2001, p. 124). In particular, Simon expressed a desire to become more similar to his American roommates and less like other international students from his homeland.

Presented by a different therapist and/or a different client, this case might simply be cast into the rather straightforward mold of assertiveness training. However, as described by Christopher (2001), Simon's presenting problem stimulated deeper personal reflection:

> I confess that initially this case placed me in a difficult position with respect to my own values. Having spent a number of years critiquing Western culture and learning about the moral visions of non-Western traditions, my tendency was to focus on the limitations of assertiveness and the individualism it manifests and supports. Moreover, I was troubled to see someone from a cultural tradition as rich as Simon's almost eager to forsake this heritage to become Western . . . . I . . . felt a sense of reservation about helping Simon with his stated goals. (p. 125)

This case illustrates an interesting potential contextual dilemma associated with cross-cultural counseling. That is, how does the therapist handle a situation in which he or she values a client's culture to a greater degree than the client?

Take some time to reflect on John Christopher's dilemma. How would you be affected by a similar situation? Are there any particular ethnocultural perspectives, philosophies, or behavior patterns that you find more desirable than your own?

ing and decision-making. Religious orientations are as varied as the countries from which Asian Americans have come, including such diverse belief systems as Buddhism, Islam, Hinduism, Christianity, Janism, and many branches in each.

Much has been written about the Western mind or worldview and the Eastern mind or worldview in religious and philosophical literature. Although the following quote may not help the interviewer with any particular Asian American client, it may serve as a guide in our quest to be more authentically multicultural:

A Cup of Tea

Nan-in, a Japanese master during the Meiji era (1868–1912), received a university professor who came to inquire about Zen. Nan-in served tea. He poured his visitor's cup full, and then kept on pouring.

The professor watched the overflow until he no longer could restrain himself. "It is overfull. No more will go in!"

"Like this cup," Nan-in said, "you are full of your own opinions and speculations. How can I show you Zen unless you first empty your cup?" (Nyogen Senzaki & Paul Reps, 1939, p. 5)

A case example of working with an Asian American client is provided in Putting It in Practice 13.5.

## OTHER DIVERSE CLIENT POPULATIONS

The groups with which we identify—the ones we claim and the ones that claim us—profoundly influence us. Our families of origin; our ethnic, cultural, and/or racial identities; and our sexual identities affect our lives continuously, both consciously and unconsciously. Further, our chosen beliefs and the experiences life brings shape our identities and the quality of our lives. The following groups of individuals are included as illustrations of this truth.

### Gay, Lesbian, Bisexual, and Transgendered People

*Mel [White, gay pastor] had no choice about being a homosexual. Believe me, if he had a choice, I know he would have chosen his marriage, his family, and his unique ministry; for Mel's values, like most gay and lesbians I know, are the same as mine and my heterosexual friends: love, respect, commitment, nurture, responsibility, honesty, and integrity. . . . We are all on this journey together and we must ensure that the road is safe for everyone, including our homosexual brothers and sisters who for far too long have been unfairly condemned and rejected. Isn't it past time that we opened our hearts and our arms to welcome them home instead of seeing them as strangers still waiting at the gate?*

—Lyla White, *Stranger at the Gates*

Sexual orientation is, of course, a very controversial topic. Many dominant world religions declare homosexuality to be sinful, although there are certainly substantial numbers of religions, and denominations within the religions, that do not take this stand (McDonald & Steinhorn, 1993). For many years, homosexuality was considered a mental disorder, and to this day, there exist treatments designed to "cure" homosexuals (Dworkin & Gutierrez, 1992).

Sexual identity and sexual orientation are intensely personal and central matters to most people. Sexual attraction is a powerful motivator of human behavior and is foundational to most people's sense of self. The longing for a soul mate is probably as old as life itself. To date, there has been no definitive explanation as to why, across time and culture, a consistent minority of humans are attracted to members of the same sex. Many theories have been offered, but, at present, it seems best to consider homosexuality, like left- or right-handedness, simply a fact of nature. Some people are attracted to opposite-sex partners for sexual intimacy, and some people are attracted to members of the same sex.

Many homosexual people report knowing they were homosexual even before kindergarten, and others report becoming aware much later in life (White, 1994). Because of stigma and lack of cultural role models, many homosexual people have, at times, struggled with their sexual orientation and tried to ignore or change it (O'Connor, 1992).

People with gender identity or sexual orientations other than heterosexual go to counselors for all the reasons heterosexual people go, and they do not necessarily identify their sexual orientations as part of the problem(s). However, many have endured verbal abuse, violence, vicious labeling, loneliness, and harsh judgments; sometimes, these experiences occurred during childhood or adolescence, while some clients report that these experiences are more recent or current. These cruelties exact a great developmental and psychological price.

Many people who are homosexual, bisexual, or transgendered do not share that information during an initial interview. In fact, many share this component of their identity with very few people. Interviewers need to listen for themes suggesting struggles with sexual identity, dating, attraction, and so on. Because many nonheterosexual people anticipate harsh judgment and rejection, some gay-friendly therapists suggest leaving homosexual-friendly pamphlets or literature in the waiting room to communicate an open attitude toward these issues (C. Van den Burg, personal communication, November 1997). It is also important that care is taken to avoid using gender-specific words indicating the assumption of heterosexuality. For example, when inquiring about intimate relationships, the word *partner* rather than *boyfriend* or *girlfriend* should be used. This allows clients to reveal the partner's gender when ready. For younger clients, or clients who are dating, it is helpful to ask general questions about romantic relationships or *romance.*

Interviewers need to be sensitive to relationship and family issues among homosexual, bisexual, and transgendered clients. Gay and lesbian couples come with all the varieties of needs and problems that trouble heterosexual couples, and more. In particular, they are often without societal and familial supports and sanctions that help and nurture heterosexual couples. In times of illness or loss, a gay or lesbian life-partner may not be recognized or accorded the same privileges of a heterosexual partner. Additionally, many such individuals experienced harsh rejection from one or more family members. These experiences may lead them to be either reluctant to admit their sexual orientation or to express their sexual orientation loudly and aggressively.

> *The day I saw a poster declaring the existence of an organization of Gay American Indians, I put my face into my hands and sobbed with relief. . . . What Americans call Gayness not only has distinct cultural characteristics, its participants have long held positions of social power in history and ritual among people all over the globe.*
>
> —Judy Grahn, *Another Mother Tongue*

## Persons with Disabilities

*But as Kit squeezed my hand, I knew that as far as she was concerned, none of these things made any difference. I was simply the man with whom she was in love. We were a man and a woman, eagerly looking forward to spending a lifetime together. Nothing else mattered, least of all my blindness . . . The waiter arrived with our drinks.*

*"Here you are mademoiselle," he said, putting Kit's bourbon and water in front of her. Then he whispered, "Where would he like his drink?"*

—Harold Krents, *To Race the Wind*

An extensive literature exists for interviewers wishing to work with clients who have physical, developmental, or emotional disabilities. In fact, there are master's- and doctoral-level training programs in special education and rehabilitation counseling and psychology. Although there are many technical aspects to various medical conditions and disabilities, in general, as with all groups of people, an open and accepting attitude is the most important prerequisite to working with people who have disabilities.

Sometimes, when interviewing a person with an obvious disability, professionals assume it is more polite to ignore crutches, missing limbs, wheelchairs, or even canes indicating blindness. However, as stated earlier with regard to race and culture, asking directly about the "difference" is usually welcomed. Such questions as "Have you used a wheelchair all your life, or is it a more recent addition?" can open the door to a candid discussion of the disability.

Facing and managing a disability affect all areas of an individual's life. However, too often, mental health professionals without rehabilitation training do not know how to calibrate the presence of the disability. The disability is either treated as the defining feature of the individual, overshadowing all else, or it is ignored; ignoring a disability implies that it really should not have any direct impact on the emotional and interpersonal functioning of the individual.

*Men who have accepted their disabilities or chronic conditions often have adopted a new set of values that replace the dominant male values in society. This process may take a good deal of time, depending upon the man's special circumstances, personality, and social situation.*

—*A Man's Guide to Coping with Disability*

## The Religiously Committed

*The challenge of ministry is to help people in very concrete situations—people with illnesses or in grief, people with physical or mental handicaps, people suffering from poverty and oppression, people caught in the complex networks of secular or religious institutions—to see and experience their story as part of God's ongoing redemptive work in the world.*

—Henri J. M. Nouwen, *The Living Reminder*

For a deeply religious person, seeking help from a secular mental health professional may feel like a contradiction of faith—or at least a very risky thing to do. Therefore, the interviewer needs to be particularly sensitive to behaviors suggesting a challenge to religious authority. Mental health issues and problems are obviously very connected to religious concerns. Finding a comfortable middle ground that denies neither perspective can be challenging. As Samuel M. Natale (1985) says in the book *Psychotherapy and the Religiously Committed Patient:*

> There are few problems more demanding in psychotherapy than dealing with a client's religious beliefs. This is so for a number of reasons, which include not only a lack of sensitivity and understanding on the part of the therapist but also a hesitation, avoidance, and even downright fear on the part of the therapist to explore distinctly religious values with a client. (p. 107)

In keeping with the trend to look at the whole picture when working with individuals, families, or couples, religion and/or spirituality can often be integrated into the counseling process (Bullis, 1996). However, although this may be true with regard to more liberal-thinking religious clients, fundamentalists and deeply committed people from most organized religions generally prefer not to seek secular help for their problems (E. Stern, 1985). Therefore, similar in some ways to working with Asian American families, the first visit may be because of a family or personal crisis. Their entry into the professional mental health world generally is not a casual inquiry into the potential use of psychotherapy to expand and grow. More likely, it is an expression of desperation. Their personal or family conflicts have become too great; and the answers, cures, or solutions within their religious framework have failed.

Because religion represents both culture and personal choice, differences between counselor and client, though not visible, can still be pronounced and unsettling (Sperry & Giblin, 1996). You might be directly asked about your religious beliefs in an initial interview. We recommend a balanced response:

- First, as a professional, it is your job to explore both the cause for concern and the concerns themselves as they relate to the client's problems and needs.
- Second, have a truthful and carefully considered answer ready. Refusing to share a brief summary of your own religious or spiritual orientation only exacerbates the concerns in most situations. After your summary, return the topic to how it feels for the client to work with you. Do not debate matters of faith.

One of our colleagues, a psychologist who is also an ordained minister, often provides religious clients with the following commentary about the relationship between religious (or spiritual) and psychological well-being:

> I understand it can be hard for a person with strong religious beliefs to consult a professional about personal problems. One way I look at it is like this: I know some people who are doing very well psychologically and very poorly when it comes to their religious adjustment. On the other hand, I know some people who are doing fine with their religious life, but they have some psychological or emotional work to do. Although many times religious and psychological well-being are highly connected, being well in one area doesn't *necessarily* mean you are feeling well in the other. I guess what I'm saying is that, if you want, I think we can work on the emotional and psychological concerns here, without violating issues of faith. (P. Bach, personal communication, March 1994)

Some mental health professionals identify their religious affiliations or beliefs in their advertising, on their cards, or in their informed consent paperwork. Others develop specific specialties in areas dealing with religious concerns (e.g., Monroe, 1997). Although a generic clinical interview includes religion as an aspect of the whole person, the interviewer must gently bring the dialogue back to problem areas and sources of distress. Also, treatment planning may certainly include consultation with religious leaders or authorities (Worthington, Kurusu, McCollough, & Sandage, 1996).

# THE IMPORTANCE OF CONTEXT

Interviewing in a multicultural setting involves a delicate balance between awareness and understanding of broad cultural group characteristics and the individual internalization and expression of those characteristics. As unique cultural beings, people must interact with an environment that exhibits its own cultural qualities and requires certain qualities of individuals. For example, a Mexican American student quickly learns that mastery of the English language is required to be successful in public schools. This is a contextual requirement that requires adaptation for success. In the process of adapting, the student makes many decisions about other aspects of his or her cultural background that either fit, don't fit, are useful or not useful, in this new context. The essential task of the interview becomes understanding the uniqueness of ethnocultural individuals within their various contexts. As Swartz-Kulstad and Martin (1999) state, ". . . the field is in need of a functional method to assess the interactive influences of all three levels—universal, group and individual—and to determine how these influences have an impact on the individual's successful adaptation to his or her psychosocial environment" (p. 283).

To address this need, Swartz-Kulstad and Martin (1999) identified five primary domains of culture and context. Taken together, the five domains provide a nice structure for building a better understanding of client issues (see Swartz-Kulstad & Martin, 1999, for a thorough discussion).

*Ethnocultural orientation* is the first domain of culture and context (Swartz-Kulstad & Martin, 1999). Ethnocultural orientation is a multidimensional domain that includes gauging the extent to which a person affiliates with his or her culture of origin and the dominant culture. This concept has also been referred to as *acculturation* (Garrett & Pichette, 2000). People born in another country who reside in the United States for more than a visit are no doubt challenged with trying to reconcile their beliefs, values, and understanding of social norms with what is required in their new home. A few words of the language creep in. The availability of familiar homeland foods is limited. The entertainment reflects and teaches the dominant culture. Obedience to the laws, education for the children, employment, housing—all require an active connection to, and understanding of, the dominant culture.

Even with the decision to engage the dominant culture, some individuals experience great stress when traditional ways of dealing with life situations do not yield predictable results. Integration requires fundamental shifts in a person's identity and behavior, thus threatening a sense of continuity and equilibrium. However, according to Swartz-Kulstad and Martin (1999), people who successfully adapt at the psychosocial level and exhibit positive mental health in a dominant culture are able to act within the expected standards of the dominant society while maintaining a clear sense of their beliefs and values. At the same time, they are able to maintain salient aspects of their culture of origin in such a way that they do not lose traditional psychosocial support systems. In other words, adaptation to the dominant culture does not require abandonment of the culture of origin, but rather flexibility in being able to employ positive aspects of both cultures in the process of adapting to a new environment.

Because it is a fluid, value-laden, and conflicted process for many people, directly asking about ethnocultural orientation is not generally advisable. There are many formal instruments to measure acculturation (Garrett & Pichette, 2000; Paniagua, 1998, Wetsit, 1992); and should this issue be central, it can be gradually addressed directly. However, in the initial interview, it is best to simply explore how strong the connections to the various cultures are and what emotions are attached to those connections.

An informal assessment of ethnocultural orientation can be obtained by listening as information emerges during the session or by asking for specific information. For example:

1. Listen for the sense of connection to the culture historically. Ask: "Did you grow up on the reservation (or in the country of origin)?" or "I know everyone's different, so I'm wondering for you personally, do you feel much connection with your culture?"

2. Listen for the relationship between the client and other members of the culture. Does the client go to cultural events? Are original cultural practices a regular part of life? Does he or she speak the original language? Ask: "What kinds of things do you celebrate?" or "Do you attend (powwows, religious services, etc.,) very often?" and "What language do you prefer to speak at home? with friends? at work?"

3. Listen for methods or style of coping with environmental demands (conscious or unconscious) Ask: "Is there anything about your work (school, home, etc.) that challenges you? How do you handle the challenges?"

4. Listen for how the person envisions life in the future. Will he or she play a role in traditional cultural ceremonies or practices? Will he or she seek a bicultural stance in life? Ask: "What things about your culture do you appreciate or not appreciate? What things about the Western culture do you appreciate, or not appreciate? How would you like your life to be in the future in terms of your culture?"

The client's cultural orientation to the past, present, and future can be very informative with regard to engagement with the dominant culture (Garrett & Pichette, 2000; Wetsit, 1992). The more culturally oriented and embedded the client is, the more important it is for the professional to seek appropriate cultural input and education to be of assistance in a culturally sensitive manner.

The second domain identified by Swartz-Kulstad and Martin (1999) is *family environment*. Because the family is a significant mechanism through which culture is transmitted, and because it is also the primary source of support for most individuals, gaining information about family dynamics is crucial. We know Russian immigrants who came to the United States during World War II who forbade their children to speak anything but English. They gave their children popular English names and pushed them full-speed into the culture. We know Laotian refugees determined that their children have the best of both: to excel at all things American and yet retain all things Laotian. We also know Iranian families in deep conflict because their children have rejected their original cultural values. In all these cases, there is variance in the degree of dependence on the family or adherence to family expectations concerning family roles and hierarchies, communication styles, individuation, and maintenance of culture. In a sense, the family can become a source of great support for an individual, while at the same time, be a cause of great stress as that individual seeks to reconcile family environmental expectations with other systems in which he or she interacts (e.g., school, work, community).

Listening to your client along the family dimension might involve covering the following:

1. What is the nature of the overall family environment? Is there a strong nuclear and/or extended family? What is the proximity to, or availability of, family sup-

port? What is the level of dependence on the family for support? Ask: "Tell me about your family. How did you grow up? What kinds of things did your parents do? How often does your whole family get together? What happens when all the grandparents and aunts and uncles get together?"

2. Listen for subtle or overt expectations for conformity to family beliefs and values. If they exist, what importance does the client place on meeting family expectations? Ask: "How would you describe the kind of life your family wants for you? What kind of life do you want for your own children? Have you ever done something that disappointed your parents? Would you tell me about it? Have you ever argued with your parents? What happened? What happens when your children argue with you?"

3. What are the discrepancies between family expectations and those of the other systems the client interacts with? Ask: "I'm wondering if you ever feel as if you have to act differently at work than you do at home or with your neighborhood friends. What happens when you act as you do at work when you're home?"

*Community environment* is the third domain of culture and context. This domain involves structural aspects of the community where the client currently lives (i.e., geographical place, social support networks, work settings, and institutional support systems). For those who have recently immigrated, it also involves comparisons with former community environments and conditions under which migration occurred (voluntary or involuntary; see Ogbu, 1992). For example, Sandhu, Portes, and McPhee (1996) reported less stress involved with voluntary migration as opposed to those who were forced to migrate, whereas involuntary minorities may view engagement with the dominant community as a threat to their identity, and thus resist accessing supportive structures (Castillo, Quintana, & Zamarripa, 2000).

The sociopolitical climate must also be considered in assessment of community environment. There is always the possibility that racism (sexism, ageism, etc.), bias, and discrimination contribute to community-related stress.

Here are some things to listen for and ask about as you gauge your client's community environment.

1. Where is the client's community? How many people of similar ethnocultural backgrounds live there? How does this community compare with the former community (rural, urban, etc.)? If the client is an immigrant, what were the conditions of his or her arrival? Is he or she in the United States legally? Ask: "How would you describe your community? How is it similar or different from your home community? How did you come to this country?" (Be very sure that a client knows about confidentiality.)

2. How are the client or the client's parents employed? What is their socioeconomic status (SES)? Ask: "What do you do for a living? How are you and your family doing financially?"

3. What parts of the community does the client perceive to be supportive? Is he or she a member of a spiritual community and, if so, what is the level of involvement? How does he or she view institutions such as government, schools, and so on? Ask: "Where do you go, or whom do you see when you need help with something? How important is spirituality to you? Do you practice any particular faith? How often do you visit with your children's teachers? Are you comfortable visiting with your children's teachers? How do you feel when you see a police officer?"

4. Are there any observable signs of racism, discrimination, or prejudice in his or her community? Does the client feel welcome or valued in the community? Ask: "Have you experienced prejudice or any racist behaviors in your community? What would you like me to know about these incidents?"

The fourth domain of culture and context is *communication style.* It includes the extent to which a person is able to send and receive accurate information as he or she interacts with his or her environment. Certainly, a great potential for difficulty exists in this domain because interpretation of verbal and nonverbal information is so dependent on cultural background. For example, direct eye contact can be interpreted as hostile and disrespectful behavior from the perspective of some cultures, while avoiding direct eye contact can be interpreted as resistant or disrespectful in others. In the same way, inability to adequately express yourself verbally to another presents difficulties. Successful adaptation to a context is greatly enhanced when an individual is reasonably sure that the messages he or she sends and gets are received and interpreted in the way they were intended.

Another component of communication style involves how a person handles misunderstandings. A person willing to ask for clarification is less likely to experience communication breakdowns than one who is not. However, some people might feel it is disrespectful to ask, or may feel ashamed or embarrassed for not understanding. For these reasons, the interviewer might consider observing for the following issues:

1. What are the person's sensitivities to nonverbal cues (i.e., proximity, facial expressions, eye contact, touch, and physical gestures)?
2. How does the client use his or her voice? What are the intonations, inflexions, voice level, and rate of speech?
3. How are the client's verbal tracking skills? Will the client ask for clarification if he or she doesn't understand something? Are there any attitudes associated with asking for clarification (shame, embarrassment, etc.)?

The final domain of cultural context involves *language usage.* It differs from communication style primarily because it is concerned with the content of what was spoken, rather than the qualitative style. Language usage is the "what," whereas communication style is the "how."

According to Castillo and associates (2000), language is associated with cultural, social, and cognitive variables. Not only does it involve the ability to communicate, but also it affects perceptions of others about the language user. For example, people can be either positively or negatively evaluated according to which language they speak (Castillo et al., 2000). People are also positively or negatively evaluated based on how well they speak their newly acquired language. Additionally, Swartz-Kulstad and Martin (1999) report that potential for ethnocultural conflict increases whenever people entering a new environment are not able to understand the language. A person's ability to communicate effectively is a good predictor of ability to successfully adapt to a given environment. Therefore, it is extremely important to understand not only the language that a person speaks in any given context, but also the level of proficiency and comprehension. Here are some questions for the interviewer to consider:

1. What is the client's preferred language? What is the language proficiency? Ask: "What languages do you speak? Which do you prefer to use at home, at

work/school, or with friends?" Keep in mind that direct questioning may not be the best way to evaluate language proficiency.
2. How do language differences affect the ability of the interviewer to communicate with the client? Ask: "What language would you prefer to use in counseling? Are you able to understand my (English, Spanish, Japanese)?" Or, if you cannot speak any other languages, ask: "How comfortable are you with my English?"

## INTERVIEWING CONTEXT AND PROCEDURES

Thus far, we have discussed counselor awareness of himself or herself as a cultural being, and the importance of knowing the cultural characteristics of the client—whether those are attributable to group, universal, or individual influences. We have also covered the importance of broad contextual elements as they interact with the individual as a unique ethnocultural being. What has been left out until now is how the actual interviewing context and procedures might impact the interviewing process.

For many people raised in many cultures, consulting with a mental health professional comes as a last resort. Seeing an outsider for personal problems goes against traditional problem-solving strategies. This means that clients from another culture may experience an enormous amount of stress or anxiety because of the counseling process—in addition to the stress that brought them in. Moreover, they have expectations for counseling that may or may not match the abilities or styles of the interviewer. Therefore, extra care should be taken to ensure that clients feel welcome, to establish credibility, and to build trust (Castillo et al., 2000). At the very least, the counselor must ensure that clients feel and believe their interests are being served without threatening their worldview.

Using standardized assessment instruments may produce anxiety, confusion, or anger in ethnoculturally different clients. For all the reasons described, standardized assessment procedures may be inappropriate for the ethnoculturally different client. In the past, testing procedures used to aid in diagnosis and treatment have been misused. Although many attempts have been made to address cultural bias in assessment instruments, such biases still exist (Paniagua, 1998).

Unfortunately, although culture-specific or culturally fair testing procedures are sometimes available, such approaches limit valuable information available to the interviewer. Culture-specific assessment limits the person's experience to membership of a particular group, thus missing the uniqueness of the individual; culturally fair assessment instruments tend to wash out the cultural influences, thus neglecting the impact culture has on a person's life (Swartz-Kulstad & Martin, 1999, 2000). While specific information regarding instrumentation is beyond the scope of this book, an interviewer working with a culturally different client should consider the following general questions:

Are there other, less culturally bound options to obtain the necessary information?

Are there ways to accommodate or ameliorate the cultural differences?

Will the use of this assessment procedure help me to understand the individual's experience as a unique cultural being?

Additional guidelines for interviewing culturally different clients are provided in Table 13.1.

**Table 13.1.   The Dos and Don'ts of Initial Sessions with Multicultural Clients**

The following are suggestions for interviewers working with clients who come from cultural, racial, ethnic, religious, or life experience backgrounds different from themselves. The applicability and relevance of each suggestion must be evaluated with the particular clinical situation at hand. Our intention is to provide a thought-provoking checklist.

**Open Inquiry**

1. Do ask about tribal, ethnic, or background differences that are obvious or are made obvious by information provided by the client.
2. Don't insist on a more thorough exploration of these differences than is offered.
3. Do realize that acculturation and cultural identity are fluid and developmental.
4. Don't assume all members of a given family group or couple have the same levels of cultural identity or the same experiences interfacing with the dominant culture.

**Family**

1. Do recognize that for many or most nondominant cultures in the United States, the role of family is central. The concept of family is often broader, more inclusive, and more definitive in a given individual's sense of identity. Therefore, be attuned to matters of family with heightened awareness and sensitivity.
2. Don't impose either your own definition of family or the definition of family you've read about with regard to the client's culture. Simply be open to the client's sense of family.
3. Do graciously allow family members to attend some part of an initial interview if they so request.
4. Don't define family strictly along biological lines.

**Communication Styles**

1. Do remember that patterns of eye contact, direct verbalization of problem areas, storytelling, and note taking all have culturally determined norms that vary widely.
2. Don't assume a chatty or overly familiar style, even if that is your predominant style. Strive to demonstrate respect.
3. Do ask for clarification if something is not clear.
4. Don't ask for clarification in a manner that suggests your lack of clarity is the client's problem.

**Religious and Spiritual Matters**

1. Do accept the client's beliefs regarding the sources of distress: ancestral disapproval, the evil eye, God's wrath, or trouble because of misbehavior in another life. A strong relationship of trust must be established before one can determine the adaptive and maladaptive aspects of such beliefs and thereby work within the frame toward healing or growth.
2. Don't assume you are being told the whole story regarding faith or belief systems early on. Most are powerful and quite private and will not be easily or fully shared.
3. Do take advantage of any possible link to meaningful spiritual or religious beliefs or connections that may help address the current distress.
4. Don't hesitate to allow input into the problem from religious or spiritual persons respected by the client.

## CULTURE-BOUND SYNDROMES

Because theories of human functioning are culture-bound, our current diagnostic system for mental health problems is heavily culturally influenced (Paniagua, 2001; D. W. Sue et al., 1996). In addition, the manifestation of mental angst and distress occurs through different culturally specific symptom complexes that change over time. For example, in contrast to Freud's era (Jones, 1955), not many women in the United States currently have vapors or fainting spells; however, eating disorders were almost unheard of a hundred years ago. Posttraumatic stress symptoms reflect at least some common human responses to trauma across cultures, but the name of the disorder has varied over many centuries. In addition, to some extent, what is actually considered traumatic is culturally specific, and what to do in the face of trauma constitutes culturally informed advice.

Simons and Hughes (1993) have coined the phrase *culture-related syndromes* to denote mental disorders or symptom complexes that are specific to a given culture. Summarizing the work of Griffith and Baker (1993); Rubel, O'Nell, and Collado-Ardon (1984); and Simons and Hughes (1993); Paniagua (1998) has compiled a list of common syndromes from various cultures. This illustrative list is provided in Table 13.2.

The information in Table 13.2 reveals many things about the broad field of mental health diagnostic systems. First, *symptoms* may be similar across cultures, but causes may be viewed very differently. (Psychotic thinking, anxiety, or depressive symptoms may be consistently described across cultures but attributed to satanic influence, bad behavior, brain disease, trauma, family patterns, learning, etc.) Second, *causes* of human distress (brain disease, trauma, exposure, grief, attachment loss or disturbance)

**Table 13.2.    Culturally Specific Mental, Emotional, and Behavioral Disorders**

| Name of Disorder | Cultural Origins | Symptoms | Cause |
|---|---|---|---|
| *Ataque de nervios* | Hispanic | Out-of-consciousness state | Evil spirits |
| Falling-out | African American | Seizure-like symptoms | Traumatic events such as robbery |
| Ghost sickness | American Indian | Weakness, dizziness | Action of witches, evil forces |
| *Hwa-byung* | Asian communities | Pain in upper abdomen, fear of death, tiredness | Imbalance between reality and anger |
| *Koro* | Asian men | Desire to grab penis | Belief that it will retract into body and cause death |
| *Mal puesto*, hex, rootwork, voodoo death | African American and Hispanic | Unnatural disease or death | Power of people who use evil spirits |
| *Susto, eapanto, pasmo, miedo* | Hispanic | Tiredness, weakness | Frightening or startling experiences |
| *Wackinko* | American Indian | Anger, withdrawal, mutism, suicide | Disappointment, interpersonal problems |
| Wind/cold illness | Hispanic and Asian | Fear of cold wind, feeling weak and susceptible to illness | Belief that natural and supernatural elements are not balanced |

may be identified similarly across cultures, but the disturbance or distress may show itself in vastly different symptoms. For a general discussion regarding issues in diagnosis, refer to Chapter 10; however, from a multicultural viewpoint, remember that much of our understanding of human distress is culture-bound, and there are many things to learn from other cultural perspectives.

## MATTERS OF ETIQUETTE

When working with ethnoculturally different clients, it helps to follow some basic rules of multicultural etiquette.

### Asking for Free Education

A gay friend of ours once told us he was sick and tired of being the source of all gay and lesbian information for his entire graduate program, including classmates, professors, and supervisors. Even more frustrating for him was the fact that his heterosexual therapist had also asked him for education about his needs as a gay client. Our friend believed such questioning revealed not only ignorance, but also laziness and lack of respect. He had a point. Relying on clients as a sole source of multicultural education is inappropriate. Each client has his or her own level of patience with a well-intended but ignorant interviewer or therapist. Clinical sensitivity is called for in determining how much is okay to ask clients directly and how much should be learned through other sources.

### Bad Education

Very few people without a sociopolitical agenda are willing to be the sole spokesperson for an entire cultural or social group. No single Vietnam veteran can speak for all Vietnam veterans; no Indian, for all Indians; no woman, for all women. Therefore, be wary of those who would purport thus to speak. To become acquainted with another culture or set of life experiences requires much exposure, reading, discussing, experiencing, thinking, and rethinking. It is a hard-earned education in which no one really gets a terminal degree. There is always more to know—even about your own culture. Single-source education is *not enough* and, as pointed out earlier, can be hazardous.

### Asking in Small Communities

Effective interviewing requires asking about very personal matters in the client's life. Small communities of humans are notorious for breaks in confidentiality among insiders and providing inaccurate or simply no information to outsiders. Being a member of a culture embedded in a different, dominant culture almost guarantees that you are a member of a small community, even if you live in a very large, urban area. Examples of such communities abound, from gay and lesbian communities to religious communities to "Indian Country," where the joke is that there are three ways to spread information: telephone, telegraph, and tell-a-cousin.

Further, many cultural groups have had the experience of being asked about their culture by persons who subsequently abused the information. Some basic cultural truths are considered sacred—not to be shared with outsiders. Persons outside the culture can easily misunderstand other truths about a given culture. Unfortunately, sometimes information is sought for less than charitable reasons.

Therefore, it should come as no surprise that, initially, sharing intimate information with a stranger has added baggage for people from small cultural communities. First, you are an outsider, at least by virtue of your profession. If you live in the community or are a member of the culture, you might be a blend of insider-outsider. If you work at an agency, relatives and friends of the client may work there or have been there as clients (Paniagua, 1998). Assumptions about who knows what and who will share what are not the same assumptions urban people from the dominant culture make. It may take patience, extra education, careful, repeated explanation, and a great deal of time to build the kind of trust that allows the depth of sharing necessary for a therapeutic relationship to develop.

## SUMMARY

This chapter addressed philosophical and practical concerns in the realm of multicultural counseling, taking the position that human reactions to interacting and working with persons of other cultures are learned reactions. Such learning begins early in life; thus, to be effective, open, and affirming of differences, the mental health professional may need to unlearn certain attitudes as well as continually add new learning, always questioning the culture-bound assumptions and blind spots in our theories and techniques. We must cultivate attitudes that allow us to learn from other cultures and other people's life experiences and differences.

General information associated with the four most populous minority cultures in the United States—American Indians, African Americans, Hispanics, and Asian Americans—were explored in this chapter. Each of these broad cultural groupings represents many distinct cultures and subcultures, and any attempts at overall generalizations fall far short of the specificity necessary to offer effective, culturally appropriate mental health assistance. Information provided in this chapter is merely a beginning in terms of what the interviewer needs to know to work effectively with individuals or families from these cultures. In addition, the chapter discussed basic parameters related to gays and lesbians, persons with disabilities, and persons who have strong religious worldviews.

Culturally different clients must be understood, not only from their cultural perspective, but also from an individually unique contextual perspective. This chapter defined and explored contextual perspectives including ethnocultural orientation, family environment, community environment, communication style, and language usage. Additionally, the clinical interview and assessment procedures were briefly examined as contextual variables that might affect culturally different clients.

Finally, the chapter reviewed culture-bound syndromes and matters of etiquette pertaining to multiculturalism.

## SUGGESTED READINGS AND RESOURCES

Comas-Díaz, L., & Griffith, E. E. H. (Eds.). (1998). *Clinical guidelines in cross-cultural mental health.* New York: John Wiley & Sons. This book offers practical guidelines for mental health practitioners who work with clients with diverse ethnocultural backgrounds. It examines ethnicity, family values, language, religion, and so on, as these issues may pertain to mental health.

Dworkin, S. H., & Gutierrez, F. J. (1992). *Counseling gay men and lesbians: Journey to the end of the rainbow.* Alexandria, VA: American Association for Counseling and Development. This is an excellent compilation of issues relevant to counselors working with homosexual people. It covers topics such as cultural issues, coming out, couples issues, violence, and ethical concerns.

McGoldrick, M., Giordano, J., & Pearce, J. K. (1996). *Ethnicity and family therapy.* New York: Guilford. This book is similar in some ways to other recommended texts. However, to the extent possible, it includes material from professionals who are also members of the culture in question and deals with recommendations for family work, addressing historically relevant facts to undergird the recommendations. It addresses a much broader range of cultures (e.g., Indonesian, Dutch, German, Jewish, and Iranian) than simply the four often addressed.

Paniagua, F. A. (1998) *Assessing and treating culturally diverse clients: A practical guide* (2nd ed.). Thousand Oaks, CA: Sage. This is a hands-on book that explores the broad generalities associated with the four largest minority groups in the United States and then makes practical sense of how to thoughtfully and professionally apply this knowledge in the context of providing ethical and effective mental health services.

Stern, M. E. (1985). *Psychotherapy and the religiously committed patient.* New York: Haworth Press. This small, edited book is a sophisticated compilation of authors who address with compassion, respect, and depth aspects of religion and spirituality as they relate to psychotherapy.

Vargas, L. A., & Koss-Chioino, J. D. (1992). *Working with culture: Psychotherapeutic interventions with ethnic minority children and adolescents.* San Francisco: Jossey-Bass. This is an insightful book that does not shy away from addressing the complexities of working with children combined with the complexities of working with persons from other cultures.

# References

Abt, I. R., & Stuart, L. E. (Eds.). (1982). *The newer therapies: A sourcebook.* New York: Van Nostrand-Reinhold.

Achebe, C. (1994). *Things fall apart.* New York: Doubleday. (Original work published 1959)

Adler, A. (1927). *Understanding human nature.* Garden City, New York: Garden City Publishing.

Adler, A. (1937). Position in family constellation influences life style. *International Journal of Individual Psychology, 3,* 211–227.

Adler, A. (1958). *What life should mean to you.* New York: Capricorn. (Original work published 1931)

Adler, G. (1996). Transitional objects, self objects, real objects, and the process of change in psychodynamic psychotherapy. In L. E. Lifson (Ed.), *Understanding therapeutic action: Psychodynamic concepts of cure* (pp. 69–84). Hillsdale, NJ: Analytic Press.

Agerbo, E., Mortensen, P. B., Eriksson, T., Qin, P., & Westergaard-Nielsen, N. (2001). Risk of suicide in relation to income level in people admitted to hospital with mental illness: Nested case-control study. *British Medical Journal, 322,* 334–335.

Ainsworth, M. D. S. (1989). Attachments beyond infancy. *American Psychologist, 44,* 709–716.

Amatea, E. S., & Brown, B. E. (1993). The counselor and the family: An ecosystemic approach. In J. Wittmer (Ed.), *Managing your school counseling program.* Minneapolis, MN: Educational Media.

American Academy of Pediatrics. Committee on Psychosocial Aspects of Child and Family Health. (1998). Guidance for effective discipline. *Pediatrics, 101,* 723–728.

American Association for Marriage and Family Therapy. (2001). *AAMFT code of ethics.* Washington, DC: Author.

American Counseling Association. (1995). *Code of ethics and standards of practice.* Alexandria, VA: Author.

American Psychiatric Association. (1994). *Diagnostic and statistical manual of mental disorders* (4th ed.). Washington, DC: Author.

American Psychiatric Association. (2000). *Diagnostic and statistical manual of mental disorders* (4th ed., text rev.). Washington, DC: Author.

American Psychological Association. (1992). Ethical principles of psychologists and code of conduct. *American Psychologist, 47,* 1597–1611.

Andersen, T. (1991). *The reflecting team: Dialogues and dialogues about the dialogues.* New York: W. W. Norton.

Anderson, R. N. (2001, Oct. 12). Deaths: Leading causes for 1999. *National Vital Statistics Reports, 49,* (11).

Anderson, R. N., Kochanek, K. D., & Murphy, S. L. (1997). Report of final mortality statistics, 1995. *Monthly vital statistics report, 45*(Suppl. 2, table 7). Hyattsville, MD: National Center for Health Statistics.

Annis, H. M., & Chan, D. (1983). The differential treatment model: Empirical evidence from a personality typology of adult offenders. *Criminal Justice and Behavior, 10,* 159–173.

Archer, R. (1992). *MMPI-A: Assessing adolescent psychopathology.* Hillsdale, NJ: Erlbaum.

Atkinson, D. R., & Hackett, G. (1998). *Counseling diverse populations* (2nd ed.). Boston: McGraw-Hill.

Augenbraum, H., & Stavans, I. (1993). *Growing up Latino.* Boston: Houghton Mifflin.

Axelson, J. A. (1999). *Counseling and development in a multicultural society* (3rd ed.). Belmont, CA: Brooks/Cole.

Axline, V. M. (1964). *Dibs: In search of self.* New York: Ballantine Books.

Bailey, J. M., Kim, P. Y., Hills, A., & Linsenmeier, J. A. (1997). Butch, femme, or straight acting? Partner preferences of gay men and lesbians. *Journal of Personality and Social Psychology, 73,* 960–973.

Balleweg, B. J. (1990). The interviewing team: An exercise for teaching assessment and conceptualization skills. *Teaching of Psychology, 17,* 241–242.

Banaka, W. H. (1971). *Training in depth interviewing.* New York: Harper & Row.

Bandler, R., & Grinder, J. (1975). *The structure of magic. I: A book about language and therapy.* Palo Alto, CA: Science and Behavior Books.

Bandler, R., & Grinder, J. (1979). *Frogs into princes.* Moab, UT: Real People Press.

Bandura, A. (1969). *Principles of behavior modification.* New York: Holt, Rinehart and Winston.

Barker, S. B., & Hawes, E. C. (1999). Eye movement desensitization and reprocessing in individual psychology. *Journal of Individual Psychology, 55,* 146–161.

Barkham, M., Rees, A., Stiles, W. B., Shapiro, D. A., Hardy, G. E., & Reynolds, S. (1996). Dose-effect relations in time-limited psychotherapy for depression. *Journal of Consulting and Clinical Psychology, 64,* 927–935.

Barkley, R. A. (1990). *Attention-deficit hyperactivity disorder: A handbook for diagnosis and treatment.* New York: Guilford Press.

Barlow, D. H., & Craske, M. G. (1994). *Mater of your anxiety and Panic II.* New York: Graywind.

Barnett, J. E. (1998). Termination without trepidation. *Psychotherapy Bulletin, 33,* 20–22.

Bartholomew, K. (1990). Avoidance of intimacy: An attachment perspective. *Journal of Social and Personal Relationships, 7,* 147–178.

Bartlett, E. E. (1996). Protecting the confidentiality of children and adolescents. In *The Hatherleigh Guide to child and adolescent therapy.* New York: Hatherleigh.

Basow, S. A. (1980). *Sex role stereotypes: Traditions and alternatives.* Monterey, CA: Brooks/Cole.

Bateson, G. (1972). *Steps to an ecology of mind.* New York: Ballantine Books.

Baucom, D. H., & Epstein, N. (1990). *Behavioral marital therapy.* New York: Brunner/Mazel.

Bauman, L. J., & Friedman, S. B. (1998). Corporal punishment. *Pediatric Clinics of North America, 45,* 403–414.

Baumrind, D. (1975). Child care practices anteceding three patterns of preschool behavior. *Genetic Psychology Monograph, 75,* 43–88.

Beahrs, J. O., & Gutheil, T. G. (2001). Informed consent in psychotherapy. *American Journal of Psychiatry, 285,* 329–333.

Beautrais, A. L. (2001). Suicides and serious suicide attempts: Two populations or one? *Psychological Medicine, 31* [Special issue], 837–854.

Beck, A. T. (1976). *Cognitive therapy and the emotional disorders.* New York: International Universities Press.

Beck, A. T., Brown, G., & Steer, R. A. (1989). Prediction of eventual suicide in psychiatric inpatients by clinical ratings of hopelessness. *Journal of Consulting and Clinical Psychology, 57,* 309–310.

Beck, A. T., Rush, A. H., Shaw, B. F., & Emery, G. (1979). *Cognitive therapy of depression.* New York: Guilford Press.

Beitman, B. D. (1983). Categories of countertransference. *Journal of Operational Psychiatry, 14,* 82–90.

Bellini, M., & Bruschi, C. (1996). HIV infection and suicidality. *Journal of Affective Disorders, 38,* 153–164.

Bem, D., & Allen, A. (1974). On predicting some of the people some of the time: The search for cross-situational consistencies in behavior. *Psychological Review, 81,* 506–520.

Benjamin, A. (1981). *The helping interview* (3rd ed.). Boston: Houghton Mifflin.

Benjamin, A. (1987). *The helping interview with case illustrations.* Boston: Houghton Mifflin.

Bennett, B. E., Bryant, B. K., VandenBos, G. R., & Greenwood, A. (1990). *Professional liability and risk management.* Washington, DC: American Psychological Association.

Bennett, C. C. (1984). Know thyself. *Professional Psychology, 15,* 271–283.

Berkhoffer, N. (1978). *The white man's Indian: Images of the American Indian from Columbus to the present.* New York: Vintage Press.

Berman, A. L., & Jobes, D. A. (1996). *Adolescent suicide: Assessment and intervention.* Washington, DC: American Psychological Association.

Bertolino, B. (1999). *Therapy with troubled teenagers.* New York: John Wiley & Sons.

Bertolino, B., & O'Hanlon, B. (2002). *Collaborative, competency-based counseling and therapy.* Needham Heights, MA: Allyn & Bacon.

Binik, Y. M., Cantor, J., Ochs, E., & Meana, M. (1997). From the couch to the keyboard: Psychotherapy in cyberspace. In S. Keisler (Ed.), *Culture of the Internet* (pp. 71–100). Mahwah, NJ: Erlbaum.

Birch, M., & Miller, T. (2000). Inviting intimacy: The interview as therapeutic opportunity. *International Journal of Social Research Methodology: Theory and Practice, 3,* 189–202.

Birdwhistell, M. L. (1952). *Introduction to kinesis: An annotation system for analysis of body motion and gesture.* Louisville: University of Louisville Press.

Birdwhistell, M. L. (1970). *Kinesics and context.* Philadelphia: University of Pennsylvania Press.

Black, L. (1996). Families of African origin: An overview. In M. McGoldrick, J. Giordano, & J. K. Pearce (Eds.), *Ethnicity and family therapy* (2nd ed., pp. 57–65). New York: Guilford Press.

Blaney, P. H. (1986). Affect and memory: A review. *Psychological Bulletin, 99,* 229–246.

Blatt, S. J., Zuroff, D. C., Bondi, C. M., Sanislow, C. A., III, & Pitkonis, P. A. (1998). When and how perfectionism impedes the brief treatment of depression: Further analyses of the National Institute of Mental Health Treatment of Depression Collaborative Research Program. *Journal of Consulting and Clinical Psychology, 66,* 423–428.

Bloom, B. L. (1992). Computer-assisted psychological intervention: A review and commentary. *Clinical Psychology Review, 12,* 169–197.

Bögels, S. M. (1994). A structured-training approach to teaching diagnostic interviewing. *Teaching of Psychology, 21,* 144–150.

Bongar, B. (1991). *The suicidal patient: Clinical and legal standards of care.* Washington, DC: American Psychological Association.

Bongar, B., & Harmatz, M. (1989). Graduate training in clinical psychology and the study of suicide. *Professional Psychology: Research and Practice, 20,* 209–213.

Bornstein, P. H., & Bornstein, M. T. (1986). *Marital therapy: A behavioral-communications approach.* New York: Pergamon Press.

Bostwick, J. M., & Pankratz, V. S. (2000). Affective disorders and suicide risk: A reexamination. *American Journal of Psychiatry, 157,* 1925–1932.

Bowlby, J. (1969). *Attachment and loss. Volume I: Attachment.* New York: Basic Books.

Bowlby, J. (1977). The making and breaking of affectional bonds. *British Journal of Psychiatry, 130,* 201–210.

Bowlby, J. (1988). *A secure base.* New York: Basic Books.

Boyer, D. (1988). *In and out of street life: A reader on interventions with street youth.* Portland, OR: Tri-County Youth Services Consortium.

Bradford, E., & Lyddon, W. J. (1994). Assessing adolescent and adult attachment: An update. *Journal of Counseling and Development, 73,* 215–219.

Brammer, L. M. (1979). *The helping relationship* (2nd ed.). Englewood Cliffs, NJ: Prentice-Hall.

Brems, C. (1993). *A comprehensive guide to child psychotherapy.* Boston: Allyn & Bacon.

Brenneis, C. B. (1994). Observations on psychoanalytic listening. *Psychoanalytic Quarterly, 63,* 29–53.

Brockington, I. (2001). Suicide in women. *International Clinical Psychopharmacology, 16* [Special issue], S7–S19.

Brockman, W. P. (1980). *Empathy revisited: The effect of representational system matching on certain counseling process and outcome variables.* Unpublished doctoral dissertation, College of William and Mary, Williamsburg, VA.

Brody, C. M. (1984). *Women therapists working with women: New theory and process of feminist therapy.* New York: Springer.

Bronfenbrenner, U. (1979). *The ecology of human development.* Cambridge, MA: Harvard University Press.

Bronfenbrenner, U. (1986). Ecology of the family as a context for human development: Research perspectives. *Developmental Psychology, 22,* 732–742.

Brown, J. H., Henteleff, P., Barakat, S., & Rowe, C. J. (1986). Is it normal for terminally ill patients to desire death? *American Journal of Psychiatry, 143,* 208–210.

Brown, L. S. (1994). *Subversive dialogues.* New York: Basic Books.

Brown, L. S., & Brodsky, A. M. (1992). The future of feminist therapy. *Psychotherapy, 29,* 51–57.

Brown, L. S., & Walker, L. E. (1990). Feminist therapy perspectives on self-disclosure. In G. Stricker & M. Fisher (Eds.), *Self-disclosure in the therapeutic relationship* (pp. 135–154). New York: Plenum Press.

Brown, T. A., Atony, M. M., & Barlow, D. H. (1995). Diagnostic comorbidity in panic disorder. *Journal of Consulting and Clinical Psychology, 63,* 408–418.

Buck, S. (1999). The function of the frame and the role of the fee in the therapeutic situation. *Women and Therapy, 22,* 37–49.

Buie, D. H. (1981). Empathy: Its nature and limitations. *Journal of the American Psychoanalytic Association, 29,* 281–307.

Bullis, R. K. (1996). *Spirituality in social work practice.* Washington, DC: Taylor & Francis.

Butcher, J. N., Dahlstrom, W. G., Graham, J. R., Tellegen, A. M., & Kaemmer, B. (1989). *MMPI-2: Manual for administration and scoring.* Minneapolis: University of Minnesota.

Campfield, K. M., & Hills, A. M. (2001). Effect of timing of critical incident stress debriefing (CISD) on posttraumatic symptoms. *Journal of Traumatic Stress, 14,* 327–340.

Cannon, W. B. (1939). *The wisdom of the body* (Rev. ed.). New York: Norton.

Capra, F. (1975). *The tao of physics.* New York: Random House.

Carkhuff, R. R. (1987). *The art of helping* (6th ed.). Amherst, MA: Human Resource Development Press.

Caspi, A., & Roberts, B. W. (2001). Target article: Personality development across the life course. *Psychological Inquiry, 12* [Special issue], 49–66.

Castillo, E. M., Quintana, S. M., & Zamarripa, M. X. (2000). Cultural and linguistic issues. In E. S. Shapiro & T. R. Kratchowill (eds.), *Conducting school-based assessments of child and adolescent behavior* (pp. 274-308). New York: Guilford Press.

Castonguay, L. G. (2000). A common factors approach to psychotherapy training. *Journal of Psychotherapy Integration, 10,* 263–282.

Chao, C. M. (1992). The inner heart: Therapy with Southeast Asian families. In L. A. Vargas & J. D. Koss-Chioino (Eds.), *Working with culture: Psychotherapeutic interventions with ethnic minority children and adolescents* (157-181). San Francisco: Jossey-Bass.

Cherpitel, C. J. (1997). Brief screening instruments for alcoholism. *Alcohol Health and Research World, 21,* 348–351.

Chessick, R. D. (1990). Psychoanalytic listening: III. *Psychoanalysis and Psychotherapy, 8,* 119–135.

Christopher, J. C. (1996). Counseling's inescapable moral visions. *Journal of Counseling and Development, 75,* 17–25.

Christopher, J. C. (2001). Culture and psychotherapy: Toward a hermeneutic approach. *Psychotherapy, 38,* 115–128.

Cialdini, R. F. (1998). *Influence: Science and practice.* New York: Talman Co.

Clark, E. M., & Teasdale, J. D. (1982). Diurnal variation in clinical depression and accessibility of memories of positive and negative experiences. *Journal of Abnormal Psychology, 91,* 87–95.

Coles, R. (1990). *The spiritual life of children.* Boston: Houghton Mifflin.

Coloroso, B. (1995). *Kids are worth it.* New York: Avon Books.

Comas-Díaz, L. (1989). Culturally relevant issues and treatment implications for Hispanics. In D. Koslow & E. P. Salett (Eds.), *Crossing cultures in mental health* (pp. 31-48). Washington, DC: Sietar.

Comas-Díaz, L., & Duncan, J. W. (1995). The cultural context: A factor in assertiveness training with mainland Puerto Rican women. *Psychology of Women Quarterly, 9,* 463–467.

Comas-Díaz, L., & Griffith, E. E. H. (Eds.). (1998). *Clinical guidelines in cross-cultural mental health.* New York: Wiley.

Constantino, M. J., Castonguay, L. G., & Schut, A. J. (2002). The working alliance: A flagship for the "scientist-practitioner" model in psychotherapy. In G. S. Tryon (Ed.), *Counseling based on process research: Applying what we know.* (pp. 81–131). Boston: Allyn & Bacon.

Conwell, Y., Duberstein, P. R., Cox, C., Herrmann, J. H., Forbes, N. T., & Caine, E. D. (1996). Relationships of age and Axis I diagnoses in victims of completed suicide: A psychological autopsy study. *American Journal of Psychiatry, 153,* 1001–1008.

Coppen, A. (1994). Depression as a lethal disease: Prevention strategies. *Journal of Clinical Psychiatry, 55,* 37–45.

Corey, G. (2001). *Theory and practice of counseling and psychotherapy* (6th ed.). Monterey, CA: Brooks/Cole.

Corey, G., Corey, M. S., & Callahan, P. (2003). *Issues and ethics in the helping professions* (6th ed.). Pacific Grove, CA: Brooks/Cole.

Cormier, W. H., & Cormier, L. S. (1998). *Interviewing strategies for helpers: Fundamental skills and cognitive behavioral interventions* (4th ed.). Monterey, CA: Brooks/Cole.

Cormier, L. S., & Nurius, P. (2003). Interviewing strategies for helpers (5th ed.). Monterey, CA: Brooks/Cole.

Corsini, R. (1989). *Current psychotherapies* (4th ed.). Itasca, IL: Peacock.

Corsini, R., & Wedding, D. (1995). *Current psychotherapies* (5th ed.). Itasca, IL: Peacock.

Costa, L., & Altekruse, M. (1994). Duty to warn guidelines for mental health counselors. *Journal of Counseling and Development, 72,* 346–350.

Dahl, R. (1977). *The wonderful story of Henry Sugar (and six more).* New York: Penguin Books.

Dana, R. H. (1993). *Multicultural assessment perspectives for professional psychology.* Boston: Allyn & Bacon.

Daniels, J. A. (2001). Managed care, ethics, and counseling. *Journal of Counseling and Development, 79,* 119–122.

Davidson, M. W., Wagner, W. G., & Range, L. M. (1995). Clinicians' attitudes toward no-suicide agreements. *Suicide and Life-Threatening Behavior, 25,* 410–414.

Davis, M., McKay, M., & Eshelman, E. R. (2000). *The relaxation and stress reduction workbook.* Oakland, CA: New Harbinger.

Dean, P. J., Range, L. M., & Goggin, W. C. (1996). The escape theory of suicide in college students: Testing a model that includes perfectionism. *Suicide and Life-Threatening Behavior, 26,* 181–186.

de Becker, G. (1997). *The gift of fear.* New York: Little, Brown.

Deloria, V., Jr. (1994). *God is red.* Golden, CO: Fulcrum Publishing.

de Rosiers, G. (1992). Primary or depressive dementia: Mental status screening. *International Journal of Neurosciences, 64,* 33–67.

de Shazer, S. (1985). *Keys to solution in brief therapy.* New York: Norton.

de Shazer, S. (1994). *Words were originally magic.* New York: Norton.

Diament, A. (1998). *Red tent.* New York: St. Martins Press.

Dickson, D., & Bamford, D. (1995). Improving the interpersonal skills of social work students: The problem of transfer of training and what to do about it. *British Journal of Social Work, 25,* 85–105.

DiGiuseppe, R., Linscott, J., & Jilton, R. (1996). Developing the therapeutic alliance in child-adolescent psychotherapy. *Applied and Preventive Psychology, 5,* 85–100.

Diller, J. V., Murphy, E., & Martinez, J. (1998). *Cultural diversity: A primer for the human services.* London: International Thomson.

Dolezal-Wood, S., Belar, C. D., & Snibbe, J. (1998). A comparison of computer assisted psychotherapy and cognitive-behavioral therapy in groups. *Journal of Clinical Psychology in Medical Settings, 5,* 103–115.

Dominguez, M. M., & Carton, J. S. (1997). The relationship between self-actualization and parenting style. *Journal of Social Behavior and Personality, 12,* 1093–1100.

Drye, R. D., Goulding, R. L., & Goulding, M. E. (1973). No-suicide decisions: Patient monitoring of suicidal risk. *American Journal of Psychiatry, 130,* 171–174.

Duan, C. (2000). Being empathic: The function of intention to empathize and nature of emotion. *Motivation and Emotion, 24,* 29–49.

Duan, C., Rose, T. B., & Kraatz, R. A. (2002). Empathy. In G. S. Tryon (Ed.), *Counseling based on process research: Applying what we know* (pp. 197–231). Boston: Allyn & Bacon.

Dunn, C., Deroo, L., & Rivara, F. P. (2001). The use of brief interventions adapted from motivational interviewing across behavioral domains: A systematic review. *Addictions, 96,* 1725–1742.

Dworkin, S. H., & Gutierrez, F. J. (1992). *Counseling gay men and lesbians: Journey to the end of the rainbow.* Alexandria, VA: American Association for Counseling and Development.

Eagen, T. (1994, January 30). A Washington city full of prozac. *New York Times,* 16.

Eagle, M. N. (1984). *Recent developments in psychoanalysis.* New York: McGraw-Hill.

Egan, G. (1986). *The skilled helper: Model, skills, and methods for effective helping* (3rd ed.). Pacific Grove, CA: Brooks/Cole.

Egan, G. (2002). *The skilled helper: Model, skills, and methods for effective helping* (7th ed.). Pacific Grove, CA: Brooks/Cole.

Eich, E. (1989). Theoretical issues in state dependent memory. In H. L. Roediger & F. I. M. Craik (Eds.), *Varieties of memory and consciousness: Essays in honour of Endel Tulving* (pp. 331-354). Hillsdale, NJ: Erlbaum.

Elliott, R. (1988). Tests, abilities, race, and conflict. *Intelligence, 12,* 333–335.

Ellis, A., Sichel, J., Yeager, R., DiMattia, D., & DiGiuseppe, R. (1989). *Rational-emotive couples therapy.* Englewood Cliffs, NJ: Alemany.

Ellis, T. E., & Newman, C. F. (1996). *Choosing to live: How to defeat suicide through cognitive therapy.* Oakland, CA: New Harbinger.

Ellison, J. M. (2001). *Treatment of suicidal patients in managed care.* Washington, DC: American Psychiatric Press.

Erickson, M. H., Rossi, E., & Rossi, S. (1976). *Hypnotic realities.* New York: Irvington.

Essandoh, P. K. (1996). Multicultural counseling as the "fourth force": A call to arms. *Counseling Psychologist, 24,* 126–137.

Evans, G., & Farberow, N. L. (1988). *The encyclopedia of suicide.* New York: Facts on File.

Everly, G. S., & Boyle, S. H. (1999). Critical incident stress debriefing (CISD): A meta-analysis. *International Journal of Emergency Mental Health, 1,* 165–168.

Fairbairn, R. (1952). *Object relations theory of the personality.* New York: Basic Books.

Falloon, B. A., & Horwath, E. (1993). Asceticism: Creative spiritual practice or pathological pursuit? *Psychiatry Interpersonal and Biological Processes, 56,* 310–316.

Falloon, I. R. H. (Ed.). (1988). *Handbook of behavioral family therapy.* New York: Guilford Press.

Fawcett, J., Scheftner, W. A., Fogg, L., Clark, D., Young, M. A., Hedeker, D., et al. (1990). Time-related predictors of suicide in major affective disorder. *American Journal of Psychiatry, 147,* 1189–1194.

Fenichel, O. (1945). *The psychoanalytic theory of neuroses.* New York: Norton.

Fenigstein, A. (1979). Self-consciousness, self-attention, and social interaction. *Journal of Personality and Social Psychology, 37,* 75–86.

Fenigstein, A., Scheier, M. F., & Buss, A. H. (1975). Public and private self-consciousness: Assessment and theory. *Journal of Consulting and Clinical Psychology, 43,* 522–527.

First, M. B., Spitzer, R. L., Gibbon, M. W., & Williams, J. B. (1995). The structured clinical interview for *DSM-III-R* personality disorders (SCID-II). I: Description. *Journal of Personality Disorders, 9,* 83–91.

Fisch, R., Weakland, J., & Segal, L. (1982). *The tactics of change: Doing therapy briefly.* San Francisco: Jossey-Bass.

Fisher, S. (1973). *Body consciousness: You are what you feel.* Englewood Cliffs, NJ: Prentice Hall.

Flanagan, D. P., Genshaft, J. L., & Harrison, P. L. (Eds.). (1997). *Contemporary intellectual assessment: Theories, tests, and issues.* New York: Guilford Press.

Florio, E. R., Hendryx, M. S., Jensen, J. E., Rockwood, T. H., Raschko, R., & Dyck, D. G. (1997). A comparison of suicidal and nonsuicidal elders referred to a community mental health center program. *Suicide and Life-Threatening Behavior, 27,* 182–193.

Foa, E., & Riggs, D. S. (1994). Posttraumatic stress disorder and rape. In R. S. Pynoos (Ed.), *Posttraumatic stress disorder: A clinical review* (pp. 133–163). Lutherville, MD: Sidran Press.

Foley, R., & Sharf, B. F. (1981). The five interviewing techniques most frequently overlooked by primary care physicians. *Behavioral Medicine, 8,* 26–31.

Folstein, M. F., Folstein, S. E., & McHugh, P. R. (1975). Mini-Mental State: A practical method for grading the cognitive state of patients for the clinician. *Journal of Psychiatric Research, 12,* 189–198.

Fones, C. S., Manfro, G. G., & Pollack, M. H. (1998). Social phobia: An update. *Harvard Review of Psychiatry, 5,* 247–259.

Fong, M. L., & Cox, B. G. (1983). Trust as an underlying dynamic in the counseling process: How clients test trust. *Personal and Guidance Journal, 62,* 163–166.

Fowers, B. J., & Richardson, F. C. (1996). Why is multiculturalism good? *American Psychologist, 51,* 609–621.

Francis, A., & Ross, R. (1996). *DSM-IV case studies: A clinical guide to differential diagnosis.* Washington, DC: American Psychiatric Press.

Frank, J. D. (1974). The restoration of morale. *American Journal of Psychiatry, 131,* 271–74.

Frank, J. D., & Frank, J. B. (1991). *Persuasion & healing: A comparative study of psychotherapy* (3rd ed.). Baltimore: Johns Hopkins University Press.

Franklin, A. J. (1993, July/August). The invisibility syndrome. *Family Therapy Networker,* 33–39.

Freud, A. (1946). *The ego and the mechanisms of defense* (C. Baines, Trans.). New York: International Universities Press.

Freud, S. (1949). *An outline of psychoanalysis.* New York: Norton. (Original work published 1940)

Freud, S. (1955). Group psychology and the analysis of the ego. In *Complete psychological works: Standard edition* (Vol. 18). London: Hogarth Press. (Original work published 1921)

Freud, S. (1957). The future prospects of psycho-analytic therapy. In J. Strachey (Ed.), *The standard edition* (Vol. 11). London: Hogarth. (Original work published 1910)

Freud, S. (1958). Recommendations to physicians practicing psychoanalysis. In J. Strachey (Ed. and Trans.), *The standard edition of the complete psychological works of Sigmund Freud* (Vol. 12, pp. 109–120). London: Hogarth Press. (Original work published 1912)

Fried, D., Crits-Christoph, P., & Luborsky, L. (1990). The parallel of the CCRT for the therapist with the CCRT for other people. In L. Luborsky & P. Crits-Christoph (Eds.), *Understanding transference: The CCRT method* (pp. 147–157). New York: Basic Books.

Friedmann, P. D., Saitz, R., Gogineni, A., Zhang, J. X., & Stein, M. D. (2001). Validation of the screening strategy in the NIAAA physicians' guide to helping patients with alcohol problems. *Journal of Studies on Alcohol, 62* [Special issue], 234–238.

Gandy, G. L., Martin, E. D., & Hardy, R. E. (1999). *Counseling in the rehabilitation process: Community services for mental and physical disabilities* (2nd ed.). Springfield, IL: Charles C. Thomas.

Garb, H. N. (1998). *Studying the clinician: Judgment research and psychological assessment.* Washington, DC: American Psychological Association.

Garcia-Preto, N. (1996). Latino families: An overview. In M. McGoldrick, J. Giordano, & J. K. Pearce (Eds.), *Ethnicity and family therapy* (2nd ed., pp. 141-154). New York: Guilford Press.

Gardner, H. (1983). *Frames of mind: The theory of multiple intelligences.* New York: Basic Books.

Gardner, H. (1999). *Intelligence reframed: Multiple intelligences for the 21st century.* New York: Basic Books.

Gardner, R. A. (1971). *Therapeutic storytelling with children: The mutual storytelling technique.* New York: Jason Aronson.

Garrett, M. T., & Pichette, E. F. (2000). Red as an apple: Native American acculturation and counseling with or without reservation. *Journal of Counseling and Development, 78,* 3–13.

Gaston, L. (1990). The concept of the alliance and its role in psychotherapy: Theoretical and empirical considerations. *Psychotherapy, 27,* 143–153.

Gaylin, N. L. (1989). Ipsative measures: In search of paradigmatic change and a science of subjectivity. *Person-Centered Review, 4,* 429–445.

Gazda, G. M., Asbury, F. S., Balzer, F. J., Childers, W. C., & Walters, R. P. (1977). *Human relations development* (2nd ed.). Boston: Allyn & Bacon.

Gazda, G. M., Asbury, F. S., Balzer, F. J., Childers, W. C., & Walters, R. P. (1984). *Human relations development: A manual for educators* (3rd ed.). Boston: Allyn & Bacon.

Geller, J. D., & Gould, E. (1996). A contemporary psychoanalytic perspective: Rogers' brief psychotherapy with Mary Jane Tilden. In B. A. Farber & D. C. Brink (Ed.), *The psychotherapy of Carl Rogers: Cases and commentary* (pp. 211–230). New York: Guilford Press.

Gelso, C. J., & Hayes, J. A. (1998). *The psychotherapy relationship: Theory, research, and practice.* New York: John Wiley & Sons.

George, R. L., & Cristiani, T. S. (1994). *Counseling: Theory and practice* (4th ed.). Boston: Allyn & Bacon.

Gibbs, J. T. (1997). African-American suicide: A cultural paradox. *Suicide and Life-Threatening Behavior, 27,* 68–79.

Gibbs, M. A. (1984). The therapist as imposter. In C. M. Brody (Ed.), *Women therapists working with women: New theory and process of feminist therapy* (pp. 22-33). New York: Springer.

Gibson, P. (1994). Gay male and lesbian youth suicide. In M. R. Feinleib (Ed.), *Report of the secretary's task force on youth suicide. Vol. 3: Preventions and interventions in youth suicide* (pp. 110–142). Rockville, MD: U.S. Department of Health and Human Services.

Gilligan, C. (1982). *In a different voice: Psychological theory and women's development.* Cambridge, MA: Harvard University Press.

Giordano, P. J. (1997). Establishing rapport and developing interviewing skills. In J. R. Matthews & C. E. Walker (Eds.), *Basic skills and professional issues in clinical psychology* (pp. 59–82). Needham Heights: Allyn & Bacon.

Glasser, W. (1998). *Choice theory: A new psychology of personal freedom.* New York: HarperCollins.

Glasser, W. (2000). *Counseling with choice theory: The new reality therapy.* New York: HarperCollins.

Goldenberg, I., & Goldenberg, H. (2000). *Family therapy: An overview* (5th ed.). Belmont, CA: Brooks/Cole.

Goldfried, M. (1990). *Psychotherapy integration: A mid-life crisis for behavior therapy.* Paper presented at the 24th annual meeting of the Association for the Advancement of behavior therapy, San Francisco.

Goldfried, M. (Ed.). (2001). *How therapists change: Personal and professional recollections.* Washington, DC: American Psychological Association.

Goldfried, M., & Davison, G. (1976). *Clinical behavior therapy.* New York: Holt, Rinehart and Winston.

Goldfried, M., & Davison, G. (1994). *Clinical behavior therapy* (exp ed.). Oxford, England: John Wiley & Sons.

Goldman, L. (1972). Tests and counseling: A better way. *Measurement and Evaluation in Guidance, 15,* 70–73.

Gordon, M. (1991). *ADHD/hyperactivity: A manual for parents and teachers.* Dewitt, NY: Gordon Systems.

Gottman, J. M., & DeClaire, J. (2001). *The relationship cure: A five-step guide for building better connections with family, friends, and lovers.* New York: Crown.

Gould, S. J. (1981). *The mismeasure of man.* New York: Norton.

Grahn, J. (1990). *Another mother tongue.* Boston: Beacon Press.

Gray, J. (1992). *Men are from Mars, women are from Venus.* New York: HarperCollins.

Green, R. J. (1996). Why ask, why tell? Teaching and learning about lesbians and gays in family therapy. *Family Process, 35,* 389–400.

Greenberg, J. R., & Mitchell, S. A. (1983). *Object relations in psychoanalytic theory.* Cambridge, MA: Harvard University Press.

Greenberg, L. S., & Safran, J. D. (1987). *Emotion in psychotherapy: Affect, cognition, and the process of change.* New York: Guilford Press.

Greenberg, M. A., Wortman, C. B., & Stone, A. A. (1996). Emotional expression and physical health: Revising traumatic memories or fostering self-regulation? *Journal of Personality and Social Psychology, 71,* 588–602.

Greenberg, R. P., & Staller, J. (1981). Personal therapy for therapists. *American Journal of Psychiatry, 138,* 1467–1471.

Greenson, R. R. (1965). The working alliance and the transference neurosis. *Psychoanalytic Quarterly, 34,* 155–181.

Greenson, R. R. (1967). *The technique and practice of psychoanalysis* (Vol. 1). New York: International Universities Press.

Greenspan, S. I., & Greenspan, N. T. (1991). *The clinical interview of the child* (2nd ed.). Washington, DC: American Psychiatric Press.

Griffith, E. E. H., & Baker, F. M. (1993). Psychiatric care of African Americans. In A. C. Gaw (Ed.), *Culture, ethnicity, and mental illness (pp. 147–173).* Washington, DC: American Psychiatric Press.

Grinder, J., & Bandler, R. (1976). *The structure of magic: II.* Palo Alto, CA: Science and Behavior Books.

Guerney, B. G. (1977). *Relationship enhancement.* San Francisco: Jossey-Bass.

Guest, J. (1982). *Ordinary people.* New York: Viking.

Gunderson, J. G., Phillips, K. A., Triebwaser, J., & Hirschfeld, R. (1994). The diagnostic interview for depressive personality. *American Journal of Psychiatry, 151,* 1300–1304.

Gurman, A. S., & Jacobson, N. S. (2002). *Clinical handbook of couple therapy* (3rd ed.). New York: Guilford.

Gustafson, J. P. (1997). *The complex secret of brief psychotherapy: A panorama of approaches.* New York: Aronson.

Gustafson, K. E., McNamara, J. R., & Jensen, J. A. (1994). Parents informed consent decisions regarding psychotherapy for their children: Consideration of therapeutic risks and benefits. *Professional Psychology: Research and Practice, 25,* 16–22.

Hack, T. F., & Cook, A. J. (1995). Getting started: Intake and initial sessions. In D. G. Martin & A. D. Moore (Eds.), *First steps in the art of intervention* (pp. 46-74). Pacific Grove, CA: Brooks/Cole.

Hadley, S. W., & Strupp, H. H. (1976). Contemporary views of negative effects in psychotherapy. *Archives of General Psychiatry, 33,* 1291–1302.

Hahn, W. K., & Marks, L. I. (1996). Client receptiveness to the routine assessment of past suicide attempts. *Professional Psychology: Research and Practice, 27,* 592–594.

Haley, J. (1973). *Uncommon therapies: The psychiatric techniques of Milton Erickson.* San Francisco: Jossey-Bass.

Hall, C. C. I. (1997). Cultural malpractice; the growing obsolescence of psychology with the changing U.S. population. *American Psychologist, 52,* 642–651.

Hall, E. T. (1966). *The hidden dimension.* Garden City, NY: Doubleday.

Hall, G. C. N., Barongan, C., Bernal, G., Comas-Díaz, L., Hall, C. C. I., LaDue, R. A., et al. (1997). Misunderstandings of multiculturalism. *American Psychologist, 52,* 654–655.

Hall, R. C., Platt, D. E., & Hall, R. C. W. (1999). Suicide risk assessment: A review of risk factors for suicide in 100 patients who made severe suicide attempts: Evaluation of suicide risk in a time of managed care. *Psychosomatics, 40,* 18–27.

Halling, S., & Goldfarb, M. (1996). The new generation of diagnostic manuals (*DSM-III, DSM-III-R,* and *DSM-IV*): An overview and a phenomenologically based critique. *Journal of Phenomenological Psychology, 27,* 49–71.

Hamilton, M. (1967). A rating scale for depression. *Journal of Neurology, Neurosurgery, and Psychiatry, 23,* 56–62.

Hammer, A. (1983). Matching perceptual predicates: Effect on perceived empathy in a counseling analogue. *Journal of Counseling Psychology, 30,* 172–179.

Hampson, R. B., & Beavers, W. R. (1996). Measuring family therapy outcome in a clinical setting: Families that do better or do worse in therapy. *Family Process, 35,* 347–361.

Handelsman, M. M., & Glavin, M. D. (1988). Facilitating informed consent for outpatient psychotherapy: A suggested written format. *Professional Psychology: Research and Practice, 19,* 223–225.

Hanna, F. J., Hanna, C. A., & Keys, S. G. (1999). Fifty strategies for counseling defiant, aggressive adolescents: Reaching, accepting, and relating. *Journal of Counseling and Development, 77,* 395–404.

Harrington, R. (1993). *Depressive disorder in childhood and adolescence.* Chichester, England: John Wiley & Sons.

Hartman, A. (1995). Diagrammatic assessment of family relationships. *Families in Society, 76,* 111–122.

Hasin, D. J., Trautman, K. D., Miele, G. M., Samet, S., Smith, M., & Endicott, J. (1998). Psychiatric research interview for substance and mental disorders (PRISM): Reliability in substance abuse. *American Journal of Psychiatry, 153,* 1195-1201.

Hatfield, E., & Walster, G. W. (1981). *A new look at love.* Reading, MA: Addison-Wesley.

Hawkins, R. L. (1992). Therapy with the male couple. In S. H. Dworkin & F. J. Guitierrez (Eds.), *Counseling gay men and lesbians: Journey to the end of the rainbow* (pp. 81–94). Alexandria, VA: American Association for Counseling and Development.

Hayes, K. F. (1999). *Working it out: Using exercise in psychotherapy.* Washington, DC: American Psychological Association.

Hazan C., & Shaver, P. R. (1987). Romantic love conceptualized as an attachment process. *Journal of Personality and Social Psychology, 59,* 270–280.

Healy, D. (2000). Antidepressant induced suicidality. *Primary Care in Psychiatry, 6,* 23–28.

Heinrich, R. K., Corbine, J. L., & Thomas, K. R. (1990). Counseling Native Americans. *Journal of Counseling and Development, 69,* 128–133.

Helstone, F. S., & van Zurren, F. J. (1996). Clinical decision making in intake interviews for psychotherapy: A qualitative study. *British Journal of Medical Psychology, 69,* 191–206.

Hendrix, H. (1988). *Getting the love you want: A guide for couples.* New York: Holt and Company.

Herman, J. L. (1992). *Trauma and recovery.* New York: Basic Books.

Herman, S. M. (1998). The relationship between therapist-client modality similarity and psychotherapy outcome. *Journal of Psychotherapy Practice and Research, 7,* 56–64.

Herring, R. (1990). Understanding Native American values: Process and content concern for counselors. *Counseling and Values, 34,* 134–136.

Herron, J., Ticehurst, H., Appleby, L., Perry, A., & Cordingley, L. (2001). Attitudes toward suicide prevention in front line health staff. *Suicide and Life-Threatening Behavior, 31,* 242–247.

Hess, E. H. (1975). *The tell-tale eye.* New York: Van Nostrand-Reinhold.

Hibbs, E. D., & Jensen, P. S. (1996). *Psychosocial treatments for child and adolescent disorders.* Washington, DC: American Psychological Association.

Hickling, L. P., Hickling, E. J., Sison G. F., & Radetsky, S. (1984). The effect of note-taking on a simulated clinical interview. *Journal of Psychology, 116,* 235–240.

Hill, C. E. (2001). *Helping skills: The empirical foundation.* Washington, D.C.: American Psychological Association.

Hillyer, D. (1996). Solution-oriented questions: An analysis of a key intervention in solution-focused therapy. *Journal of American Psychiatric Nurses Association, 2,* 3–10.

Hines, P., & Boyd-Franklin, N. (1996). African American families. In M. McGoldrick, J. Giordano, & J. K. Pearce (Eds.), *Ethnicity and family therapy* (2nd ed., pp. 66–84). New York: Guilford Press.

Ho, M. K. (1992). *Minority children and adolescents in therapy.* Newbury Park, CA: Sage.

Ho, M. K. (1993). *Family therapy with ethnic minorities.* Newbury Park, CA: Sage.

Hodges, K. (1985). *Manual for the child assessment schedule.* Unpublished manuscript, University of Missouri-Columbia.

Holt, R. R. (1969). *Assessing personality.* New York: Harcourt Brace Jovanovich.

Hood, A. B., & Johnson, R. W. (1997). *Assessment in counseling.* Alexandria, VA: American Counseling Association.

Horowitz, M., Marmar, C., Krupnick, J., Wilner, N., Kaltreider, N., & Wallerstein, R. (1984). *Personality styles and brief psychotherapy.* New York: Basic Books.

Horsley, G. C. (1997). In-laws: Extended family therapy. *American Journal of Family Therapy, 25,* 18–27.

Hoyt, M. F. (1996). Welcome to possibilityland: A conversation with Bill O'Hanlon. In M. Hoyt (Ed.), *Constructive therapies* (Vol. 2, pp. 87–123). New York: Guilford Press.

Hrdy, S. B. (1999). *Mother nature: A history of mothers, infants, and natural selection.* New York: Pantheon Books.

Hubble, M. A., Duncan, B. L., & Miller, S. D. (1999). *The heart and soul of change: What works in therapy.* Washington, DC: American Psychological Association.

Hughes, C. C. (1993). Culture in clinical psychiatry. In A. C. Gaw (Ed.), *Culture, ethnicity, and mental illness* (pp. 3–41). Washington, DC: American Psychiatric Press.

Hughes, D. A. (1998). *Building the bonds of attachment.* Northvale, NJ: Jason Aronson.

Hughes, D. H. (1996). Suicide and violence assessment in psychiatry. *General Hospital Psychiatry, 18,* 416–421.

Hughes, J. N., & Baker, D. B. (1990). *The clinical child interview.* New York: Guilford Press.

Hutchins, D. E., & Cole, C. G. (1997). *Helping relationships and strategies* (3rd ed.). Monterey, CA: Brooks/Cole.

Huxley, A. (1932). *Brave new world.* New York: Harper & Row.

Hyman, I. A. (1997). *The case against spanking.* New York: Jossey-Bass.

Igartua, K. J. (1998). Therapy with lesbian couples: The issues and the interventions. *Canadian Journal of Psychiatry, 43,* 391–396.

International Association of Marriage and Family Counselors. (1993). Ethical code for the International Association of Marriage and Family Counselors. *Family Journal: Counseling and Therapy for Couples and Families, 1,* 73–77.

Isaacs, M. L. (1997). The duty to warn and protect: Tarasoff and the elementary school counselor. *Elementary School Guidance and Counseling, 31,* 326–348.

Ivey, A. E., D'Andrea, M., Ivey, M. B., & Simek-Morgan, L. (2002). *Theories of counseling and psychotherapy: A multicultural perspective* (5th ed.). Boston: Allyn & Bacon.

Ivey, A. E., & Ivey, M. (1999). *Intentional interviewing and counseling* (4th ed.). Pacific Grove, CA: Brooks/Cole.

Izard, C. E. (1977). *Human emotions.* New York: Plenum Press.

Izard, C. E. (1982). *Measuring emotions in infants and children.* New York: Cambridge University Press.

Jacobson, N. (1996). *Integrative couples therapy: Promoting acceptance and change.* New York: Norton.

Jobes, D. A., & Berman, A. L. (1993). Suicide and malpractice liability: Assessing and revising policies, procedures, and practice in outpatient settings. *Professional Psychology: Research and Practice, 24,* 91–99.

Jones, E. (1955). *The life and work of Sigmund Freud* (Vol. II). New York: Basic Books.

Jongsma, A. E. (2001). *The adult psychotherapy progress notes planner.* New York: John Wiley & Sons.

Jongsma, A. E., & Peterson, L. M. (1995). *The complete psychotherapy treatment planner.* New York: John Wiley & Sons.

Jongsma, A. E., & Peterson, L. M. (1999). *The complete adult psychotherapy treatment planner.* New York: John Wiley & Sons.

Jongsma, A. E., Peterson, L. M., & McInnis, W. P. (1996). *The child and adolescent psychotherapy treatment planner.* New York: John Wiley & Sons.

Jongsma, A. E., Peterson, L. M., & McInnis, W. P. (2000a). *The adolescent psychotherapy treatment planner.* New York: John Wiley & Sons.

Jongsma, A. E., Peterson, L. M., & McInnis, W. P. (2000b). *The child psychotherapy treatment planner.* New York: John Wiley & Sons.

*Journal of the American Academy of Child and Adolescent Psychiatry.* (2001). Summary of the practice parameters for the assessment and treatment of children and adolescents with suicidal behavior. *Author, 40,* 495-499.

Juhnke, G. A. (1996). The adapted-SAD persons: A suicide assessment scale designed for use with children. *Elementary School Guidance and Counseling, 30,* 252–263.

Kabat-Zinn, J. (1995). *Wherever you go, there you are: Mindfulness meditation in everyday life.* New York: Hyperion.

Kachur, S. P., Potter, L. B., James, S. P., & Powell, K. E. (1995). *Suicide in the United States* (Violence Surveillance Summary Series, No. 1). Atlanta, GA: National Center for Injury Prevention and Control.

Kaplan, M. L., Asnis, G. M., Sanderson, W. C., Keswani, L., De Lecuona, J. M., & Joseph, S. (1994). Suicide assessment: Clinical interview vs. self-report. *Journal of Clinical Psychology, 50,* 294–298.

Karon, B. P. (2000). The clinical interpretation of the Thematic Apperception Test, Rorschach, and other clinical data: A reexamination of statistical versus clinical prediction. *Professional Psychology, 31,* 230–233.

Kaye, N. S., & Soreff, S. M. (1991). The psychiatrist's role, responses, and responsibilities when a patient commits suicide. *American Journal of Psychiatry, 148,* 739–743.

Kaysen, S. (1993). *Girl, interrupted.* New York: Vintage Books.

Kazdin, A. E. (1979). Fictions, factions, and functions of behavior therapy. *Behavior Therapy, 10,* 629–656.

Kazdin, A. E. (1995). *Conduct disorders in childhood and adolescence* (2nd ed.). Thousand Oaks, CA: Sage.

Keats, D. M. (2000). *Interviewing: A practical guide for students and professionals.* Buckingham, England: Open University Press.

Kelly, F. D. (1997). *The clinical interview of the adolescent: From assessment and formulation to treatment planning.* Springfield, IL: Charles C. Thomas.

Kelly, G. A. (1955). *The psychology of personal constructs* (2 vols.). New York: Norton.

Kendall, P. C., & Bemis, K. M. (1983). Thought and action in psychotherapy: The cognitive-behavioral approaches. In M. Hersen, A. E. Kazdin, & A. S. Bellack (Eds.), *The clinical psychology handbook* (pp. 565-592). New York: Pergamon Press.

Kernberg, O. F. (1976). *Object relations theory and clinical psychoanalysis.* New York: Jason Aronson.

Kihlstrom, J. F. (1985). Hypnosis. *Annual Review of Psychology, 36,* 385–418.

King, R., Riddle, M., Chappell, P., Hardin, M., Anderson, G., Lombroso, P., et al. (1991). Emergence of self-destructive phenomena in children and adolescent during fluoxetine treatment. *Journal of the American Academy of Child and Adolescent Psychiatry, 30,* 171–176.

Kishi, Y., Robinson, R. G., & Kosier, J. T. (2001). Suicidal ideation among patients during the rehabilitation period after life-threatening physical illness. *Journal of Nervous and Mental Diseases, 189,* 623–628.

Kitano, H. L. (1969). *Japanese Americans: The evolution of a subculture.* Englewood Cliffs, NJ: Prentice Hall.

Kivlighan, D. M., Jr. (2002). Transference, interpretation, and insight. In G. S. Tryon (Ed.), *Counseling based on process research: Applying what we know* (pp. 166–196). Boston: Allyn & Bacon.

Kleepsies, P. M. (1993). Stress of patient suicidal behavior: Implications for interns and training programs in psychology. *Professional Psychology, 24,* 477–482.

Klein, P. D. (1997). Multiplying the problems of intelligence by eight: A critique of Gardner's theory. *Canadian Journal of Education, 22,* 377–394.

Klerman, G. (1984). The advantages of the *DSM-III. American Journal of Psychiatry, 141,* 539–542.

Knapp, M. L. (1972). *Nonverbal communication in human interaction.* New York: Holt, Rinehart and Winston.

Knickmeyer, S. (1996). Media coverage of suicides. *Suicide and Life-Threatening Behavior, 26,* 269–271.

Kohut, H. (1972). *The analysis of the self.* New York: International Universities Press.

Kohut, H. (1977). *The restoration of the self.* New York: International Universities Press.

Kohut, H. (1984). *How does analysis cure?* London: University of Chicago Press.

Koocher, G. P., Goodman, G. S., White, C. S., & Fredrick, W. N. (1996). Psychological science and the use of anatomically detailed dolls in child sexual abuse assessments. *Annual Progress in Child Psychiatry and Child Development, 1996,* 367–425.

Korchin, S. J. (1976). *Modern clinical psychology.* New York: Basic Books.

Kovacs, M., & Paulaukas, S. L. (1984). Developmental stage and the expression of depressive disorders in children: An empirical analysis. *New Directions for Child Development, 26,* 59–80.

Kposowa, A. J. (2001). Unemployment and suicide: A cohort analysis of social factors predicting suicide: A Longitudinal Mortality Study. *Psychological Medicine, 31,* 127–138.

Kramer, P. D. (1993). *Listening to prozac.* New York: Viking.

Krents, H. (1972). *To race the wind.* Toronto, Ontario, Canada: Longmans Canada Limited.

Kronenberger, W. G., & Meyer, R. G. (1996). *The child clinician's handbook.* Boston: Allyn & Bacon.

Krumboltz, J. D., & Thoresen, C. E. (Eds.). (1976). *Counseling methods.* New York: Holt, Rinehart and Winston.

Krupnick, J. L., Stosky, S. M., Simmens, S., Moyer, J., Elkin, I., Watkins, J., et al. (1996). The role of the therapeutic alliance in psychotherapy and pharmacotherapy outcome: Findings in the National Institute of Mental Health Treatment of Depression Collaborative Research Program. *Journal of Consulting and Clinical Psychology, 64,* 532–539.

Kurdek, L., & Smith, J. P. (1987). Partner monogamy in married, heterosexual, cohabitating, gay, and lesbian couples. *Journal of Sex Research, 23,* 212–232.

Kushner, H. I. (1991). *American suicide: A psychocultural exploration.* New Brunswick, NJ: Rutgers University Press.

Kutchins, H., & Kirk, S. A. (1997). *Making us crazy. DSM: The psychiatric bile and the creation of mental disorders.* New York: Free Press.

Laing, R. D. (1982). *The voice of experience.* New York: Pantheon Books.

Lambert, M. J. (1989). The individual therapist's contribution to psychotherapy process and outcome. *Clinical Psychology Review, 9,* 469–485.

Lambert, M. J., & Bergin, A. K. (1994). The effectiveness of psychotherapy. In A. K. Bergin & S. L. Garfield (Eds.), *Handbook of psychotherapy and behavior change* (4th ed., pp. 143–189). New York: John Wiley & Sons.

Lambert, M. T., & Fowler, D. R. (1997). Suicide risk factors among veterans: Risk management in the changing culture of the Department of Veterans Affairs. *Journal of Mental Health Administration, 24,* 350–358.

Landreth, G. L., & Lobaugh, A. F. (1998). Filial therapy with incarcerated fathers: Effects on parental acceptance of child, parental stress, and child adjustment. *Journal of Counseling and Development, 76,* 157–165.

Langs, R. (1973). *The technique of psychoanalytic psychotherapy.* New York: Jason Aronson.

Langs, R. (1986). *Unconscious communication and the technique of psychotherapy.* Continuing education seminar, Syracuse, NY.

Lankton, S. R., Lankton, C. H., & Matthews, W. J. (1991). Ericksonian family therapy. In A. S. Gurman & D. P. Kniskern (Eds.), *Handbook of family therapy* (Vol. 2, pp. 239–283). New York: Brunner/Mazel.

Lansky, M. R. (1986). Marital therapy for narcissistic disorders. In N. S. Jacobson & A. S. Gurman (Eds.), *Clinical handbook of marital therapy* (pp. 562-584). New York: Guilford Press.

Lazarus, A. A. (1976). *Multimodal behavior therapy.* New York: Springer.

Lazarus, A. A. (1981). *The practice of multimodal therapy.* New York: McGraw-Hill.

Lazarus, A. A. (1994). How certain boundaries and ethics diminish therapeutic effectiveness. *Ethics and Behavior, 4,* 255–261.

Lazarus, A. A. (1997). *Brief but comprehensive psychotherapy: The multimodal way.* New York: Springer.

Lazarus, A. A., Beutler, L. E., & Norcross, J. C. (1992). The future of technical eclecticism. *Psychotherapy, 29,* 11–20.

Leahy, R. L., & Holland, S. J. (2000). *Treatment plans and interventions for depression and anxiety disorders.* New York: Guilford Press.

Lee, E. (1996). Asian American families: An overview. In M. McGoldrick, J. Giordano, & J. K. Pearce (Eds.), *Ethnicity and family therapy* (2nd ed., pp. 227-248). New York: Guilford Press.

Lee, S., Wright, S., Sayer, J., Parr, A.–M., Gray, R., & Gournay, K. (2001) Physical restraint training for nurses in English and Welsh psychiatric intensive care and regional secure units. *Journal of Mental Health, 10* [Special issue], 151–162.

Le Guin, U. K. (1969). *The left hand of darkness.* New York: Ace Books.

Lennon, S. J., & Davis, L. L. (1990). Categorization in first impressions. *Journal of Psychology, 123,* 439–446.

Lester, D. (1996). *Patterns of suicide & homicide in the world.* Huntington, NY: Nova Science Publishers.

Leve, R. M. (1995). *Child and adolescent psychotherapy.* Boston: Allyn & Bacon.

Levitt, E. A. (1964). The relationship between abilities to express emotional meanings vocally and facially. In J. R. Davis (Ed.), *The communication of emotional meaning.* New York: McGraw-Hill.

Lieberman, M. A., Yalom, I. D., & Miles, M. B. (1973). *Encounter groups: First facts.* New York: Basic Books.

Linehan, M. (1993). *Cognitive-behavioral treatment of borderline personality disorder.* New York: Guilford Press.

Linehan, M. (1999). Standard protocol for assessing and treating suicidal behaviors for patients in treatment. In D. G. Jacobs (Ed.), *The Harvard Medical School guide to suicide assessment and intervention* (pp. 146–187). San Francisco: Jossey-Bass.

Litman, R. E. (1995). Suicide prevention in a treatment setting. *Suicide and Life-Threatening Behavior, 25,* 134–142.

Locke, E. A., Shaw, K. N., Saari, L. M., & Latham, G. P. (1981). Goal setting and task performance: 1969–1980. *Psychological Bulletin, 90,* 125–152.

Loftus, E. F. (2001). Imagining the past. *Psychologist* (Special Issue: After the facts), *14,* 584-587.

Lovett, J. (1999). *Small wonders: Healing childhood trauma with EMDR.* New York: Simon & Schuster.

Lowry, J. L., & Ross, M. J. (1997). Expectations of psychotherapy duration: How long should psychotherapy last? *Psychotherapy, 34,* 272–277.

Luborsky, L. (1984). *Principles of psychoanalytic psychotherapy: A manual for supportive-expressive treatment.* New York: Basic Books.

Luborsky, L., Singer, B., & Luborsky, L. (1975). Comparative studies of psychotherapies. *Archives of General Psychiatry, 32,* 995–1008.

Luquet, W. (1996). *Short term couples therapy: The imago model in action.* New York: Brunner/Mazel.

Lynn, S. J., Martin, D. J., & Frauman, D. C. (1996). Does hypnosis pose special risks for negative effects? *International Journal of Clinical and Experimental Hypnosis, 44*, 7–19.

Maag, J. W. (2001). Rewarded by punishment: Reflections on the disuse of positive reinforcement in schools. *Exceptional Children, 67,* 173–186.

Macaskill, N., & Macaskill, A. (1992). Psychotherapists-in-training evaluate their personal therapy: Results of a U.K. survey. *British Journal of Psychotherapy, 9,* 133–138.

MacDonald, B. (1947). *Mrs. Piggle-Wiggle.* New York: Scholastic.

Machover, K. (1949). *Personality projection in the drawings of the human figure.* Springfield, IL: Thomas.

Mahalik, J. R. (2002). Understanding client resistance in therapy: Implications from research on the counseling process. In G. S. Tryon (Ed.), *Counseling based on process research: Applying what we know* (pp. 66–80). Boston: Allyn & Bacon.

Maholick, L. T., & Turner, D. W. (1979). Termination: That difficult farewell. *American Journal of Psychotherapy, 33,* 583–591.

Mahoney, M. J. (1990). *Developmental psychotherapy.* Workshop presented at the annual meeting of the Association for the Advancement of Behavior Therapy, San Francisco.

Mahoney, M. J. (1991). *Human change processes.* New York: Basic Books.

Mallinckrodt, B. (1991). Client's representation of childhood emotional bonds with parents, social support, and formation of the working alliance. *Journal of Counseling Psychology, 38,* 401–409.

Marcus, S. V., Marquis, P., & Sakai, C. (1997). Controlled study of treatment of PTSD using EMDR in an HMO setting. *Psychotherapy, 34,* 307–315.

Margulies, A. (1984). Toward empathy: The uses of wonder. *American Journal of Psychiatry, 141,* 1025–1033.

Marin, G., & Marin, B. V. (1991). *Research with Hispanic populations.* Newbury Park, CA: Sage.

Martin, D. G., & Moore, A. D. (1995). *First steps in the art of intervention: A guidebook for trainees in the helping professions.* Pacific Grove, CA: Brooks/Cole.

Maslow, A. H. (1970). *Motivation and personality* (2nd ed.). New York: Harper & Row.

Matarazzo, J. D. (1983). The reliability of psychiatric and psychological diagnosis. *Clinical Psychology Review, 3,* 103–145.

Matthews, J. R., & Walker, C. E. (1997). *Basic skills and professional issues in clinical psychology.* Boston: Allyn & Bacon.

Maurer, R. E., & Tindall, J. H. (1983). Effect of postural congruence on client's perception of counselor empathy. *Journal of Counseling Psychology, 30,* 158–163.

Mayerson, N. (1984). Preparing clients for group therapy: A critical review and theoretical formulation. *Clinical Psychology Review, 4,* 191–213.

McCarthy, P. R., & Foa, E. (1990). Obsessive-compulsive disorder. In M. E. Thase, B. A. Edelstein, & M. Hersen (Eds.), *Handbook of outpatient treatment of adults: Nonpsychotic mental disorders* (pp. 209-234). New York: Plenum Press.

McDaniel, J., Purcell, D., & D'Augelli, A. R. (2001). The relationship between sexual orientation and risk for suicide: Research findings and future directions for research and prevention. *Suicide and Life-Threatening Behavior, 31*(Suppl.), 84–105.

McDonald, H. B., & Steinhorn, A. I. (1993). *Understanding homosexuality: A guide for those who know, love, or counsel gay and lesbian individuals.* New York: Crossroad.

McDonnell, T. P. (Ed.). (1974). *A Thomas Merton Reader.* New York: Doubleday.

McGoldrick, M., Garcia-Preto, N., Hines, P., & Lee, E. (1989). Ethnicity and women. In M. McGoldrick, D. Anderson, & F. Walsh (Eds.), *Women in families* (169-199). New York: Norton.

McGoldrick, M., & Gerson, R. (1985). *Genograms in family assessment.* New York: Norton.

McGoldrick, M., Giordano, J., & Pearce, J. K. (1996). *Ethnicity and family therapy* (2nd ed.). New York: Guilford Press.

McIntosh, J. L. (1991). Epidemiology of suicide in the United States. In A. A. Leenaars (Ed.), *Life span perspectives of suicide* (pp. 55–69). New York: Plenum Press.

McKenzie, I., & Wurr, C. (2001). Early suicide following discharge from a psychiatric hospital. *Suicide and Life-Threatening Behavior, 31,* 358–363.

McLean, P. D., & Woody, S. R. (2001). *Anxiety disorders in adults: An evidence-based approach to psychological treatment.* London: Oxford University Press.

McNeilly, R. B. (2000). *Healing the whole person: A solution-focused approach to using empowering language, emotions, and actions in therapy.* New York: John Wiley & Sons.

Mead, M. A., Hohenshil, T. H., & Singh, K. (1997). How the *DSM* system is used by clinical counselors: A national study. *Journal of Mental Health Counseling, 19,* 383–401.

Meador, B., & Rogers, C. R. (1984). Person-centered therapy. In R. J. Corsini (Ed.), *Current psychotherapies* (pp. 155-194). Itasca, IL: Peacock.

Mearns, D. (1997). *Person-centred counselling training.* Thousand Oaks, CA: Sage.

Meehl, P. E. (1954). *Clinical versus statistical prediction: A theoretical analysis and a review of the evidence.* Twin Cities: University of Minnesota Press.

Meehl, P. E. (1986). Causes and effects of my disturbing little book. *Journal of Personality Assessment, 50,* 370–375.

Meichenbaum, D. (1997). The evolution of a cognitive-behavior therapist. In J. K. Zeig (Ed.), *The evolution of psychotherapy: The third conference* (pp. 96-104). New York: Brunner/Mazel.

Meier, S. T., & Davis, S. R. (2001). *The elements of counseling* (4th ed.). Pacific Grove, CA: Brooks/Cole.

Meissner, W. W. (1991). *What is effective psychotherapy: The move from interpretation to relation.* New York: Aronson.

Mersky, H. (1996). Influences of the media: A powerful what? *Lancet, 347,* 416.

Mezzich, J. E., & Shea, S. C. (1990). Interviewing and diagnosis. In M. E. Thase, B. A. Edelstein, & M. Hersen (Eds.), *Handbook of outpatient treatment of adults: Nonpsychotic mental disorders* (pp. 3-18). New York: Plenum Press.

Miller, J. B. (1986). *Toward a new psychology of women* (2nd ed.). Boston: Beacon Press.

Miller, M. (1985). *Information center: Training workshop manual.* San Diego, CA: The Information Center.

Miller, P. H. (1995). *Theories of developmental psychology* (3rd ed.). San Francisco: Freeman.

Miller, W. R. (1983). Motivational interviewing with problem drinkers. *Behavioural Psychotherapy, 11,* 147-172.

Miller, W. R. (2000). Motivational interviewing. IV: Some parallels with horse whispering. *Behavioral and Cognitive Psychotherapy, 28* [Special issue], 285–292.

Miller, W. R., & Rollnick, S. (1991). *Motivational interviewing: Preparing people to change addictive behavior.* New York: Guilford Press.

Miller, W. R., & Rollnick, S. (1998). *Motivational interviewing* (Vols. 1–7) [Professional training videotape series, produced by Theresa B. Moyers]. Albuquerque, NM: Horizon West Productions.

Miller, W. R., & Rollnick, S. (2002). *Motivational interviewing: Preparing people for change.* New York: Guilford Press.

Minuchin, S., & Fishman, H. C. (1981). *Family therapy techniques.* Cambridge, MA: Harvard University Press.

Minuchin, S., Rosman, B. L., & Baker, L. (1978). *Psychosomatic families: Anorexia nervosa in context.* Oxford: Harvard University Press.

Mischel, W. (1968). *Personality and assessment.* New York: John Wiley & Sons.

Mitchell, J., & Everly, G. S. (1993). *Critical incidence stress debriefing.* New York: Chevron Publishing.

Molnar, B. E., Berkman, L. F., & Buka, S. L. (2001). Psychopathology, childhood sexual abuse and other childhood adversities: Relative links to subsequent suicidal behavior in the U.S. *Psychological Medicine, 31,* 965–977.

Monroe, P. G. (1997). Building bridges with biblical counselors. *Journal of Psychology and Theology, 25,* 28–37.

Moos, R. H., & Moos, B. S. (1986). *Family environment scale manual.* Palo Alto, CA: Consulting Psychologists Press.

Moras, K., & Strupp, H. H. (1982). Pretherapy interpersonal relations, patients' alliance and outcome in brief therapy. *Archives of General Psychiatry, 39,* 405–409.

Morgan, H. (1996). An analysis of Gardner's theory of multiple intelligence. *Roeper Review, 18,* 263–269.

Moris, R. (1990). *Forensic suicidology.* Paper presented at the meeting of the American Psychological Association, Boston.

Morrison, J. (1993). *The first interview.* New York: Guilford Press.

Morrison, J. (1994). *The first interview* (revised for the *DSM-IV*). New York: Guilford Press.

Morse, G. G. (1997). Effect of positive reframing and social support on perception of perimenstrual changes among women with premenstrual syndrome. *Health Care Women International, 18,* 175–193.

Morshead, L. L. (1990). *Psychotherapists' responses to anger manifested by female clients.* Paper presented at the meeting of the American Psychological Association, Boston.

Mosak, H. H. (1989). Adlerian psychotherapy. In R. J. Corsini & D. Wedding (Eds.), *Current psychotherapies* (4th ed., pp. 65–116). Itasca, IL: Peacock.

Moscicki, E. K. (1997). Identification of suicide risk factors using epidemiologic studies. *Psychiatric Clinics of North America, 20,* 499–517.

Moursund, J. (1992). *The process of counseling and therapy* (3rd ed.). Englewood Cliffs, NJ: Prentice Hall.

Muehrer, P. (1995). Suicide and sexual orientation: A critical summary of recent research and directions for future research. *Suicide and Life-Threatening Behavior, 25,* 72–81.

Murphy, B. C. (1992). Counseling lesbian couples: Sexism, heterosexism, and homophobia. In S. H. Dworkin & F. J. Guitierrez (Eds.), *Counseling gay men and lesbians: Journey to the end of the rainbow* (pp. 63–79). Alexandria, VA: American Association for Counseling and Development.

Murphy, G. E., & Wetzel, R. D. (1990). The lifetime risk of suicide in alcoholism. *Archives of General Psychiatry, 47,* 383–392.

Murphy, J. (1997). *Solution-focused counseling in middle and high schools.* Alexandria, VA: American Counseling Association.

Murphy, K. R., & Davidshofer, C. O. (1988). *Psychological testing.* Englewood Cliffs, NJ: Prentice Hall.

Myers, D. G. (1989). *Psychology* (2nd ed.). New York: Worth.

Myers, I. B. (1962). *Manual: The Myers-Briggs Type Indicator.* Princeton, NJ: Educational Testing Service.

Myers, I. B., & McCaulley, M. H. (1985). *Manual: A guide to the development and use of the Myers-Briggs Type Indicator.* Palo Alto, CA: Consulting Psychologists.

Nash, L. (1996). The delusion of infection with HIV. *Australian and New Zealand Journal of Psychiatry, 30,* 467–471.

Natale, S. M. (1985). Confrontation and the religious beliefs of a client. In E. M. Stern (Ed.), *Psychotherapy and the religiously committed patient.* New York: Haworth Press.

Nathan, P. E. (1998). Practice guidelines: Not yet ideal. *American Psychologist, 53,* 290–299.

Nathan, P. E., & Gorman, J. M. (1998). *A guide to treatments that work.* New York: Oxford Press.

National Association of Social Workers. (1996). *Code of ethics.* Washington, DC: Author.

Neeleman, J., Wessely, S., & Lewis, G. (1998). Suicide acceptability in African and White Americans: The role of religion. *Journal of Nervous and Mental Disease, 186,* 12–16.

Neff, J. A., & Hoppe, S. K. (1993). Race/ethnicity, acculturation, and psychological distress: Fatalism and religiosity as cultural resources. *Journal of Community Psychology, 21,* 3–20.

Nelson, M. L., & Neufeldt, A. (1996). Building on an empirical foundation: Strategies to enhance good practice. *Journal of Counseling and Development, 74,* 609–615.

Norcross, J. C. (2000). Psychotherapist self-care: Practitioner-tested, research-informed strategies. *Professional Psychology, 31,* 710–713.

Norman, M. G., Davies, F., Nicholson, I. R., Cortese, L., & Malla, A. K. (1998). The relationship of two aspects of perfectionism with symptoms in a psychiatric outpatient population. *Journal of Social and Clinical Psychology, 17,* 50–68.

North, C. S., Smith, E. M., & Spitznagel, E. L. (1993). Is antisocial personality a valid diagnosis among the homeless? *American Journal of Psychiatry, 150,* 578–583.

Noshpitz, J. D. (1994). Self-destructiveness in adolescence: Psychotherapeutic issues. *American Journal of Psychotherapy, 48,* 347–362.

Nouwen, H. J. M. (1977). *The living reminder.* New York: Seabury Press.

Nutt, R. L., Hampton, B. R., Folks, B., & Johnson, R. J. (1990). *Applying feminist principles to supervision.* Paper presented at the meeting of the American Psychological Association, Boston.

O'Brien, S. (1989). *American Indian tribal governments.* Norman: University of Oklahoma Press.

O'Connor, M. F. (1992). Psychotherapy with gay and lesbian adolescents. In S. H. Dworkin & F. J. Gutierrez (Eds.), *Counseling gay men and lesbians: Journey to the end of the rainbow* (pp. 3-22). Alexandria, VA: American Association for Counseling and Development.

Odell, M., & Campbell, C. E. (1998). *The practical practice of marriage and family therapy: Things my training supervisor never told me.* New York: Hawthorne Press.

Ogbu, J. U. (1992). Understanding cultural diversity and learning. *Educational Researcher, 21,* 5–14.

O'Hanlon, B., & Bertolino, B. (1998). *Even from a broken web: Brief, respectful solution-oriented therapy for sexual abuse and trauma.* New York: John Wiley & Sons.

Ohberg, A., Vuori, E., Ojanpera, I., & Loenngvist, P. (1996). Alcohol and drugs in suicides. *British Journal of Psychiatry, 169,* 75–80.

O'Kelly, J. G., Piper, W. E., Kerber, R., & Fowler, J. (1998). Exercise groups in an insight-oriented, evening treatment program. *International Journal of Group Psychotherapy, 48,* 85–98.

Okun, B. F. (1997). *Effective helping: Interviewing and counseling techniques* (5th ed.). Monterey, CA: Brooks/Cole.

Olson, M. E. (2000). *Feminism, community, and communication.* Binghamton, New York: Haworth Press.

Osman, A., Bagge, C. L., & Gutierrez, P. M. (2001). The Suicidal Behaviors Questionnaire—Revised (SBQ-R): Validation with clinical and nonclinical samples. *Assessment, 8,* 443–454.

Oster, G. D., & Gould, P. (1987). *Using drawings in assessment and therapy.* New York: Brunner/Mazel.

Othmer, E., & Othmer, S. C. (1994). *The clinical interview using DSM-IV. Vol. 1: Fundamentals.* Washington, DC: American Psychiatric Press.

Overholser, J. C., Freiheit, S. R., & DiFilippo, J. M. (1997). Emotional distress and substance abuse as risk factors for suicide attempts. *Canadian Journal of Psychiatry, 42,* 402–408.

Paniagua, F. A. (1998). *Assessing and treating culturally diverse clients: A practical guide* (2nd ed.). London: Sage.

Paniagua, F. A. (2001). *Diagnosis in a multicultural context: A casebook for mental health professionals.* Thousand Oaks, CA: Sage.

Papp, P. (1976). Family choreography. In P. J. Guerin Jr. (Ed.), *Family therapy: Theory and practice* (pp. 276-299). New York: Gardner Press.

Parrott, L. (1992). Earliest recollections and birth order: Two Adlerian exercises. *Teaching of Psychology, 19,* 40–42.

Patterson, C. H. (1996). Multicultural counseling: From diversity to universality. *Journal of Counseling and Development, 74,* 227–231.

Patterson, C. H., & Watkins, C. E. (1996). *Theories of psychotherapy.* New York: HarperCollins.

Patterson, J., Williams, L., Grauf-Grounds, C., & Charmow, L. (1998). *Essential skills in family therapy: From the first interview to termination.* New York: Guilford Press.

Patterson, W. M., Dohn, H. H., Bird, J., & Patterson, G. A. (1983). Evaluation of suicidal patients: The SAD PERSONS scale. *Psychosomatics, 24,* 343–349.

Paunonen, S. V. (2001). Inconsistencies in the personality consistency debate. *Psychological Inquiry, 12* [Special issue], 91–93.

Pearlman, L. A., & Mac-Ian, P. S. (1995). Vicarious traumatization: An empirical study of the effec' of trauma work on trauma therapists. *Professional Psychology Research and Practice, 26,* 558–565.

Pearn, J. (2000). Traumatic stress disorders: A classification with implications for prevention and management. *Military Medicine, 165,* 434–440.

Peck, M. S. (1978). *The road less traveled.* New York: Simon & Schuster.

Pedersen, P. (1996). The importance of both similarities and differences in multicultural counseling: Reaction to C. H. Patterson. *Journal of Counseling and Development, 74,* 236–237.

Pedersen, P., Draguns, J., Lonner, J., & Trimble, J. (1996). *Counseling across cultures* (4th ed.). Honolulu: University of Hawaii Press.

Pennebaker, J. W. (1995). *Emotions, disclosure and health.* Washington, DC: American Psychological Association.

Pennebaker, J. W. (2000). The effects of traumatic disclosure on physical and mental health: The values of writing and talking about upsetting events. In J. M. Violanti & D. Paton (Eds.), *Posttraumatic stress intervention: Challenges, issues, and perspectives* (pp. 97–114). Springfield, IL: Charles C. Thomas.

Peterson, J. V., & Nisenholz, B. (1987). *Orientation to counseling.* Boston: Allyn & Bacon.

Phares, E. J. (1988). Clinical Psychlogy (3rd. ed.). Chicago: Dorsey Press.

Piersma, H. L., & Boes, J. L. (1997). The GAF and psychiatric outcome: A descriptive report. *Community Mental Health Journal, 33,* 35–41.

Pietrofesa, J. J., Hoffman, A., & Splete, H. H. (1984). *Counseling: An introduction* (2nd ed.). Boston: Houghton Mifflin.

Pipes, R. B., & Davenport, D. S. (1999). *Introduction to psychotherapy: Common clinical wisdom* (2nd ed.). Englewood Cliffs, NJ: Prentice Hall.

Pizer, B. (1997). When the analyst is ill: Dimensions of self-disclosure. *Psychoanalytic Quarterly, 66,* 450–469.

Plaud, J. J., & Eifert, G. H. (1998). *From behavior theory to behavior therapy.* Boston: Allyn & Bacon.

Plotkin, R. (1981). When rights collide: Parents, children, and consent to treatment. *Journal of Pediatric Psychology, 6,* 121–130.

Poe, E. A. (1985). Silence: A fable. In *Works of Edgar Allan Poe.* New York: Avenel Books.

Polanski, P. J., & Hinkle, J. S. (2000). The mental status examination: Its use by professional counselors. *Journal of Counseling and Development, 78,* 357–364.

Ponterotto, J. G., Rivera, L., & Sueyoshi, L. A. (2000). The career-in-culture interview: A semistructured protocol for the cross cultural intake interview. *Career Development Quarterly, 49,* 85–96.

Pope, K. S. (1990). Therapist-patient sex as sex abuse: Six scientific, professional and practical dilemmas in addressing victimization and rehabilitation. *Professional Psychology: Research and Practice, 21,* 227–239.

Priestley, G., & Pipe, M. E. (1997). Using toys and models in interviews with young children. *Applied Cognitive Psychology, 11,* 69–87.

Prochaska, J. O., & DiClemente, C. C. (1984). *The transtheoretical approach: Crossing traditional boundaries of therapy.* Homewood, IL: Dow Jones/Irwin.

Puig-Antich, J., Chambers, W., & Tabrizi, M. A. (1983). The clinical assessment of current depressive episodes in children and adolescents: Interviews with parents and children. In D. Cantwell & G. Carlson (Eds.), *Childhood depression* (pp. 157–179). New York: Spectrum.

Random House. (1993). *Random House unabridged dictionary* (2nd ed.). New York: Author.

Rapoport, J. L., & Ismond, D. R. (1996). *DSM-IV training guide for diagnosis of childhood disorders.* New York: Brunner/Mazel.

Raue, P. J., Castonguay, L. G., & Goldfried, M. (1993). The working alliance: A comparison of two therapies. *Psychotherapy Research, 3,* 197–207.

Raue, P. J., Goldfried, M., & Barkham, M. (1997). The therapeutic alliance in psychodynamic-interpersonal and cognitive-behavioral therapy. *Journal of Consulting and Clinical Psychology, 65,* 582–587.

Read, J., Agar, K., Barker-Collo, S., Davies, E., & Moskowitz, A. (2001). Assessing suicidality in adults: Integrating childhood trauma as a major risk factor. *Professional Psychology: Research and Practice, 32,* 367–372.

Reischauer, E. (1988). *The Japanese today: Change and conformity.* Cambridge, MA: Belknap.

Renik, O. (1995). The ideal of the anonymous analyst and the problem of self-disclosure. *Psychoanalytic Quarterly, 64,* 466-495.

Renik, O. (1999). Playing one's cards face up in analysis: An approach to the problem of self-disclosure. *Psychoanalytic Quarterly, 68,* 521-530.

Resnik, H. L. P. (1980). Suicide. In H. I. Kaplan & B. J. Sadock (Eds.), *Comprehensive textbook of psychiatry* (3rd ed.). Baltimore: Williams & Wilkins.

Richardson, B. (2001). *Working with challenging youth: Lessons learned along the way.* Philadelphia: Brunner-Routledge.

Ricks, D. F. (1974). Supershrink: Methods of a therapist judged successful on the basis of adult outcomes of adolescent patients. In D. F. Ricks, M. Roff, & A. Thomas (Eds.), *Life history research in psychopathology* (pp. 324-343). Minneapolis: University of Minnesota Press.

Riley, P. (Ed.). (1993). *Growing up Native American: An anthology.* New York: Morrow.

Rilke, R. M. (1992). *Letters to a young poet* (J. Burnham, Trans.). San Rafael, CA: New World Library.

Robins, E. (1985). Psychiatric emergencies. In H. I. Kaplan & B. J. Sadock (Eds.), *Comprehensive textbook of psychiatry* (3rd ed.). Baltimore: Williams & Wilkins.

Robinson, B. E. (1997). Guideline for initial evaluation of the patient with memory loss. *Geriatrics, 52,* 30–32.

Robinson, D. J. (2001). *Brain calipers: Descriptive psychopathology and the psychiatric mental status examination* (2nd ed.). Port Huron, MI: Rapid Psychler Press.

Robinson, F. (1950). *Principles and procedures in student counseling.* New York: Harper & Row.

Rodolfa, E. R., Kraft, W. A., & Reilley, R. R. (1988). Stressors of professionals and trainees at APA-approved counseling and VA medical center internship sites. *Professional Psychologist: Research and Practice, 19,* 43–49.

Rogers, C. R. (1942). *Counseling and psychotherapy.* Boston: Houghton Mifflin.

Rogers, C. R. (1951). *Client-centered therapy.* Boston: Houghton Mifflin.

Rogers, C. R. (1957). The necessary and sufficient conditions of therapeutic personality change. *Journal of Consulting Psychology, 21,* 95–103.

Rogers, C. R. (1958). The characteristics of a helping relationship. *Personnel and Guidance Journal, 37,* 6–16.

Rogers, C. R. (1961). *On becoming a person.* Boston: Houghton Mifflin.

Rogers, C. R. (1962). The interpersonal relationship: The core of guidance. *Harvard Educational Review, 32,* 416–429.

Rogers, C. R. (1969). *Freedom to learn: A view of what education might become.* Columbus, OH: Merrill.

Rogers, C. R. (1972). *Carl Rogers on counseling, a personal perspective at 75.* Corona Del Mar, CA: Psychological and Educational Films.

Rogers, C. R. (1977). *Carl Rogers on personal power.* New York: Delacorte.

Rogers, C. R. (1983). *Freedom to learn for the 80's.* Columbus, OH: Merrill.

Rogers, R. (2001). *Handbook of diagnostic and structured interviewing.* New York: Guilford Press.

Rollnick, S., & Bell, A. (1991). Brief motivational interviewing for use by the nonspecialist. In W. R. Miller & S. Rollnick (Eds.), *Motivational interviewing* (pp. 203–213). New York: Guilford Press.

Rollnick, S., & Miller, W. R. (1995). What is motivational interviewing? *Behavioral and Cognitive Psychotherapy, 23,* 325–334.

Rosenberg, J. I. (1999). Suicide prevention: An integrated training model using affective and action-based interventions. *Professional Psychology, 30,* 83–87.

Rosenberg, J. I. (2000). The complexities of suicide prevention and intervention training: A response to Sommers-Flanagan, Rothman, and Schwenkler. (2000). *Professional Psychology, 31,* 100–101.

Rosenthal. L. D., Zorick, F. J., & Merlotti, L. (1990). Signs and symptoms associated with cataplexy in narcolepsy patients. *Biological Psychiatry, 27,* 1057-1060.

Rosenthal, R., & Akiskal, H. S. (1985). Mental status examination. In M. Hersen & S. M. Turner (Eds.), *Diagnostic interviewing* (25-52). New York: Plenum Press.

Rossau, C. D., & Mortensen, P. B. (1997). Risk factors for suicide in patients with schizophrenia: Nested case-control study. *British Journal of Psychiatry, 171,* 355–359.

Roth, A., & Fonagy, P. (1996). *What works for whom?* New York: Guilford Press.

Rothbaum, B. O. (1997). A controlled study of eye movement desensitization and reprocessing for posttraumatic stress disordered sexual assault victims. *Bulletin of the Menninger Clinic, 61,* 317–334.

Roukema, R. W. (1998). *What every patient, family, friend, and caregiver needs to know about psychiatry.* Washington, DC: American Psychiatric Press.

Roy, A. (1989). Suicide. In H. Kaplan & B. Sadock (Eds.), *Comprehensive textbook of psychiatry* (5th ed.). Baltimore: Williams & Wilkins.

Rubel, A. J., O'Nell, C. W., & Collado-Ardon, R. (1984). *Susto: A folk illness.* Berkeley: University of California Press.

Russell, S. T., & Joyner, K. (2001). Adolescent sexual orientation and suicide risk: Evidence from a national study. *American Journal of Public Health, 91,* 1276–1281.

Rutter, M., & Rutter, M. (1993). *Developing minds.* New York: Basic Books.

Saint Exupery, A. de. (1971). *The little prince.* New York: Harcourt Brace Jovanovich.

Sandhu, D. S., Portes, P. R., & McPhee, S. A. (1996). Assessing cultural adaptation: Psychometric properties of the Cultural Adaptation Pain Scale. *Journal of Multicultural Counseling and Development, 24,* 15-25.

Sanua, V. D. (1996). The myth of organicity of mental disorders. *Humanistic Psychologist, 24,* 55–78.

Sarles, R. M. (1994). Transference-countertransference issues with adolescents: Personal reflections. *American Journal of Psychotherapy, 48,* 64–74.

Satir, V. (1967). *Conjoint family therapy.* Palo Alto, CA: Science and Behavior Books.

Sattler, J. M. (1992). *Assessment of children* (2nd ed.). San Diego, CA: Author.

Scarf, M. (1995). *Intimate worlds.* New York: Random House.

Schact, T. E., Binder, J. L., & Strupp, H. H. (1984). The dynamic focus. In H. H. Strupp & J. L. Binder (Eds.), *Psychotherapy in a new key* (pp. 56-109). New York: Basic Books.

Schmidt, H. G., Norman, G. R., & Boshuizen, H. P. (1990). A cognitive perspective on medical expertise. *Academic Medicine, 65,* 611–621.

Seay, T. A. (1978). *Systematic eclectic therapy.* Jonesboro, TN: Pilgrimage Press.

Segal, D. L. (1997). Structured interviewing and DSM classification. In S. M. Turner & M. Hersen (Eds.). *Adult psychopathology and diagnosis* (3rd ed., pp. 24-57). New York: John Wiley & Sons.

Segal, H. (1993). Countertransference. In A. Alexandris & G. Vaslamatzis (Eds.). *Countertransference: Theory, technique, teaching.* Northvale, NJ: Jason Aronson.

Segal, J. (1993). Against self-disclosure. In W. Dryden (Ed.). *Questions and answers on counselling in action* (pp. 11–18). London: Sage.

Selekman, M. D. (1993). *Pathways to change.* New York: Guilford Press.

Seligman, L. (1996). *Diagnosis and treatment planning in counseling* (2nd ed.). New York: Plenum Press.

Seligman, L. (1998). *Selecting effective treatments* (rev. ed.). San Francisco, CA: Jossey-Bass/Pfeiffer.

Seligman, M. E. P. (1995). The effectiveness of psychotherapy: The *Consumer Report* study. *American Psychologist, 50,* 965–974.

Seligman, M. E. P., & Levant, R. F. (1998). Managed care policies on inadequate science. *Professional Psychology, 29,* 211–212.

Senzaki, N., & Reps, P. (1939). *101 Zen stories.* Philadelphia: David McKay.

Seppae, K., Lepistoe, J., & Sillanaukee, P. (1998). Five-Shot questionnaire on heavy drinking. *Alcoholism: Clinical and Experimental Research, 22,* 1788–1791.

Shapiro, F. (1995). *Eye movement desensitization and reprocessing: Basic principles, protocols, and procedures.* New York: Guilford Press.

Shapiro, F. (2001). *Eye movement desensitization and reprocessing: Basic principles, protocols, and procedures* (2nd ed.). New York: Guilford Press.

Sharpley, C. F. (1984). Predicate matching in NLP: A review of research on the preferred representational system. *Journal of Counseling Psychology, 31,* 238–248.

Shea, S. C. (1998). *Psychiatric interviewing: The art of understanding* (2nd ed.). Philadelphia: Saunders.

Shea, S. C. (1999). *The practical art of suicide assessment: A guide for mental health professionals and substance abuse counselors.* New York: John Wiley & Sons.

Shea, S. C., & Mezzich, J. E. (1988). Contemporary psychiatric interviewing: New directions for training. *Psychiatry, 51,* 385–397.

Sheitman, B. B., Lee, H., Strauss, R., & Lieberman, J. A. (1997). The evaluation and treatment of first-episode psychosis. *Schizophrenia Bulletin, 23,* 653–661.

Sheline, J. L., Skipper, B. J., & Broadhead, W. E. (1994). Risk factors for violent behavior in elementary school boys: Have you hugged your child today? *American Journal of Public Health, 84,* 661–663.

Shirk, S., & Harter, S. (1996). Treatment of low self-esteem. In M. A. Reineke, F. M. Dattilio, & A. Freeman (Eds.), *Cognitive therapy with children and adolescents: A casebook for clinical practice* (pp. 175–198). New York: Guilford Press.

Shneidman, E. S. (1980). Psychotherapy with suicidal patients. In T. B. Karasu & L. Bellak (Eds.), *Specialized techniques in individual psychotherapy* (pp. 306-328). New York: Brunner/Mazel.

Shneidman, E. S. (1981). *Suicide thoughts and reflections, 1960–1980.* New York: Guilford Press.

Shneidman, E. S. (1984). Aphorisms of suicide and some implications for psychotherapy. *American Journal of Psychotherapy, 38,* 319–328.

Shneidman, E. S. (1996). *The suicidal mind.* New York: Oxford University Press.

Siassi, I. (1984). Psychiatric interview and mental status examination. In G. Goldstein & M. Hersen (Eds.), *Handbook of psychological assessment* (pp. 259-275). New York: Pergamon Press.

Sifneos, P. E. (1987). *Short-term dynamic psychotherapy.* New York: Plenum Press.

Silverman, C. (1968). The epidemiology of depression—A review. *American Journal of Psychiatry, 124,* 883–891.

Silverman, W. (1987). *Anxiety disorders interview schedule for children (ADIS).* Albany, NY: Graywind.

Simon, R. I. (1999). The suicide prevention contract: Clinical, legal, and risk management issues. *Journal of the American Academy of Psychiatry and the Law, 27,* 445–450.

Simon, R. I. (2000). Taking the "Sue" out of suicide: A forensic psychiatrist's perspective. *Psychiatric Annals, 30,* 399–407.

Simonds, S. L. (1994). *Bridging the silence: Nonverbal modalities in the treatment of adult survivors of childhood sexual abuse.* New York: Norton.

Simons, R. C., & Hughes, C. C. (1993). Cultural-bound syndromes. In A. C. Gaw (Ed.), *Culture, ethnicity, and mental illness* (pp. 75–93). Washington, DC: American Psychiatric Press.

Skerrett, K. (1996). From isolation to mutuality: A feminist collaborative model of couples therapy. In M. Hill & E. D. Rothblum (Eds.), *Feminist perspectives* (pp. 93–105). New York: Harrington Park Press.

Skinner, B. F. (1972). *Walden two.* New York: Knopf.

Smail, D. (1997). *Illusion and reality: The meaning of anxiety.* London: Constable.

Smail, D. (2000, July). *Helping with distress.* Presented at the annual conference of the Central England Region of Cruse, Kettering, United Kingdom.

Smith, M. L., Glass, G. V., & Miller, T. I. (1980). *The benefits of psychotherapy.* Baltimore: Johns Hopkins University Press.

Smith-Hanen, S. S. (1977). Effects of nonverbal behaviors on judged levels of counselor warmth and empathy. *Journal of Counseling Psychology, 24,* 87–91.

Snyder, D. K. (1979). Multidimensional assessment of marital satisfaction. *Journal of Marriage & the Family, 41,* 813-823.

Snyder, D. K. (1981). *Marriage satisfaction inventory manual.* Los Angeles: Western Psychological Services.

Snyder, M. (1974). Self-monitoring of expressive behavior. *Journal of Personality and Social Psychology, 30,* 526–537.

Soisson, E. L., VandeCreek, L., & Knapp, S. (1987). Thorough record keeping: A good defense in a litigious era. *Professional Psychology: Research and Practice, 18,* 498–502.

Sommers, J. (1986). *Psychiatric and familial sabotage in a case of obsessive-compulsive disorder.* Paper presented at the meeting of the Western Psychological Association. Seattle, WA.

Sommers-Flanagan, J. (1998, February 16). Tough kids may feel the bite of conscience. *The Missoulian,* C12.

Sommers-Flanagan, J., & Means, J. R. (1987). Thou shalt not ask questions: An approach to teaching interviewing skills. *Teaching of Psychology, 14,* 164–166.

Sommers-Flanagan, J., Rothman, M., & Schwenkler, R. (2000). Training psychologists to become competent suicide assessment interviewers: Commentary on Rosenberg's. (1999). suicide prevention training model. *Professional Psychology, 31,* 99–100.

Sommers-Flanagan, J., & Sommers-Flanagan, R. (1989). A categorization of pitfalls common to beginning interviewers. *Journal of Training and Practice in Professional Psychology, 3,* 58–71.

Sommers-Flanagan, J., & Sommers-Flanagan, R. (1995a). Intake interviewing with suicidal patients: A systematic approach. *Professional Psychology, 26,* 41–47.

Sommers-Flanagan, J., & Sommers-Flanagan, R. (1995b). Rapid emotional change strategies with difficult youth. *Child and Family Behavior Therapy, 17,* 11–22.

Sommers-Flanagan, J., & Sommers-Flanagan, R. (1996). The Wizard of Oz metaphor in hypnosis with treatment-resistant children. *American Journal of Clinical Hypnosis, 39,* 105–114.

Sommers-Flanagan, J., & Sommers-Flanagan, R. (1997). *Tough kids, cool counseling: User-friendly approaches with challenging youth.* Alexandria, VA: American Counseling Association.

Sommers-Flanagan, J., & Sommers-Flanagan, R. (1998). Assessment and diagnosis of conduct disorder. *Journal of Counseling and Development, 76,* 189–197.

Sommers-Flanagan, J., Sommers-Flanagan, R., & Palmer, C. (2001). Counseling interventions for children with disruptive behaviors. In E. R. Welfel & R. E. Ingersoll (Eds.), *The mental health desk reference* (pp. 205–212). New York: John Wiley & Sons.

Sommers-Flanagan, R., Elander, C. D., & Sommers-Flanagan, J. (2000). *Don't divorce us!: Kids' advice to divorcing parents.* Alexandria, VA: American Counseling Association.

Sommers-Flanagan, R., Elliot, D., & Sommers-Flanagan, J. (1998). Exploring the edges: Boundaries and breaks. *Ethics and Behavior, 8,* 37–48.

Sonne, J. L., & Pope, K. S. (1991). Treating victims of therapist-patient sexual involvement. *Psychotherapy, 28,* 174–187.

Spanier, G. B. (1976). Measuring dyadic adjustment: New scales for assessing the quality of marriage and similar dyads. *Journal of Marriage & the Family, 38,* 15-28.

Speight, S. L., & Vera, E. M. (1997). Similarity and difference in multicultural counseling: Considering the attraction and repulsion hypotheses. *Counseling Psychologist, 25,* 280–298.

Sperry, L., & Giblin, P. (1996). Marital and family therapy with religious persons. In E. P. Shafranske (Ed.), *Religion and the clinical practice of psychology* (pp. 511–532). Washington, DC: American Psychological Association.

Spiegal, S. (1989). *An interpersonal approach to child therapy.* New York: Columbia University Press.

Spitzer, R. L., Forman, J., & Nee, J. (1979). *DSM-III* field trials. I: Initial interrater diagnostic reliability. *American Journal of Psychiatry, 136,* 818–820.

Sporakowski, M. J., Prouty, A. M., & Habben, C. (2001). Assessment in couple and family counseling. In E. R. Welfel & R. E. Ingersoll (Eds.), *The mental health desk reference* (pp. 372–378). New York: John Wiley & Sons.

Staats, A. W. (1996). *Behavior and personality: Psychological behaviorism.* New York: Springer.

Steenbarger, B. (1994). Duration and outcome in psychotherapy: An integrative review. *Professional Psychology: Research and Practice, 25,* 111–119.

Steffens, D. C., & Morgenlander, J. C. (1999). Initial evaluation of suspected dementia. Asking the right questions. *Postgraduate Medicine, 106,* 72–76, 79–80, 82–83.

Stephan, W. G., Diaz-Loving, R., & Duran, A. (2000). Integrated threat theory and intercultural attitudes: Mexico and the United States. *Journal of Cross-Cultural Psychology, 31,* 240–249.

Stern, E. M. (1985). *Psychotherapy and the religiously committed patient.* New York: Haworth Press.

Stern, S. (1993). Managed care, brief therapy, and therapeutic integrity. *Psychotherapy, 30,* 162–175.

Sternberg, R. J. (1985). *Beyond IQ: A triarchic theory of human intelligence.* New York: Cambridge University Press.

Sternberg, R. J., & Wagner, R. K. (Eds.). (1986). *Practical intelligence: Origins of competence in the everyday world.* New York: Cambridge University Press.

Stiles, W. B., Shapiro, D. A., & Elliot, R. (1986). Are all psychotherapies equivalent? *American Psychologist, 41,* 165–180.

Straus, M. A., Sugarman, D. B., & Giles-Sims, J. (1997). Spanking children and subsequent antisocial behavior of children. *Archives of Pediatric Adolescent Medicine, 151,* 761–767.

Strean, H. S. (1985). *Resolving marital conflict: A psychodynamic perspective.* New York: John Wiley & Sons.

Stricker, G., & Fisher, M. (Eds.). (1990). *Self-disclosure in the therapeutic relationship.* New York: Plenum Press.

Strong, B., & DeVault, C. (1989). *The marriage and family experience* (4th ed.). St. Paul, MN: West.

Strong, S. R. (1968). Counseling: An interpersonal influence process. *Journal of Counseling Psychology, 15,* 215–224.

Strub, R. L., & Black, F. W. (1977). *The mental status examination in neurology.* Philadelphia: Davis.

Strub, R. L., & Black, F. W. (1999). *The mental status examination in neurology* (4th ed.). Philadelphia: Davis.

Strupp, H. H. (1955). The effect of the psychotherapist's personal analysis upon his techniques. *Journal of Consulting Psychology, 19,* 197–204.

Strupp, H. H. (1983). Psychoanalytic psychotherapy. In M. Hersen, A. E. Kazdin, & A. S. Bellack (Eds.), *The clinical psychology handbook* (471–488). New York: Pergamon Press.

Strupp, H. H., & Binder, J. L. (1984). *Psychotherapy in a new key.* New York: Basic Books.

Strupp, H. H., & Hadley, S. W. (1979). Specific vs. nonspecific factors in psychotherapy: A controlled study of outcome. *Archives of General Psychiatry, 36,* 1125–1136.

Stuart, R. B., & Stuart, F. (1975). *Premarital counseling inventory manual.* Ann Arbor, MI: Compuscore.

Sue, D. W., Arredondo, P., & McDavis, R. J. (1992). Multicultural counseling competencies and standards: A call to the profession. *Journal of Counseling and Development, 70,* 477–486.

Sue, D. W., Ivey, A. E., & Pedersen, P. B. (1996). *A theory of multicultural counseling & therapy.* Pacific Grove, CA: Brooks/Cole.

Sue, D. W., & Sue, D. (1999). *Counseling the culturally different* (3rd ed.). New York: John Wiley & Sons.

Sue, D. W., & Sue, S. (1987). Cultural factors in the clinical assessment of Asian Americans. *Journal of Consulting and Clinical Psychology, 55,* 479–487.

Sue, S. (1998). In search of cultural competence in psychotherapy and counseling. *American Psychologist, 53,* 440–448.

Sullivan, H. S. (1970). *The psychiatric interview.* New York: Norton.

Susser, I., & Patterson, T. C. (Eds.). (2000). *Cultural diversity in the U.S.: A critical reader.* London: Blackwell.

Sutton, C. T., & Broken Nose, M. A. (1996). American Indian families: An overview. In M. McGoldrick, J. Giordano, & J. K. Pearce (Eds.), *Ethnicity and family therapy* (2nd ed., pp. 31–44). New York: Guilford Press.

Swartz-Kulstad, J. L., & Martin, W. E., Jr. (1999). Impact of culture and context on psychosocial adaptation: The cultural and contextual guide process. *Journal of Counseling and Development, 77,* 281–293.

Swartz-Kulstad, J. L., & Martin, W. E., Jr. (2000). Culture as an essential aspect of person-environment fit. In W. E. Martin Jr. & J. L. Swartz-Kulstad (Eds.), *Person-environment psychology and mental health: Assessment and intervention* (pp.169-195). Mahwah, NJ: Erlbaum.

Szajnberg, N. M., Moilanen, I., Kanerva, A., & Tolf, B. (1996). Munchausen-by-proxy syndrome: Countertransference as a diagnostic tool. *Bulletin of the Menninger Clinic, 60,* 229–237.

Szasz, T. S. (1961). *The myth of mental illness.* New York: Hoeber-Harper.

Szasz, T. S. (1970). *The manufacture of madness: A comparative study of the inquisition and the mental health movement.* New York: McGraw-Hill.

Szasz, T. S. (1986). The case against suicide prevention. *American Psychologist, 41,* 806–812.

Takushi, R., & Uomoto, J. M. (2001). The clinical interview from a multicultural perspective. In L. A. Suzuki & J. G. Ponterotto (Eds.), *Handbook of multicultural assessment.* San Francisco: Jossey-Bass.

Tamburrino, M. B., Lynch, D. J., Nagel, R., & Mangen, M. (1993). Evaluating empathy in interviewing: Comparing self-report with actual behavior. *Teaching and Learning in Medicine, 5,* 217–220.

Tannen, D. (1990). *You just don't understand: Women and men in conversation.* New York: Morrow.

Tarasoff v. Regents of the University of California, 118 Cal. Rptr. 129, 529 P. 2d 533 (1974).

Teicher, M., Glod, C., & Cole, J. (1990). Emergence of intense suicidal preoccupation during fluoxetine treatment. *American Journal of Psychiatry, 147,* 207–210.

Teo, T., & Febbraro, A. R. (1997). Norm, factuality, and power in multiculturalism. *American Psychologist, 52,* 656–657.

Teyber, E. (1997). *Interpersonal process in psychotherapy: A guide for clinical training.* Pacific Grove, CA: Brooks/Cole.

Thomas, L. (1974). *The lives of a cell.* New York: Bantam Books.

Thompson, M., Kaslow, N., Kingree, J., Puett, R., Thompson, N., & Meadows, L. (1999). Partner abuse and posttraumatic stress disorder as risk factors for suicide attempts in a sample of low-income, inner-city women. *Journal of Traumatic Stress, 12,* 59–72.

Thomson, M. (1989/1997). *On art and therapy: An exploration.* London: Free Association Books.

Thoresen, C. E., & Mahoney, M. J. (1974). *Behavioral self-control.* New York: Holt, Rinehart and Winston.

Timonen, M., Viilo, K., Hakko, H., Vaeisaenen, E., Raesaenen, P., & Saerkioja, T. (2001). Psychiatric disorders are more severe among suicide victims of higher occupational level. *British Medical Journal, 323,* 232.

Toates, F. M. (2001). *Biological psychology: An integrative approach.* Boston: Pearson Education.

Tracey, T., Hays, K. A., Malone, J., & Herman, B. (1988). Changes in counselor response as a function of experience. *Journal of Counseling Psychology, 35,* 119–126.

Trilling, L., & Marcus, S. (1961). *The life and work of Sigmund Freud.* New York: Basic Books.

Trull, R. J., & Phares, E. J. (2001). *Clinical psychology: Concepts, methods, and profession* (6th ed). Belmont, CA: Wadsworth/Thomson.

Ullmann, L. P., & Krasner, L. (1965). *Case studies in behavior modification.* New York: Holt, Rinehart and Winston.

U.S. Bureau of the Census. (1992). *1992 census of population.* Washington, DC: U.S. Government Printing Office.

U.S. Bureau of the Census. (2001). *2000 Census of the population.* Washington, DC: U.S. Government Printing Office.

Vacc, N. A., & Juhnke, G. A. (1997). The use of structured clinical interviews for assessment and counseling. *Journal of Counseling and Development, 75,* 470–480.

Vacc, N. A., Wittmer, J., & DeVaney, S. B. (1988). *Experiencing and counseling multicultural and diverse populations.* Muncie, IN: Accelerated Development.

Van Wagoner, S. L., Gelso, C. J., Hayes, J. A., & Diemer, R. A. (1991). Countertransference and the reputedly excellent therapist. *Psychotherapy, 28,* 411–421.

Vontress, C. E., Johnson, J. A., & Epp, L. R. (1999). *Cross-cultural counseling: A casebook.* Alexandria, VA: American Counseling Association.

Wagner, L., Davis, S., & Handelsman, M. M. (1998). In search of the abominable consent form: The impact of readability and personalization. *Journal of Clinical Psychology, 54,* 115–120.

Wakefield, J. C. (1997). Diagnosing *DSM-IV*—Part II: Eysenck (1986) and the essentialist fallacy. *Behavioural Research and Therapy, 35,* 651–665.

Walters, R. P. (1980). *Amity: Friendship in action. Part I: Basic friendship skills.* Boulder, CO: Christian Helpers.

Warwick, L. L. (1999). What is necessary and what is right? Feminist dilemmas in community mental health. *Women and Therapy, 22,* 39–51.

Watkins, C. E. (1995). And then there is psychotherapy supervision, too. *American Journal of Psychotherapy, 49,* 313.

Watkins, C. E., & Watts, R. E. (1995). Psychotherapy survey research studies: Some consistent findings and integrative conclusions. *Psychotherapy in Private Practice, 13,* 49–68.

Watkins, J. G. (1978). *The therapeutic self.* New York: Human Sciences Press.

Watkins, J. G. (1992). *Hypnoanalytic techniques: Clinical hypnosis.* New York: Irvington.

Watkins, J. G., & Watkins, H. H. (1997). *Ego states.* New York: Norton.

Watzlawick, P., Weakland, J., & Fisch, R. (1974). *Change: Principles of problem formation and problem resolution.* New York: Norton.

Wax, E. (2001, May 30). Lesson plans becoming obsolete: Cultural differences require broader teaching methods. *The Washington Post,* A-9.

*Webster's ninth new collegiate dictionary.* (1985). Springfield, MA: Author.

Wechsler, D. (1958). *The measurement and appraisal of adult intelligence* (4th ed.). Baltimore: Williams & Wilkins.

Wechsler, D., & Stone, C. P. (1945). *Wechsler Memory Scale manual.* New York: Psychological Corporation.

Weinberg, G. (1984). *The heart of psychotherapy: A journey into the mind and office of the therapist at work.* New York: St. Martin's Press.

Weiner, I. B. (1975). *Principles of psychotherapy.* New York: John Wiley & Sons.

Weiner, I. B. (1997). *Psychodiagnosis in schizophrenia.* Mahwah, NJ: Erlbaum. (Original work published 1966)

Weiner, I. B. (1998). *Principles of psychotherapy* (2nd ed.). New York: John Wiley & Sons.

Weiss, A. R. (1986). Teaching counseling and psychotherapy skills without access to a clinical population: The short interview method. *Teaching of Psychology, 13,* 145–147.

Welfel, E. R. (2002). *Ethics in counseling and psychotherapy: Standards, research, and emerging issues* (2nd ed.). Pacific Grove, CA: Brooks/Cole.

Welfel, E. R., & Heinlen, K. T. (2001). The responsible use of technology in mental health practice. In E. R. Welfel & R. E. Ingersoll (Eds.), *The mental health desk reference* (pp. 484–489). New York: John Wiley & Sons.

Wells, A. (1997). *Cognitive therapy of anxiety disorders: A practice manual and conceptual guide.* New York: John Wiley & Sons.

Westefeld, J. S., & Furr, S. R. (1987). Suicide and depression among college students. *Professional Psychology, 18,* 119–123.

Wetsit, D. (1992). *Counseling preferences of American Indian students at the University of Montana.* Unpublished dissertation, University of Montana, Missoula.

Whitaker, C. A., & Burnberry, W. M. (1988). *Dancing with the family: A symbolic experiential approach.* New York: Brunner/Mazel.

White, M. (1994). *Stranger at the gate.* New York: Simon & Schuster.

Widiger, T. A. (1997). Mental disorders as discrete clinical conditions: Dimensional versus categorical classification. In S. M. Turner & M. Hersen (Eds.), *Adult psychopathology and diagnosis* (pp. 3–23). New York: John Wiley & Sons.

Widiger, T. A., & Clark, L. A. (2000). Toward *DSM-V* and the classification of psychopathology. *Psychological Bulletin, 126,* 946–963.

Wiger, D. (1999). *The clinical documentation sourcebook with disk.* New York: John Wiley & Sons.

Wilkes, T. C. R., Belsher, G., Rush, A. J., & Frank, E. (1994). *Cognitive therapy with depressed adolescents.* New York: Guilford Press.

Wilkinson, S., & Kitzinger, C. (Eds.). (1996). *Representing the other: A feminism & psychology reader.* London: Sage.

Williams, T. T. (1991). *Refuge: An unnatural history of family and place.* New York: Random House.

Willie, C. (1981). Dominance in the family: The Black and White experience. *Journal of Black Psychology, 7,* 91–97.

Willock, B. (1986). Narcissistic vulnerability in the hyper-aggressive child: The disregarded (unloved, uncared-for) self. *Psychoanalytic Psychology, 3,* 59–80.

Willock, B. (1987). The devalued (unloved, repugnant) self: A second facet of narcissistic vulnerability in the aggressive, conduct-disordered child. *Psychoanalytic Psychology, 4,* 219–240.

Wilmot, W. W., & Hocker, J. L. (1997). *Interpersonal conflict.* New York: McGraw-Hall.

Wilson, M. N., Phillip, D., Kohn, L. P., & Curry-El, J. A. (1995). Cultural relativistic approach toward ethnic minorities in family therapy. In J. F. Aponte, R. Y. Rivers, & J. Wohl (Eds.), *Psychological interventions and cultural diversity* (pp. 92–108). Boston: Allyn & Bacon.

Winslow, F. (1895). Suicide as a mental epidemic. *Journal of the American Medical Association, 25,* 471–474.

Witt, S. D. (1997). Parental influence on children's socialization to gender roles. *Adolescence, 32,* 253–259.

Witvliet, C. V. O., Ludwig, T. E., & Vander Laan, K. L. (2001). Granting forgiveness or harboring grudges: Implications for emotion, physiology, and health. *Psychological Science, 12,* 117–123.

Wolberg, B. (1995). *Technique of psychotherapy* (4th Rev. ed., Parts 1 & 2). New York: Grune & Stratton.

Wollersheim, J. P. (1974). The assessment of suicide potential via interview methods. *Psychotherapy, 11,* 222–225.

Worell, J., & Johnson, N. G. (1997). *Shaping the future of feminist psychology: Education, research, and practice.* Washington, DC: American Psychological Association.

World Health Organization. (1997a). *Multiaxial classification of child and adolescent psychiatric disorders: The ICD-10 classification of mental and behavioural disorders in childhood and adolescence.* London: Cambridge University Press.

World Health Organization. (1997b). *The multiaxial presentation of the ICD-10 for use in adult psychiatry.* London: Cambridge University Press.

Worthington, E. L., Kurusu, T. A., McCollough, M. E., & Sandage, S. J. (1996). Empirical research on religion and psychotherapeutic processes and outcomes: A 10-year review and research prospectus. *Psychological Bulletin, 119,* 448–487.

Wright, J. H., & Davis, D. (1994). The therapeutic relationship in cognitive-behavioral therapy: Patient perceptions and therapist responses. *Cognitive and Behavioral Practice, 1,* 25–45.

Yalom, I. (1989). *Love's executioner: And other tales of psychotherapy.* New York: Basic Books.

Yalom, I. (1995). *The theory and practice of group psychotherapy* (3rd ed.). New York: Basic Books.

Yalom, I. (1997). *Lying on the couch: A novel.* New York: Perennial.

Young-Eisendrath, P. (1993). *You're not what I expected: Learning to love the opposite sex.* New York: Morrow.

Yu, M. M., & Watkins, T. (1996). Group counseling with DUI offenders: A model using client anger to enhance group cohesion and movement. *Alcoholism Treatment Quarterly, 14,* 47–57.

Zaro, J. S., Barach, R., Nedelman, D. J., & Dreiblatt, I. S. (1977). *A guide for beginning psychotherapists.* New York: Cambridge University Press.

Zeer, D. (2000). *Office yoga: Simple stretches for busy people.* San Francisco: Chronicle Books.

Zetzel, E. R. (1956). Current concepts of transference. *International Journal of Psycho-Analysis, 37,* 369-375.

Zuckerman, E. L. (2000). *Clinician's thesaurus: The guidebook for writing psychological reports* (5th ed.). New York: Guilford Press.

Zuckerman, M. (1990). Some dubious premises in research and theory on racial differences: Scientific, social, and ethical issues. *American Psychologist, 45,* 1297–1303.

Zuckerman, M. (2000). *Vulnerability to psychopathology: A biosocial model.* Washington, DC: American Psychological Association.

# Author Index

# Subject Index

## *About the Authors*

**John Sommers-Flanagan** is a clinical psychologist specializing in treating difficult youth. He is also the executive director of Families First, a private, nonprofit organization dedicated to parent education and support. John is an active member of both the American Psychological Association and the American Counseling Association and teaches and supervises graduate students from a number of different disciplines. He also has a strong interest teaching healthy psychological skills to the general public through the media. During his spare time he enjoys reading, gardening, exercise of any kind, eating oat bran pancakes on Saturday mornings, and hanging out with the family.

**Rita Sommers-Flanagan** is a clinical psychologist, professor in counselor education, and a past rehabilitation counselor. Besides an ongoing interest in effective clinical interviewing, Rita teaches and publishes in applied ethics, theories of counseling and psychotherapy, and feminist therapy. Opportunities to teach in Belize, C.A., and in England have increased her concerns regarding mental health issues at the global level.

Both John and Rita are widely sought after workshop leaders and speakers. They have co-written many professional articles and four books, including *Tough Kids, Cool Counseling* and *Problem Child or Quirky Kid.* A fifth book—*Theories and Techniques of Counseling Psychotherapy*—is soon to be published by John Wiley and Sons.